INSTITUTIONAL

CHANGE

AND

HEALTHCARE

ORGANIZATIONS

INSTITUTIONAL CHANGE *and* HEALTHCARE ORGANIZATIONS

From Professional Dominance to Managed Care

W. RICHARD SCOTT
MARTIN RUEF
PETER J. MENDEL
CAROL A. CARONNA

THE UNIVERSITY OF CHICAGO PRESS
CHICAGO AND LONDON

W. RICHARD SCOTT is professor of sociology, organizational behavior, education, and health research and policy at Stanford University. His books include *Hospital Structure and Performance* (1987, with Ann Flood), *Institutions and Organizations* (1995), and *Organizations: Rational, Natural, and Open Systems,* 4th ed. (1998).

MARTIN RUEF is an assistant professor of sociology at the University of North Carolina. His research interests include organization theory, the sociology of the professions, quantitative methodology, and the sociology of culture.

PETER J. MENDEL is a doctoral candidate in sociology at Stanford University. His interests focus on comparative institutional and organizational analysis.

CAROL A. CARONNA is a doctoral candidate in sociology at Stanford University. Her research interests are organizations, social psychology, and gender.

The University of Chicago Press, Chicago 60637
The University of Chicago Press, Ltd., London
© 2000 by The University of Chicago
All rights reserved. Published 2000
Printed in the United States of America
09 08 07 06 05 04 03 02 01 00   1 2 3 4 5

ISBN: 0-226-74309-8 (cloth)
ISBN: 0-226-74310-1 (paper)

Library of Congress Cataloging-in-Publication Data

Institutional change and healthcare organizations : from professional dominance to managed care / W. Richard Scott . . . [et al.].
   p.   cm.
   Includes bibliographical references and index.
   ISBN 0-226-74309-8 (cloth : alk. paper)—ISBN 0-226-74310-1 (paper : alk. paper)
   1. Health services administration—California—San Francisco Bay Area—History—20th century.   2. Medical care—California—San Francisco Bay Area—History—20th century.
3. Medicine—California—San Francisco Bay Area—History—20th century.   I. Scott, W. Richard.

R172.S24 I57   2000
362.1'09764'6—dc21
                                                                99-048850

Contents

Figures and Tables

TABLES

Case Illustrations

Students of organizations have recently accorded renewed attention to the ways in which institutional environments shape organizational forms, structures, and processes. The importance of cultural-cognitive, normative, and regulative frameworks as constraints on and enablers of organizations is increasingly recognized. But much less attention has been given to examining the ways in which institutional environments change or to the effects of these changes on constituent organizations and organizing processes.

The field of healthcare services, particularly in the United States and during recent decades, presents a marvelous opportunity to examine an institutional arena undergoing rapid, even "profound," change. We observe much evidence of new rules, new belief systems, and new modes of governance and, simultaneously, many examples of new types of healthcare organizations and new modes of financing, managing, and delivering services. Traditional organizations, like hospitals, are declining in numbers, strength, and centrality, and newer organizational forms, like health maintenance organizations, are on the rise.

Other arenas, for example, publishing and financial services, have also undergone rapid change during the late decades of the twentieth century. What makes the changes in healthcare so interesting is the contrast between today's chaos and the stability evidenced by previous institutional arrangements. For over fifty years, from the early 1920s well into the 1960s, the healthcare arena was a well-ordered field, ruled over by a firmly entrenched medical establishment. Organized medicine, backed by the power of the state, exercised hegemonic control over healthcare, determining who could perform which services and how these were to be delivered and financed. How was it that this stable, professionally dominated complex of institutionalized arrangements came apart? Why were some actors and practices delegitimated, and how did new claimants and modes of thinking and acting arise?

To address these questions, we have carried out an empirical study of changes occurring over half a century in the healthcare delivery system of one metropolitan region, the San Francisco Bay Area. While we limit our investigation to explaining developments in a single large, but geographically limited, region, we search for explanations far and wide, exploring the effects of changes occurring beyond the boundaries of the Bay Area, in the State of California, and in the United States more generally. The effects of institutional environments are not restricted to local arenas; many of the forces we study—laws, the actions of professional associations, court decisions, the content of media—influence behavior in distant and remote locations. Thus, while the Bay Area provides our empirical case, our larger topic is change in healthcare institutions and organizations.

Our research was conducted during the mid-1990s, a period of great turbulence in U.S. healthcare. The pace of change was sufficiently rapid, and the level of confusion among participants and observers sufficiently high, that we decided it would be prudent not to restrict our study to the present time period but to take a longer, more deliberative stance. We elected to study change processes over a fifty-year period, from the end of World War II in 1945 to the present.[1] We believe this design choice affords us a better vantage point from which to understand and comment on more recent changes.

The primary changes we attempt to explain are transformations in the types, numbers, and activities of healthcare organizations. For many readers, this may seem a strange and remote subject. Where are the individual patients and their concerns? Where are the data on mortality, morbidity, and patient satisfaction? Most studies focus on these individual patient outcomes, but we have elected not to do so. Our interest is in the mortality and morbidity of healthcare organizations. We ask, which types of organizations are failing and which flourishing? How have the types of interdependence and linkages among these organizations undergone change? How have these changes come about? In our view, such questions are of fundamental importance. Organizations not only provide contexts within which work is carried out but themselves take action as significant collective social actors. In either case—as contexts or actors—they profoundly influence what goals are sought and what actions are undertaken to accomplish them. Organizations are the "medium," but the medium is often the message.

---

1. The ending date for our study varies by topic and was set largely by the availability of data. Some of the larger data sets only cover the period through the early 1990s. In other cases, our observations extend to 1999.

While much of our effort is devoted to studying changes over time in selected types of healthcare organizations, or "organizational populations," we employ case studies of individual organizations in order to understand better the ways in which organizations not only react to but take action to influence their environments. Too often institutional analysts treat organizations as passive foils, reflecting external forces. We attempt to redress this bias in our approach.

Our work is targeted primarily to students of organizations and institutions, on the one hand, and to those interested in healthcare systems, on the other. The volume deals with complex issues and contains some quantitative analyses, but we have labored to produce an account that will be accessible to the general, interested reader. As individual consumers, all of us have a stake in healthcare, and some knowledge of the changes affecting this institutional complex should be useful and of interest to many.

A comment on terminology. We routinely employ the term "healthcare" to describe the field of study. We deliberately chose this term, which is gaining in popularity, as appropriate for describing the organizational field now under construction. There appears to be movement away from such older terms as "medical care" or "medical services," designed to distinguish between health and medicine. "Healthcare," for us, connotes the new emphasis on health (in contrast to illness), is inclusive of preventive and health maintenance services as well as acute care, and breaks away from the physician-dominated control of "medical" functions.

The world of healthcare is also plagued with many acronyms and abbreviations. To assist the reader through the thicket of alphabetized labels, we provide a glossary of such terms used throughout the book.

In these final paragraphs, the senior author has chosen to follow the example of his own former professor, Otis Dudley Duncan, with whom he collaborated in the writing of his first book while still a doctoral student at the University of Chicago. Duncan explained in the preface to *Metropolis and Region* that he exercised "the prerogative of speaking for himself alone in order to speak more enthusiastically about the work of his collaborators than would be modest in a collective statement."[2] My co-authors have each made invaluable contributions to this volume. All have been engaged in all phases of the project from design, data collection, and analysis to final manuscript preparation.

Martin Ruef provided much of the technical prowess required to carry out the event-history analyses, from formatting and data entry to the

2. Otis Dudley Duncan, W. Richard Scott, Stanley Lieberson, Beverly Duncan, Hal H. Winsborough, *Metropolis and Region* (Baltimore: Johns Hopkins University Press, 1960).

generation, testing, and interpretation of hypotheses. In addition, he is primarily responsible for our analysis of the two components of change—adaptive and ecological processes—and he helped to design and carry out tests of legitimation effects on organizational survival. Peter Mendel was indispensable as he indefatigably and imaginatively assembled much of the data employed to chart changes in the institutional and material-resource environments; and he designed and executed the factor analyses to test our arguments concerning institutional change and its effects on organizational populations at the field level. It is largely due to Carol Caronna's persistence and persuasiveness that the case studies play such a large role in our study. She insisted on the importance of organizations as actors, not simply as carriers of institutional logics, and she prepared most of the case illustrations employed throughout the volume. Carol was also responsible for compiling and organizing information on healthcare systems.

There developed, then, a kind of rough division of labor among us, and each of us took particular responsibilities for some phases of the work. In this respect, as a group, we enjoyed the benefits of "distributed learning," each of us being expert in some different area and all of us relying on that expertise. But specialization as a basis of collaboration was replaced during the final months of manuscript preparation. All four of us became generalists and worked tirelessly and equally to improve and integrate the arguments, analyses, and illustrations throughout the book. Both moments were effective and gratifying. It is difficult to imagine a more cooperative team atmosphere or a more satisfying professional experience than this project has afforded. If it gives my co-authors the same running start on their scholarly careers that my collaboration with Dudley Duncan gave me 38 years ago, I will be most pleased.

Stanford, California
October 1998

Acknowledgments

This project could not have been carried out without the generous assistance of a grant from the Robert Wood Johnson Foundation. The grant, provided by their Investigator Initiated Awards Program, allowed us to carry out a project of our own choosing and enabled us to design and complete a much more ambitious project than would otherwise have been feasible. We are grateful for their financial assistance.

The research was conducted between 1994 and 1998. In addition to three of the co-authors, a number of other doctoral students participated in various phases of the research. These students included Bobai Li, Kathy Kuipers, and Elaina Kyrouz. Four other doctoral students made substantial contributions. Randi Cohen was active in the early design discussions and was particularly helpful in crafting the case study element of the project. Seth Pollack took an active part in shaping our conceptualization of institutional environments and helped Peter Mendel in the early phases of data collection, focusing particularly on creating the policy maps (Tables 6.8a and 6.8b). Seth was also largely responsible for charting the history of the successive planning regimes (Case Illustration 6.A) and contributed in the gathering of organizational case research, especially for the Palo Alto Medical Clinic. Sammie Speigner played a leading role in helping to select and collect some of the organizational population data sets. He also was active in designing the study of healthcare systems, and he took the lead in devising instruments to assess the extent of centralization of decision-making in these multiorganizational systems. And Junko Takagi helped to design and carry out the discourse analysis reported in chapter 6. All of these participants were doctoral students in the Department of Sociology at Stanford University with the exception of Seth Pollack, who was completing his doctoral degree in the School of Education, also at Stanford.

In order to allow undergraduate and master's level students to become more familiar with healthcare issues and to obtain research experience, *xxi* we conducted several quarter-long departmental workshops on the orga-nization of medical care. In addition, a sophomore seminar called Trans-formation of Healthcare Organizations was offered, and students in this course assisted with collection of data on healthcare systems in the Bay Area. Still other students became involved by taking courses in directed research. Students participating in one or more of these courses and, hence, contributing to the project included: Erikka Ahn, Darren Allaway, Ian Bachrach, Samuel Brasch, Ray Carey, Nina Chinosornvatana, Lindsey Cole, Jene Elzie, Eric Ferguson, Ari Fernandez, Karen Hertz, Chris Krare, Brian Kucer, Kane Lai, Richard Lee, Erin Mosher, Kristin Pasquini, Carolyn Repa, Lara Shean, David Sherman, Anne Sonka, Katie Stokes, Micah Tep-per, Nancy Tseng, Derek Weatherford, and Jennifer Williams. Four such students—Lianne Chun, Khahn Doan, Michael Elisofon, and Jacqueline Shen—made exceptional contributions and provided much appreciated yeoman service on a host of specific research tasks.

Two other students at this level were particularly active in and devoted to the project. Tari B. Vickery was heavily involved in data entry and in collecting and analyzing case histories of hospitals in the Bay Area. Matthew D. Solomon assisted with the historical study of the Palo Alto Medical Clinic and the Stanford Medical Center.

A number of individual scholars made important contributions in our effort to obtain organizational or environmental data. Alan D. Meyer (College of Business, University of Oregon) and David B. Starkweather (School of Public Health, University of California, Berkeley) had each conducted previous studies of hospitals in the San Francisco Bay Area and generously shared their data and insights with us. Douglas R. Wholey (School of Management, University of Minnesota) made available to us his machine-readable data on HMOs in the Bay Area. Ed Pearlstien assisted us in locating relevant materials in our study of San Jose Hospital. And Andrew E. Newman (Department of Sociology, University of Michigan) allowed us to employ data from his dissertation relevant to the growth of administrative agencies in the State of California.

In the course of collecting and interpreting our data, we took advantage of the expertise of many individuals who were willing to consult with us. Their names, and affiliations at that time, are listed below:

Jeffrey A. Alexander, Professor of Health Management and Policy, School of Public Health, University of Michigan
Elizabeth Armstrong, doctoral candidate, Department of Sociology, University of California, Berkeley

Linda Bergthold, Senior Researcher, Lewin Group

Dr. Lawrence P. Casalino, doctoral candidate, School of Public Health, University of California, Berkeley

Shelley Correll, doctoral candidate, Department of Sociology and University Statistical Applications Consulting, Stanford University

Don Cram, doctoral candidate, Department of Finance, Graduate School of Business, Stanford University

Carroll L. Estes, Director of Institute of Health and Aging and Professor of Sociology, Department of Social and Behavioral Sciences, School of Nursing, University of California, San Francisco

Peter N. Grant, General Counsel for the Hospital Council for Northern and Central California

Merwyn R. Greenlick, Faculty Director, Oregon Health Policy Institute

Maureen Humphreys, Associate Director of VA, Palo Alto Healthcare System

John R. Kimberly, Professor of Management, Healthcare Systems, and Sociology, The Wharton School, University of Pennsylvania

Dr. R. Hewlett Lee, retired Executive Director, Palo Alto Medical Clinic

Dr. Sharon Levine, Associate Director for Physician and Professional Support Services, The Permenente Medical Group

Donald W. Light, Professor of Comparative Healthcare Systems and Director of the Division of Social and Behavioral Medicine, School of Medicine and Dentistry of New Jersey

Karen Lincolns, doctoral candidate, University of California, San Francisco

Alan D. Meyer, Professor of Management, Lundquist College of Business, University of Oregon

Kathleen Montgomery, Assistant Professor of Organizations and Management, Anderson Graduate School of Management, University of California, Riverside

Barbara Norish, doctoral candidate, School of Public Health, University of California, Berkeley

James O'Leary, Senior Data Analyst, California Medical Review, Inc.

Donald A. Palmer, Professor of Organizational Behavior, Graduate School of Management, University of California, Davis

James C. Robinson, Professor of Economics, School of Public Health, University of California, Berkeley

Thomas G. Rundall, Professor and Director, Graduate Program in Health Sciences Management, School of Public Health, University of California, Berkeley

Stephen M. Shortell, Professor, Kellogg School of Management, Northwestern University

Dr. Marvin Smoller, President, Smoller Healthcare Consulting and retired member, The Permanente Medical Group

David B. Starkweather, Professor Emeritus, School of Public Health, University of California, Berkeley

Jay Thorwaldson, Director of Public Affairs, Palo Alto Medical Foundation

Andrew Van de Ven, Professor, Carlton School of Management, University of Minnesota, Minneapolis

Kim Weeden, doctoral candidate, Department of Sociology, Stanford University

A number of our students and colleagues read and made constructive comments on earlier drafts of this volume. We are indebted to the following (as well as to a number of anonymous reviewers) for helpful suggestions in improving the manuscript:

Sanford M. Dornbusch, Professor of Sociology, Emeritus, Stanford University

Michael Elisofon, masters student, Stanford University

Mary L. Fennell, Professor of Sociology, Brown University

Walter W. Powell, Professor of Sociology, Arizona University

Teresa L. Scheid, Associate Professor of Sociology, University of North Carolina, Charlotte

Paul Wong, masters student, Stanford University

In addition, we have been blessed with the bountiful library and information resources of the San Francisco Bay Area, including those of three venerable research institutions—Stanford University, University of California at Berkeley, and University of California at San Francisco. Four librarians at Stanford were especially helpful in locating research materials in collections here and elsewhere: Richard B. Fitchen, of Green Library's Reference Services; Betty Y. Lum, of the Jonsson Library of Government Documents' Reference Desk; Sonia Moss, of Interlibrary Borrowing Services, and Heather E. Murapa, of Branner Earth Sciences Library.

Finally, our quest for information on healthcare systems at the local, state, and national levels brought us in touch with many people who gather and maintain an invaluable amount and variety of data. Those generously sharing their stores of archival knowledge, both small and large, as well as the expertise to help interpret them properly, included:

Carolyn Anderson, Analyst, California Office of Statewide Health
Planning and Development

Julie Baitty, Health Resources and Services Administration, U.S.
Department of Health and Human Services

Phyllis Barnhourse, Medical Care Statistics Section, California Department
of Health Services

Bob Bennenfield, Housing and Household Economics Statistics, U.S.
Bureau of the Census

Mark Desio, Public Affairs Office, California Public Employees'
Retirement System

Catherine Direen, Director of Communications, California Medical
Review, Inc.

Jan Drexler, Bureau of Data Management and Strategy, U.S. Health Care
Financing Administration

Inga Franklin, Bureau of Health Professions, U.S. Department of Health
and Human Services

Mark Gemmell, Health Care Division, Services Employees International
Union

Ruth Given and Sally Roberts, California Medical Association

Penny Havlicek, Department of Professional Activities Information,
American Medical Association

Jim Hirbayashi and Bill Brown, U.S. Patent and Trademark Office

Emma Hoo, Director of Negotiating Alliance, Pacific Business Group on
Health

Jane Kenamore, Archivist, American Medical Association

Carl Martin, Director of Marketing, Health Insurance Plan of California

Judy Rochell, Membership Director, American College of Physician
Executives

Marc Rogers, Director of Research, American Managed Care and Review
Association

Gail Royster, Federation of Chiropractic Licensing Boards

Jeff White, Librarian, Medical Group Management Association

Maureen Wise, Membership Coordinator, Santa Clara County Medical
Association

Charlene Wolfe, Public Information Services, California Department of
Consumer Affairs

Henry Wulf and Donna Hirsch, Governments Division, U.S. Bureau of
the Census

For all of these varied and helpful contributions, we are grateful.

One

A World in Transition

THE CHANGES IN MEDICAL service delivery that have occurred within the lifetime of adult Americans are truly remarkable. After years, even decades, of watching an industry that exhibited "dynamics without change" (Alford 1972), "the world in which the independent, solo practitioner in combination with the independent, voluntary hospital were the dominant forms of service provision has 'gone with the wind'" (Scott 1993: 271). In the 1990s, we are confronted with much that is new: new technologies, new ways of delivering services, new mechanisms of paying for care, new types of healthcare organizations and cooperative and competitive relations between them, new regulatory systems (as well as deregulatory processes), new players in the sector, and new assumptions and beliefs governing healthcare. Indeed, current observers refer to the medical care sector as undergoing a period of "hyperturbulence": a time of revolutionary change within the industry (Meyer, Goes, and Brooks 1993).

But not everything has changed. To a surprising extent, old forms and practices coexist alongside the new. Community hospitals, for example, are still regarded by many as central, civic, almost sacred institutions with long and honorable traditions. Presiding over some of our most fateful life crises, they remain in important respects the cathedrals of contemporary communities. With structures and practices buttressed by the power of professionals and community leaders, they do not easily adapt to new ideas and new ways. Change is not instantaneous in social systems: these structures exhibit much—perhaps, desirable—recalcitrance and inertia.

The current scene, then, reflects contradictory forces: rapid change in a sector noted for its highly institutionalized character. In an arena such as healthcare, change does not come easily, but when it does—when the existing structures and beliefs are undermined or severely challenged—profound change can occur quite rapidly (Greenwood and Hinings 1996).

OVERVIEW OF STUDY

In this study, we examine the nature and extent of changes in medical care delivery systems during the past several decades. We rely on the insightful works of Starr (1982) and Stevens (1989), but do not attempt to provide yet another social history of the American medical system. Instead, as a means of illuminating broader societal changes, we explore in detail developments in one large metropolitan region in the United States, the San Francisco Bay Area, over the fifty years from 1945 to 1995. The Bay Area is by no means presented as a representative microcosm of the American healthcare system, but, we argue, many of the features that differentiate the Bay Area are also those that place it on the cutting edge of change in medical institutions. It is farther along than most other areas of the United States in exhibiting the trends we are attempting to chart and explain.

Our study focuses on organizations as the principal players in the changes we wish to track. In modern society, organizations are influential not simply as contexts affecting individual behavior, but as actors themselves—as *collective actors* possessing resources, rights, and distinctive capabilities and limitations. Most of us continue to buy into the liberal conceit that individual persons are the primary actors in modern society and, if we attend to organizations at all, it is to regard them as instruments—as agents—we construct to aid us in pursuing our goals. We neglect the extent to which all of us are more often the agents of organizations, working to achieve not our own personal but organizational objectives (or, more accurately, achieving the means to our personal objectives, such as obtaining wages or a salary, by pursuing organizational objectives). Thus significant individuals enter into our study primarily in their role as the agents of organizations, including professional groups and associations.

Five types of organizations that deliver medical care services form the centerpiece of our investigation. They are hospitals, health maintenance organizations (HMOs), home health agencies (HHAs), end-stage renal disease centers (ESRDCs), and multihospital or integrated healthcare systems. The first two forms represent, respectively, the traditional and the newly emerging template for dispensing generalized medical services. HHAs and ESRDCs represent selected instances of a range of more specialized providers, also including surgicenters, urgent care services, and hospices, that have arisen in the past few decades as alternatives to more diffuse and multipurpose forms. Multihospital systems and integrated healthcare systems have emerged as entities linking previous forms, but also themselves constitute a new, complex organizational form. We treat these five types as organizational *populations,* with each individual organization considered a member of a distinct species.

We have also singled out for detailed attention four specific organizations in the Bay Area: Kaiser Permanente Medical Care Program (Northern California Region), Palo Alto Medical Clinic, Stanford University Hospital, and San Jose Hospital. We selected these cases to represent both innovative and traditional actors in the region. The study of these organizations allows us to examine in more detail than is possible via the study of organizational populations whether and how specific organizations responded (or failed to respond) to environmental events of apparent significance. We also wish to document the fact that organizations and their leaders are not simply passive reactors to environmental changes, but active players, attempting— sometimes with success—to influence the course of events.

We view these organizations and populations as responding to changes in their environments: local, regional, and national. We categorize these external forces into two types of environments: the material resource and the institutional. The *material-resource environment* refers to factors affecting healthcare organizations viewed as technical, production systems—as systems using resources to produce services. We consider factors affecting the demand for medical services (e.g., the sociodemographic characteristics of the human populations in the local areas served) and its supply (e.g., numbers of physicians and public funding for medical systems and services) as part of this environment.

The *institutional environment* encompasses the cultural belief systems, normative frameworks, and regulatory systems that provide meaning and stability to a sector. Although institutions provide stability in social life, they are also subject to change. One of the primary objectives of our study is to attempt to conceptualize and assess transformations of the institutional environment. We frame these transformations by three historical eras, marked by distinctive institutional arrangements and belief systems, and examine the effects of these eras on the various organizational populations. We elaborate our conception of environments later in this chapter.

Our hope is to shed light on developments in healthcare systems generally by examining how various organizations in one geographically defined region respond to forces operating both in the immediate area and at the broader societal level. A central theme we develop is that much of the transformation in the nature of medical services is reflected in the nature of the medical organizations providing those services. Thus, change in the numbers and types of organizations, and linkages among them, is our central focus and provides our principal dependent variables.

We assume that these changes are related to other subjects of interest—to services provided and outcomes experienced by providers and clients—but we do not pursue these connections here. Instead, we subscribe to the ecological-evolutionary thesis that the diversity of organizations is itself a subject of significance. As Hannan and Freeman (1989) point out, organizational diversity might seem to be a matter of only academic interest, but it has important bearing on broader societal issues. Because it "constitutes a repository of alternative solutions" to problems, organizational diversity affects "the capacity of a society to respond to uncertain future changes" (p. 7). Moreover, within a given field, such as healthcare services, the diversity of organizations signifies the changing profile of routinized collective competence for dealing with medical problems.

Several conceptions of organizational change guide our study. First, ecologists note that organizational change occurs in two quite different ways: by changes that occur as existing organizations do new things or old things in new ways (*adaptation*) and by changes that occur because existing organizations are replaced by new types of organizations (*ecological change*). We explore how hospitals adapt in a variety of ways to changes in their environments: adding services, forming alliances, joining systems, and merging. We also examine new types of organizations coming into existence, such as HMOs and ESRDCs. We will observe changes over time in the characteristics of hospitals and home health agencies but also changes in the numbers of organizations of each type, as hospitals decline in number over the period of study while more specialized forms increase.

Second, we differentiate between *incremental* and *discontinuous* change. Much change occurs gradually and almost imperceptibly, as organizational forms add and subtract personnel, subunits, and services or products. But sometimes change occurs abruptly and in such a manner that the situation is greatly altered. Greenwood and Hinings (1993) suggest that it is useful to assume that organizations conform to certain underlying patterns or *archetypes* that provide templates for organizing (see also, Miller and Friesen 1980). Incremental change involves the development of organizational structures and systems within the constraints imposed by the existing archetype; discontinuous change involves the addition of a second archetype or the substitution of one archetype for another. The emergence of HMOs (described in chap. 2) exemplifies such a new archetype. In our view, discontinuous change rarely occurs within the boundaries of existing organizations. Since it requires the substitution of one template for another or the combining of templates, it is more likely to occur by selection than by adaptation, leading to the creation of a new organizational population.

To examine these types of change, we use a variety of archival sources. For each of the five organizational populations, we created a data base that records, on an annual basis, when individual organizations entered and left each of these populations as well as changes over time in some of their basic characteristics, such as size, number of services, ownership, and licensure. We employ these data in longitudinal analyses to ascertain whether and when these organizational populations underwent various types of change. An important emphasis of our study is the interdependence of the changes observed (e.g., how transformations in one population relate to those in others) resulting in *coevolution* of organizational populations. We also collected qualitative data on each of the four organizational cases to examine their experiences in light of these changes.

Our study documents the vast transformations of the healthcare sector during the past half century. It also situates, for one large metropolitan region, what, when, and where these changes were manifested and provides a framework within which it is possible to better understand how and why they occurred. In this manner we hope to contribute to an improved understanding of the development of the healthcare sector, the nature of the forces affecting it specifically, and, more generally, the changing shape of the welfare state.

THEORETICAL FRAMEWORK

Precursor Studies

There is no lack of social science research on healthcare organizations and systems. Early studies, mostly by sociologists, examined professional behavior within clinics and hospitals or conducted case studies of individual organizations. These studies (e.g., Georgopoulos 1972; Goss 1961; Freidson 1975) stressed the uniqueness of the organizational arrangements associated with medical forms as physicians successfully resisted subordinate roles within administrative structures. Employing larger samples of organizations, research by Roemer and Friedman (1971) and Flood and Scott (1987), among others, examined the effects of medical staff organization and organizational structures within hospitals on quality of care. Other studies documented the effectiveness of associations, such as the American Medical Association, in restricting competition and defending the autonomy of professional providers (e.g., Garceau 1941; *Yale Law Journal* 1954; Freidson 1970a; Kessel 1970). Most studies conducted as late as the 1970s focused on the distinctive aspects of this professionally dominated sector.

Similarly, early studies of medical services by economists emphasized that market transactions in this sector did not conform well to conventional economic models. A number of factors were recognized as reducing the efficiency of market behavior (see Arrow 1963; Klarman 1965). First, because there is high uncertainty surrounding the provision of medical care, preferred outcomes cannot be guaranteed and quality of care received is difficult to assess, particularly by the consumer. Second, much of the demand for care is not directly determined by patients' needs or choices. Rather, physicians act as intermediate agents, exerting substantial influence over medical services, including the type and amount of service and organizational locus of care (Fuchs 1974). Third, the effects on prices of restraint of trade exercised by near-monopoly providers—in the form of both community hospitals and a restricted supply of physicians—were duly noted (e.g., Feldstein 1971; Kessel 1970).

From the 1960s onward, social scientists attended to the rapid expansion and shifting nature of political intervention in the healthcare sector. First, public agencies attempted to improve and rationalize healthcare services by creating structures to enable and encourage health planning. Then, to assure more equitable access to care, these agencies purchased services for senior citizens and the indigent. More recently, they have pursued a variety of strategies to effect cost containment. Political scientists and policy analysts examined the processes involved in the creation of these regulatory and funding systems and, together with economists, have also examined the effects—both intended and unintended—of these reform attempts. May (1967) reviewed attempts to develop planning regimes for hospitals, and Marmor (1970) and Somers and Somers (1967) examined the politics of Medicare. Effects of governmental initiatives on healthcare systems were investigated by numerous researchers, including Davis (1975), who studied the benefits and costs of Medicare, and Stevens and Stevens (1974), who studied the impact of Medicaid. For the most part, these studies have focused on specific policies or regulatory processes and, in assessing outcomes, generally emphasized effects on only one type of provider organization, usually the hospital.

Several more recent studies by sociologists are grounded in the organizational ecology framework (Hannan and Freeman 1977, 1989), which examines factors affecting the founding, growth, and eventual decline of aggregates of organizations, or *organizational populations*, exhibiting the same general form. Ecologists study the effects on population dynamics of environmental factors such as availability of material resources and political support. Populations of healthcare organizations previously studied include hospitals (Alexander and Amburgey 1987), HMOs (Christianson et al. 1991; Strang 1995), and HHAs (Estes et al. 1992). To date, no investigators have examined the effects of changes in one population of providers on changes in others, whether these are positive through mutualistic processes or negative through competitive processes, although Wholey and Burns (1993) have studied such effects as they operate among three subtypes of HMOs.

Finally, a few studies have examined the interactions and interconnections among a collection of healthcare organizations, typically hospitals, usually focusing on organizations operating in the same geographical area. Early research by Levine and White (1961) emphasized interdependence as mediated by the exchange of resources, principally information and patients. Milner (1980) examined the social processes that created a differentiated system of services and clientele and maintained status-ordered relations among 25 healthcare facilities in a single community (although primary attention was focused on three hospitals and a comprehensive health center). Fennell (1980) conducted a longitudinal study examining the division of labor among "clusters" of hospitals in 15 U.S. cities. She found stronger associations between provider (physician) diversity and range of services offered by hospital clusters than between patients' needs and services. More recent studies have examined the structure and effectiveness of networks created by federal agencies to link hospitals and research centers in order to conduct clinical trials and diffuse technical innovations (see Fennell and Warnecke 1988; Kaluzny and Warnecke 1996).

Three studies are particularly relevant to our own research. Starkweather (1990; see also, Starkweather and Carman 1987) examined competitive and integrative behavior among a collection of hospitals located in three California communities, one of which was in the San Francisco Bay Area. The study focuses on the period 1980–87—although Starkweather provides brief historical background for each of the seven hospitals included in his study.

Meyer, Goes, and Brooks (1993; Meyer, Brooks, and Goes 1990) carried out a longitudinal study of 30 hospitals randomly selected from 55 hospitals located in four counties in the San Francisco Bay Area during the period 1975 to 1989. Although their plan had been to study strategic change on the part of these individual hospitals, they quickly discovered that changes were sufficiently dramatic that it became necessary to shift attention away from the individual hospitals (organization level) up to the level of the organization field (or industry level) in order to observe more clearly the changing connections between hospitals and the new types of collective action.

The third study, conducted by Van de Ven and Grazman (1994), examined the evolution of medical organization forms in Minneapolis–St. Paul over 140 years (1853–1993). Their historical study documents the "genealogies" of four major healthcare systems now supplying over 80 percent of the medical services for this county and provides a systematic account of changes occurring over time in these delivery forms.

Limitations That Point the Way

This brief overview reveals that while there has been no dearth of social science research examining the macro-organizational aspects of medical delivery systems, there remain important neglected areas, a number of which we have explored here. First, with the exception of the population ecology studies and the handful of areawide studies just reviewed, little of the research in the healthcare area takes a longitudinal perspective, examining in a systematic manner how medical systems are changing over time. Excluding descriptive case studies or general historical accounts, much of the empirical research is cross-sectional. Second, there are few studies that isolate a single geographically defined area and attempt to examine the variety of changes transpiring in the organization of medical services in that area and the ways in which these processes affect each other. With the exception of the study by Van de Ven and Grazman, all of the recent areawide studies of healthcare organizations—by Milner, Starkweather, and Carman, and Meyer and colleagues—are largely descriptive and cover relatively short periods. These studies are theoretically informed (and the research by Meyer and colleagues examines interlevel effects) but seek to generate hypotheses rather than to test them.

Third, there are no studies that systematically examine the interrelations among several populations of healthcare organizations, ascertaining the extent to which the dynamics of one population are interdependent with those of another. Do hospitals shrink in size or numbers when HMOs enter their service areas? Do HHAs compete with hospitals, or are they mutually supportive? We know of no studies of these types of questions. Fourth, there are only a few studies that simultaneously consider the effects on healthcare organizations of both material-resource environments and institutional environments. The studies by Wholey and Burns (1993) of factors affecting HMO founding and failures is an exception to this general conclusion, but there are few others. Fifth and finally, there are no studies that simultaneously take into account both local factors, such as the concentration of organizations in the same service area, and broader influences stemming from actions by public and private entities, such as professional associations, at the county, state, and national levels. The contexts within which organizations operate are "nested" in the sense that areas are contained within counties and counties within states, and so on. These nests are not airtight containers but open sieves that allow wider influences to penetrate more local arenas.

Our study is designed to address all of these neglected areas. It involves the longitudinal examination of the evolution of five organizational populations located within a single, large metropolitan area, as well as the effects of changes in these populations on each other and the effects of the material-resource and institutional environments at various levels, ranging from the service area to the nation-state. From a sociological perspective, fifty years is not a long time,[1] but the period we have chosen is one that witnessed quite fundamental changes in our common understanding of how medical care should be delivered and financed and who has the legitimate right to make these decisions. We examine the repercussions of these changes on the organizational services in the San Francisco Bay Area.

The design of our study has been informed by a number of recent developments in organizational research. Before describing further details of our study area and design, we discuss the theoretical roots of our work.

Integrating Levels and Perspectives

During the past three decades, a flurry of theoretical activity has enriched and enlivened the study of organizations (for comprehensive reviews, see Pfeffer 1997; Scott 1998; for applications to healthcare organizations, see Fennell and Alexander 1993; Scott 1993). For many years, investigators of organizations restricted attention to the activities and processes occurring inside them, studying leadership, group morale and productivity, and variations in structural arrangements. During the 1960s, general systems theory—a broad intellectual movement affecting many sciences—invaded the domain of organization studies and transformed it by calling attention to the pervasive importance of the broader context—the environment—within which organizations operate. At first, investigators paid attention

---

1. Previous studies dealing with organizational populations suggest that a period of 100 to 200 years is required in order to encompass the full evolutionary trajectory, from birth to demise (see Carroll 1984, Singh and Lumsden 1990, Baum 1996).

only to local environments affecting organizational activities, for example, the immediate suppliers or competitors, but, over time, the focus of investigation moved "up and out"—up to encompass broader and more comprehensive phenomena affecting organizations and out to incorporate more aspects or facets of the environment.

As the levels at which organizations were studied moved higher, the number of theoretical perspectives multiplied. Three of these levels and their associated perspectives are relevant to our study: the organization set, the organizational population, and the organizational field. We define each and briefly review the most important theories associated with each.

Organization Set

The organization set is defined as encompassing a given organization of interest—the focal organization—together with its relations to other organizations that are critical to its functioning and survival (see Blau and Scott 1962; Evan 1966). The environment is seen from the vantage point of the focal organization, and attention is directed to how it views its environment, how its relations with other organizations influence its structure and performance, and how it strategically manages these relations. Several competing theoretical perspectives have developed that are applicable at this level. The earliest and still the most popular perspective is *contingency theory*, which proposes that those organizations are most successful that are able to adapt their structures to fit their environments (Lawrence and Lorsch 1967; Thompson 1967; Donaldson 1996). A related economic approach focuses on *transaction costs*, arguing that organizations design their structures to minimize the costs of negotiating and enforcing contracts among participants (Williamson 1975, 1985). Both of these approaches rest on the assumption that organizational participants are engaged in rational (or at least, "boundedly rational" [March and Simon 1958]) behavior: activities are designed to achieve goals with minimal costs.

Other perspectives applicable to this same level of analysis emphasize that participants may not share similar goals and that much behavior is governed by power struggles within the organization or power contests between organizations. Thus, the *resource dependence* perspective (Pfeffer and Salancik 1978) and the *strategic management* approach (Mintzberg 1983) point out that economic dependence can give rise to political processes—both inside and outside the organization—as participants seek to gain strategic advantage in competitive situations.

We employ this level of analysis and these perspectives primarily in chapter 8, where we examine the factors associated with a specific hospital's decision about whether to enter a multihospital system and whether to provide particular services itself or contract with other organizations for their provision. We also use this level of analysis and implicitly employ many of these perspectives in the case illustrations when we discuss how our various organizational cases react to changes in their environment.

Organizational Population

The organizational population, first introduced in the pioneering work of Hannan and Freeman (1977) and Aldrich (1979), has emerged as an important new level of analysis. Organizational populations are "specific time-and-space instances of organizational forms. That is, an organizational population consists of the set of organizations with a particular form within a (bounded) social system" (Hannan and Carroll 1995: 29). While the notion of population is closely related to that of industry, the latter term places more definitional emphasis on consumer choice within a market— including firms producing close substitutes even if using quite different materials and methods—while the former term emphasizes similarity in the production process and accompanying organizational form.

The *population ecology* approach is particularly suited to examining how specific organizational forms arise, grow in numbers up to some maximum—the "carrying capacity" of the environment—and then level out or decline. Attention is focused on the effects of population size, competition among forms, and capacity constraints on the relative numbers of organizational births and deaths. A considerable variety of organizational populations has been surveyed, which generally reflect a fairly regular convex pattern of growth and decline (for reviews, see Carroll 1984; Singh and Lumsden 1990; Baum 1996). Ecologists have proposed that the early stages of development, when the population is growing increasingly rapidly, reflect the effects of a process of legitimation, by which the form is becoming increasingly recognized, accepted, and taken-for-granted (Carroll and Hannan 1989). This "cognitive" type of legitimation is one of the important ways in which institutional forces shape organizational processes (Scott 1995). As the density of the organizations of the same type increases, however, the positive effects of legitimation are outweighed as competitive pressures begin to dominate population processes.

An important assumption underlying the ecological approach is that organizations find it difficult and dangerous to make marked changes in their forms or ways of doing business. Change is difficult because both internal sunk costs in equipment and personnel as well as external commitments and constraints prevent organizations from changing quickly or easily; thus organizations are characterized by inertia (Hannan and Freeman 1984). If this is a general characteristic of most rank-and-file organizations, think how much more difficult it is for organizations such as hospitals, staffed by professional employees, filled with specialized equipment, and embedded in community relations, to undertake significant transformations. Moreover, attempting to change is dangerous because it takes time to master new ways of thinking and working and because, in their early stages, many more innovations fail than succeed (see March 1990).

To date, most of the research on organizational populations has focused on the processes at work in shaping a single population, examining density-dependence effects (e.g., the effect of the total number of existing organizations of the same type on the probability that a new organization will survive) as well as the influence of environmental forces, such as resource availability and regulatory constraints. But population ecologists have also attended to subpopulation effects, for example, the relative success of specialists versus generalists or competition among variants of the same form. And, as noted, they have investigated the interdependence in the growth patterns of four subtypes of HMOs—staff, group, independent practice associations (IPAs), and network forms (see Christianson et al. 1991; Strang 1995).

Although ecologists have called for studies conducted at the "community ecology" level (Astley 1985; Hannan and Freeman 1989), to date, few such studies have been conducted (for an example, see Brittain 1994). At this level, the interdependence of several related populations is examined. And, it is only at this level that the creation of new populations or the erosion of the boundaries of existing populations can be observed. These processes are of obvious importance, and we propose to examine them in this study, but in our schema, we treat them as taking place at the level of the organization field.[2]

Organizational populations are a major focus in our research. Beginning in chapters 2 and 3, we provide descriptive accounts of four of our five populations (hospitals, HMOs, HHAs, and ESRDCs) and discuss their evolution over the past half century. Chapter 4 deals with population

---

2. We treat the organizational field as encompassing the community ecology level. The latter emphasizes multiple, interdependent populations but limits attention to a relatively restricted geographical area. By contrast, the field level, as described below, directs attention to broader and more distant forces as well as to local conditions.

dynamics as we attempt to disentangle the contribution of ecological and adaptation processes to evolutionary change. The fifth population, healthcare systems, is described in chapter 8.

Organization Field

A third and, for our purpose, the most useful level of analysis to emerge in recent years is that of the organization field. An *organization field* encompasses: "those organizations that, in the aggregate, constitute a recognized area of institutional life: key suppliers, resource and product consumers, regulatory agencies, and other organizations that produce similar services or products" (DiMaggio and Powell 1983: 148). So defined, fields incorporate both organization sets—individual organizations and their exchange partners and competitors—and organization populations—aggregates of organizations exhibiting similar forms and providing similar or related services. Moreover, fields include critical "vertical" relations: ownership ties that link headquarter offices to local establishments or professional and governmental actors that establish the rules and norms governing practice. Thus, the boundaries of fields are not geographical, but cultural and functional: "the notion of field connotes the existence of a community of organizations that partake of a common meaning system and whose participants interact more frequently and fatefully with one another than with actors outside the field" (Scott 1994: 207–8). As described, we focus attention on selected populations of provider organizations, but we also take into account changes in three other categories of organizations in the healthcare field: (1) purchasers, such as individual patients or their employers; (2) intermediaries, such as commercial insurance companies and health plans; and (3) governing bodies, such as professional associations and government regulators (see chap. 2). We treat these related organizational populations both as participants in the field and also as important elements in the environment of the populations of provider organizations.

While fields provide a framework for locating and bounding the phenomena of interest, we must not assume that they are nonproblematic and unchanging. We examine how the field of medical services has changed over time, involving different players and responding to different rules and logics (see also Gamm 1992). Conflicts concerning what the field is about and who is to be regarded as a legitimate participant are an important focus of our investigation. Fields are constantly being constructed and reconstructed by a changing cast of participants. Forces shaping fields are both external and endogenous, that is, the result of actions taken by field participants.

The two sets of theoretical ideas most relevant to examining the field level are the *community ecology* perspective and *institutional theory.* Community ecology examines the ways in which similar and dissimilar populations interact in a common territorial environment, attending in particular to the ways in which they develop collective modes of adaptation to the environment (Hawley 1950; Carroll 1984) and to the emergence of new kinds of organizational forms (Astley 1985; Hunt and Aldrich 1998). Institutional theory is principally concerned with examining the ways in which belief and rule systems affect social behavior and structure—in our case, organizational behavior and structure. We expand on these arguments later, in our discussion of environments (see also chap. 6).

At the field level, we concentrate on four key processes: the creation of new populations of organizations, the development of organizational linkages, boundary changes in organizational forms, and changes in the boundary of the field itself.

Creation of new populations. In 1945, of the five populations of organizations we study, only hospitals and an early version of home health agencies existed. The other, more comprehensive (integrated healthcare systems) or specialized forms (ESRDCs) came into existence during the later decades. Thus, as we emphasize, change occurs through the decline in numbers and eventual disappearance of existing forms (although our study period is not sufficiently long to permit the observation of the extinction of an existing population) as well as through the creation and growth of new forms. Some forms, such as ESRDCs, represent the splitting off of existing personnel or operations and their repackaging into new organizational units. Others, such as the HMOs, represent a more fundamental change in that two functions previously organizationally segregated—financial risk bearing, traditionally assumed by insurance firms, and service provision, traditionally assumed by medical providers—are combined in the same organizational form. In all of our cases, we examine the conditions giving rise to new forms, their growth patterns, and the effect of these patterns on those of other, competing populations (see chaps. 3 and 5). This latter process, which involves the dependence of the growth and decline rate of one type of organization on what is happening to other types, is termed *coevolution* (see Barnett 1994; Baum and Singh 1994). To understand the changing face of healthcare delivery systems, it is essential that we consider the shifting division of labor among a collection of related but different organizational populations.

Organizational linkages. We have been taught by resource dependency theorists, such as Pfeffer and Salancik (1978), that one of the primary ways that organizations deal with strong competitive pressures or interdependencies is to develop linkages with relevant organizations. Early types of linkages in the healthcare domain typically involved either the more extreme step of a change in ownership, including takeovers or mergers, or the development of looser and more limited connections, such as membership in common associations or interlocks among boards of directors. We lack the data to examine systematically all of the possible modes of connection among our organizations, but we will examine factors accounting for two important types of linkage among healthcare organizations: contracts and vertical integration, or ownership ties (see chap. 8).

Recently, another type of linkage, the strategic alliance, has become highly prevalent in the medical sector (see Kaluzny, Zuckerman, and Ricketts 1995; Brown 1996). Alliances are preferred because they eliminate much of the need for capital investment or organizational restructuring while at the same time allow independent organizations to coordinate their efforts formally. Alliances provide the primary foundation for the rapid development of "integrated healthcare systems"—the newest form of choice in the medical world (Dowling 1995). These "systems" are, at present, highly diverse, some combining only service units, others including purchasers, financing mechanisms, and/or physicians; some are built around hospitals as the central units, others around physician or medical groups. Their organizational connections may involve vertical or horizontal integration, or combinations of a wide variety of looser linking mechanisms—"virtual" integration—including contracts, exclusive or preferred relationships, alignment of incentives, and integrated information systems. Various types of systems have arisen in the San Francisco region during the latter part of the period under study.

When did these systems—both vertical and "virtual"—arise, how are they organized, and what difference, if any, do they make in the life chances of their organizational members? A number of studies of multihospital systems have been conducted (e.g., Zuckerman and Weeks 1979; Morrisey and Alexander 1987; Shortell, Morrison, and Friedman 1990; Shortell et al. 1996), and we will draw on their arguments and findings as we examine these developments in the Bay Area in chapter 8.

Changes in population boundaries. Two kinds of boundary changes are of interest: (1) changes in the boundaries separating one organizational population from another; and (2) changes in the boundaries of the organizational field itself. First, we devote much energy to tracking changes in several populations of organizations over a long period of time. The changing prevalence of one or another archetypal form is, we believe, an important indicator of changes in the larger system of services. But another type of change is also taking place. Ecologists recognize that organizational boundaries are not as firmly fixed as those that mark the differences in biological populations. Social boundaries separating one from another type of organization are subject to "blending" and "segregating" processes (Hannan and Freeman 1989). Some social forces, for example stable technologies and strong regulatory systems, work to maintain organizational forms as discrete, easily recognized entities.

By contrast, other forces cause boundaries among forms in the same field to erode and become blurred; organizational types that were once clearly distinguishable become more interpenetrated and alike. Alternatively, two different patterns or archetypes may be combined in a new hybrid form. Among our populations, the HMO best exemplifies this development. Changing transaction costs, deregulation, and entrepreneurial effort are among the processes that may cause an erosion of conventional boundaries segregating forms and give rise to new or hybrid forms.

Particularly during the past decade, blending processes have created a rich and complex mixture of organizational forms in the healthcare sector. Such changes, while affecting individual populations, can best be studied at the field level, where it is possible to examine interdependencies among populations. While we will not attempt to examine these changes in population boundaries in any systematic way, we describe the types of changes we observe (see chap. 3).

Changes in field boundaries. The relatively clear distinctions and boundaries that characterized the field of healthcare at midcentury in this country have eroded considerably in recent decades. Physicians and other medical personnel increasingly share power with managers and with public officials at both state and local levels. Physicians have a less secure claim to speak with unchallenged authority now than before. This is due in part to their internal fragmentation as well as to the rise of the consumer movement and the increasing prevalence and popularity of "non-Western" and alternative medical models (see chap. 6).

Healthcare organizations themselves are increasingly likely to provide a broader array of services unrelated to medical care and are more likely to be components of multidivisional corporations engaged in a variety of business activities. The managers of medical organizations are less likely to have been trained in specialized programs emphasizing the distinctive characteristics of healthcare, for example schools of hospital administration or public health, and more likely to come from more conventional business settings and training programs. General business ideologies and practices—for example, an emphasis on product lines, cost centers, and strategic planning—which would have seemed out of place if not illegitimate to earlier participants are now widely accepted as normal ways of thinking about and conducting healthcare. Our study provides evidence regarding all of these important changes (see chaps. 6 and 7).

The organizational field is the level at which most of our analysis takes place. It is, we believe, a highly suitable vehicle for supporting the investigation of long-term change processes occurring in complex societal sectors. The field provides an important intermediate unit connecting the study of individual organization structure and functioning on the one hand and societal level processes on the other. As DiMaggio (1986: 337) suggests: "the organizational field has emerged as a critical unit bridging the organizational and societal levels in the study of social and community change."

For these reasons we believe the organizational field level is especially well suited to inform public policy decisions. Policy-relevant studies typically examine the effects of some particular policy on a single type of organization, but policies have unintended as well as intended effects. Policies directed at hospitals, for example, may have effects on HMOs and vice versa. A focus on the broader field level increases attention to and awareness of these unanticipated effects, interdependencies, and tradeoffs. In addition, the effects of policies are usually mediated by the actions of various field-level systems, for example, professional and trade associations, and it is important to take these intermediate structures into account in designing and implementing reforms.

We have arbitrarily restricted the scope of the field of organizations studied to the San Francisco Bay region, but this geographical limitation applies only to the dependent variables: the populations of organizations and individuals whose behavior is to be explained. The causal forces that account for the changes observed—the independent variables—are not restricted to the immediate area but include wider influences at the state and national level. We turn now to discuss the principal categories of these environmental factors.

Environments

The environmental level is defined as including structures and processes, which, though not themselves the subject of explanation, are expected to shape or influence that subject. But when the subject is an organizational field, we must recognize that many environmental elements and processes are endogenous to the field. For example, the changing number and nature of hospitals is an important contextual factor shaping HMOs, and vice versa. Other environmental forces, such as funding and regulatory decisions occurring in Sacramento or in Washington, D.C., however, are clearly outside the focal field, although they both influence local events and may themselves be influenced by local actors.

Environmental factors vary in terms of their spatial and temporal scope as well as in their salience to particular field participants (Scott, Mendel, and Pollack, forthcoming). In terms of spatial factors, some events or forces operate at national or even international levels, whereas others are much more restricted. In considering the many factors affecting healthcare organizations, it is frequently difficult to decide whether it is better to employ a local or a more general indicator. For example, should the alternative health movement be assessed at the national or more local level? Similarly, temporal factors weigh heavily when the study period is of long duration and involves many changes in climate and mood. We are careful throughout to specify when particular events occurred and how long they continued to exercise influence. Finally, some variables are of critical importance to some actors but of little significance to others. We need to take into account the variable salience of environmental factors for different types of organizations.

Two broad categories of environmental variables are distinguished: the material-resource environment and the institutional environment. Theories drawn from organizational ecology and from economics—industrial organization economics, in particular—are relevant to the material-resource environment. Institutional theory, of which there are several variants, helps us to conceptualize and understand the institutional environment and provides the primary foundation of our theoretical approach.

Material-Resource Environments

All organizations require resources from the environment, and all organizations are engaged in production processes by which inputs are transformed into outputs through the application of energy, information and skills. The material-resource environment is that facet of the environment most directly relevant to viewing the organization as a production system depending on and transforming scarce resources. This environment is conceptualized as comprised of four sets of factors: (1) demand-side factors, (2) supply-side factors, (3) technologies employed by field participants, and

(4) the structure of the industry as it affects the flow of resources among organizations.

Demand-side factors. As economists have long recognized, medical care is not a conventional market arena. Demand is not steady, but irregular and unpredictable; consumers cannot readily evaluate the likelihood of obtaining benefits from treatment or even evaluate the appropriateness of their care (Arrow 1963). Physicians, as intermediaries, shape patients' choices. Patients differ, particularly in California, in the extent to which they look to conventional Western healers for their care. Cost of treatment received is typically borne by third-party payors so that demand is relatively inelastic, being insensitive to price differences. All of these and related factors shape demand for medical care (Aday et al. 1993).

Supply-side factors. The structure of factors affecting the supply of medical services similarly departs in many important respects from a competitive market. More than in most arenas, entry to practice is restricted by licensing and certification requirements. And, for practitioners such as physicians, training is prolonged and expensive and access to medical schools remains severely restricted. Until relatively recently, most U.S. physicians followed what Bennett (1977:127) has referred to as the " 'technological imperative,' the belief that every physician in every hospital should have available for his patients all the technologies of medicine, regardless of cost, questions of priority, or the optimal allocation of resources." Physicians provided whatever services were needed and third-party payors provided full reimbursement for charges. Moreover, emphasis was placed on acute services rather than preventive measures. Not until the 1980s have mechanisms been put into place to provide incentives to providers—both individuals and institutions—to treat earlier and as little as required.

Technologies. Organizational theories define the concept of technology broadly to include not only the hardware but also the skills and knowledge utilized by field participants to transform inputs into desired outputs. The healthcare sector relies heavily on technologies of all sorts, including highly specialized personnel and elaborate diagnostic and treatment mechanisms to achieve desired outcomes—in particular, reduced pain, improved functioning, and longer life. Improved healthcare and information-processing technologies during the past half century have both stimulated the demand for medical services and greatly affected their mode of delivery, supporting the creation of new, specialized organizational forms.

Industry structure. Medical markets vary greatly, even in the same geographical region, in terms of distribution of providers and the concentration of service organizations. In some areas, there is a high density of practitioners and organizations; in others, there are few alternatives. For many years, governmental policy included attempts by planners to devise more rational delivery systems and, during the 1960s, to impose restrictions on reimbursement rates, which were increasing faster than inflation (Payton and Powsner 1980). Structures also vary on the purchasing side. During the early period of our study, and in many areas up to the present, consumers of services were relatively unorganized, and purchasing remained an individual decision. But more recently, many large employers have organized themselves into purchasing groups that collect and share information on price and quality differences among available providers and, increasingly, bargain directly with providers for lower prices and higher quality (see Bergthold 1990). As we will discuss, one of the most effective of these purchasing groups has been active in the San Francisco region.

Institutional Environments

The institutional environment is composed of regulative, normative, and cultural-cognitive structures that operate to provide coherence, meaning, and stability to a field (Scott 1995). The institutional environment plays a central role in the story we have to tell. The last half century has witnessed dramatic changes in the rules governing healthcare systems and in our beliefs regarding medical care and its delivery. We emphasize three components of particular importance: (1) institutional logics, (2) institutional actors, and (3) governance systems.

Institutional logics are sets of "material practices and symbolic constructions which constitute [a field's] organizing principles and which are available to organizations and individuals to elaborate" (Friedland and Alford 1991: 248). These logics are the cognitive maps, the belief systems carried by participants in the field to guide and give meaning to their activities.

Institutional actors function both as carriers and creators of institutional logics. The institutional environment contains a variety of such actors, either individuals or organizations. Actors participate in the material-resource environment—as consumers or suppliers of medical services—but also participate in the institutional environment—possessing institutionally defined identities, capacities, rights, and responsibilities (Krasner 1988). An institutional change is signaled in the healthcare field, for example, when hospital managers once trained in schools of hospital administration are replaced by healthcare executives trained in business schools. We systematically track such changes across several categories of individual and organizational actors, defined and illustrated in chapter 2.

Governance systems are those "arrangements which support the regularized control—whether by regimes created by mutual agreement, by legitimate hierarchical authority or by non-legitimate coercive means—of the actions of one set of actors by another" (Scott, Mendel, and Pollack, forthcoming). Each societal sector or field is characterized by a somewhat distinctive governance system, composed of some combination of public and private actors employing both regulatory and normative controls over the activities conducted within that field. In the healthcare arena, three sets of principal players have participated in governance. Professionals, particularly physicians, but also others, have constructed normative frameworks that provide much of the foundation for the stable conduct of practice. During the early period, governmental agencies used their regulatory powers to enforce professional hegemony, but by the 1960s they were increasingly attempting to exercise more independent regulatory controls. The most recent period has witnessed the rise of corporate managers who create organizational frameworks to integrate and manage care providers. Changes in the nature of governance arrangements are expected to have a strong influence on which organizational forms are advantaged and the ways in which competitive forces operate.

Corresponding with the three periods of governance systems just outlined, we believe that it is possible to identify three distinctive eras during which a predominant logic prevailed and different types of actors were privileged in the healthcare field.[3]

- The era of *professional dominance*, 1945–65. During this period, professional bodies supported by state authority dominated the arena. The central value governing service provision was medical care *quality* as determined by professional providers.

- The era of *federal involvement*, 1966–82. Symbolized by the passage of the Medicare and Medicaid programs, the federal government became a major player in healthcare services during the period, initially providing funds and then increased regulation throughout the period. The central value governing the logic dominant during this period was a concern with *equity* of access to services.

3. Ruggie (1996, chap. 4) identifies a similar set of "phases" in her discussion of changes in the U.S. healthcare sector.

- The era of *managerial control and market mechanisms,* 1983–present. Beginning in the early 1980s, governmental policies shifted toward deregulation and a reliance on market forces, and large corporate groups entered the field. The central value governing institutional practice during this period is *efficiency* of service provision.

The identification of these three eras provides, at best, a crude delineation of the major types of change that have occurred in the field of healthcare in the U.S. during the last half of this century. We devote considerable effort, in chapters 6 and 9, both to justifying the appropriateness of this periodization as well as to examining the ways in which the forces at work operate across the temporal boundaries. In general, however, we believe that understanding the workings of these three eras can help us better account for the more basic changes that underlie much of the turbulence of the field.

Limitations of our Research

No single study can do everything, or even do the things it attempts to do as completely as one would like. Our work has limitations that should be acknowledged. We call attention to some obvious deficiencies; our readers will, no doubt, discover others. First, studies of organizational populations are more convincing, and analytic techniques are more powerful, if the time span selected includes the period when the populations were first founded (see Hannan and Freeman 1989). The data sets available did not permit us to meet this criterion with respect to three of the populations— hospitals, home health agencies, and integrated healthcare systems. Our systematic data on hospitals began in 1945, omitting the founding and early development period of this form by more than 75 years. We were able to ascertain when our study hospitals were founded, but we lack other relevant data on the period prior to 1945. In the jargon of the ecologist, our data set is "left-censored." We also lack data on the beginnings of the HHA population, although our data set does encompass the second major wave of growth in this form. And, a few church-related and secular nonprofit hospital systems were already in place in 1945 in the Bay Area, although most of the growth in multihospital systems occurred during the period of our study. The remaining two populations, HMOs and ESRDCs, were founded in or after 1945, and we are able to represent the full history of their evolution up to the present time.

A second, related problem with our population data is that, although we have a fairly sizable number of cases, we sometimes lack sufficient "events" to carry out definitive analyses. Among the critical events we wish to track are organizational births, deaths, mergers, and various types of transformations, for example, changes in location or in ownership form. Such events are sufficiently rare, even in volatile periods such as the one studied, that it takes many cases or long periods of time to assemble an adequate number to support statistical analyses. Some of our discussions of population events, therefore, are confined to a descriptive mode.

Third, some readers will no doubt be concerned that so much of our data has been compiled from secondary, archival sources, such as the annual surveys of the American Hospital Association or the annual statistics compiled by the California Office of Statewide Health Planning and Development (OSHPD). We are less concerned about the quality of these data largely because the variables we use—various measures of size, numbers and types of accreditations, ownership status—are reasonably straightforward, nonsensitive, and easily reported. We would have much less confidence, for example, if we were dealing with measures of health quality or health costs. We are also less worried about the problem of nonresponse or missing data because most of the respondents are required by public authorities to report these data in an accurate and timely fashion, and there are real penalties for noncompliance. The organizations making up our sample, including those that are privately owned and operated for profit, provide services viewed as critical to public health and safety and hence are subject to more strict reporting requirements than are most types of organizations.

A final concern and possible limitation of our research for some may well be our decision to focus primary attention on the subset of outcomes selected: organizational birth, death, and transformation. Most studies of medical services ignore what happens to individual medical organizations in order to focus on what existing medical organizations do: the types of patient served, the types of service provided, and the cost and quality of the work performed. Who is served, at what cost, and with what effects are obviously vital questions to pursue. But, we believe, it is also important to examine which types of organizations provide the services and how the mix of these organizations is changing over time. The organizations selected for study represent different combinations of services, providers, and functions. We think it matters, for example, that patients are being treated in their homes by HHAs rather than in hospital beds. The organization form affects what medical services are provided and how they are delivered. Changes in the number and types of provider organizations reflect changes in our beliefs and ideas about what kind of service healthcare is and how it should be provided.

The Larger Issues

Many questions are posed by this study, many types of approaches are employed, and many and varied data sets are assembled, but it is important that we not lose sight of the main theoretical issues addressed. We seek a better understanding of the nature and causes of institutional change by attending closely to the processes of destructuration and restructuration of an organizational field.

Profound Institutional Change

At the most general theoretical level, we view our study as examining an instance of profound institutional change.[4] While we intend to consider a number of processes and to examine a variety of types of organizations, we also view our effort as a single, complex case study depicting the transformations of a field of healthcare organizations. We consider these changes "profound" because and to the extent that they meet the following criteria:

1. *Multi-level.* Change occurs at the level of individual actors, in the development of new roles and individual identities affecting behavior and attitudes, but also at the wider levels of individual organizations as they take on new characteristics and pursue different strategies. At the level of populations, new types of organizations appear and older forms grow in numbers more slowly and eventually disappear. At the field level, some existing populations disappear, and some are combined into new configurations.

2. *Discontinuous.* Rather than representing only "first order," gradual or incremental change in the behavior and attributes of the actors being studied, we observe evidence of "second order," fundamental, radical change.

3. *New rules and governance mechanisms.* Rules governing the behavior of actors in the field are altered. The governance structures, including regulatory systems enforced by public agencies as well as more informal structures enforced by the normatively oriented behavior of various participants, undergo important modifications.

---

4. Alexander, D'Aunno, and Succi (1996) employ a related concept of "profound organizational change" to refer to changes occurring at the organizational level in rural hospitals, which increasingly must either undergo conversion (for example, into extended care facilities) or close down.

4. *New logics.* The logics that direct, motivate, and legitimate the behavior of actors in the field are changed. The types of ends pursued and/or the means-ends chains that guide action undergo change, as do the types of justifications that are given for action.

5. *New actors.* New types of social actors, both individual and collective, appear, sometimes representing new combinations or hybrids of existing forms, sometimes representing new entrants from other fields. Existing actors may transform their identities. The cast of characters undergoes change.

6. *New meanings.* The meanings associated with the attributes or behavior of actors in the field or the effects associated with them (that is, changes in the causal relations among variables) are modified. The "same" attributes are viewed in different ways or are observed to have different effects.

7. *New relations among actors.* The nature and extent of relations among actors in the field, including, in particular, exchange and power relations, are transformed. New types of linkages are created and the relational structure of the field exhibits substantial alterations.

8. *Modified population boundaries.* Boundaries once containing and separating organizational populations, organizations, customary activities, and personnel blend and blur.

9. *Modified field boundaries.* The borders of the field are expanded, reduced, or realigned. New definitions determine what types of activities and which types of actors are legitimate and which are more or less central or peripheral players.

Among the tasks we undertake in this study are to clarify the meaning of these types of change, describe the ways in which they are taking place in our empirical case, and explain to the extent possible how and why they are occurring in this time and place. In order to address these tasks, we examine change within a framework that recognizes the dynamic relationships between and among levels of analysis. Changes in logics and governance structures may occur at the field level, but how do these changes influence organizations and individual actors? Similarly, how does the emergence of a new type of social actor affect field-level logics and structures? Do these changes primarily reproduce existing rules and structures or modify the characteristics of higher-level systems (Giddens 1979, 1984; Greenwood and Hinings 1996)?

Many factors mediate these processes of influence between and among levels of analysis. We emphasize the importance of two: the degree of congruence between the levels and the extent of field structuration.

Congruence

Congruence is the extent to which a social actor embodies or reflects the rules, norms, and beliefs extant in its context. A social actor that, at a given time, embodies the rules and logics of the field may be more likely to reproduce them at a later time than a social actor that embodies logics distinctive from the field. Likewise, the field may have more direct influence on a congruent social actor than a distinctive one. On the other hand, field participants may pay more attention to the distinctive actor in an attempt to force compliance, while ignoring those social actors already congruent. In a field experiencing profound social change, are congruent social actors at a disadvantage? Under what conditions do noncongruent actors' models of organizing and beliefs become the basis for new, challenging logics that may in time dominate the field? These are among the questions we can explore because we have assembled data at multiple levels.

Structuration

While not a felicitous term, the master process on which this study attempts to shed light is that of *structuration.* As developed by Giddens (1979, 1984; see also Sewell 1992), the concept of structuration is employed to remind us that social structure involves the patterning of social activities and relations over time and space. Social structures only exist to the extent that they are continually produced and reproduced by social action. Hence, "structure" is too static a term to employ for a phenomenon that is actually a process. Giddens emphasizes also the "duality" of structure and action: ongoing patterns constraining and shaping action at the same time that action creates and modifies structure. We emphasize this meaning of structuration particularly in our use of the organizational case studies, viewing a specific organization as operating within, constrained by, and responding to a structural context at the same time that the organization's behavior reinforces or modifies this context.

DiMaggio and Powell (1983; see also DiMaggio 1983) employ the concept of structuration at the organizational field level to refer to the extent to which the behavior of organizations in the field constitutes (creates) a coherent structure or pattern of interaction as revealed by increasing interaction rates, amount of shared information, mutual awareness, and shared governance arrangements. Most empirical studies of field structuration have emphasized the process by which an orderly social structure is constructed over time by the interactions of a shifting set of collective and individual actors. Examples are provided by DiMaggio's (1991) study of the emergence of the field of art museums, Stern's (1979) account of the development of the governance powers of the National Collegiate Athletic Association, Leblebici and Salancik's (1982) discussion of the evolution of the Chicago Board of Trade, Suchman's (1995a) analysis of the development of standardized venture capital financing contracts in the emergence of the Silicon Valley semiconductor industry, and Dezalay and Garth's (1996) description of the construction of a transnational legal order to support international commercial arbitration. Our own study is not well suited to capture the early structuration of the field of healthcare, which took place in the U.S. primarily during the first half of the twentieth century.

Rather, given the time period of our study, we examine later phases of the structuration process, observing what we view as tendencies toward *de*structuration: the breakdown of traditional organizational forms and patterns of behavior, the dislodging of belief systems and the dismantling of governance structures dominant in earlier periods. We also look for signs of *re*structuration: attempts to put into place new organizational players, new logics, and new systems of governance. Only a few studies of these phases of structuration have been conducted to date. Previous studies include Davis, Diekmann and Tinsley's (1994) account of the "deinstitutionalization" of the conglomerate form and attempts to reinstate the more integrated firm, and Thornton's (1995) study of the reorganization of the U.S. college publishing industry involving the corporate restructuring of an earlier, stable field of independent publishing houses.

Fields that are undergoing destructuration and restructuration processes present challenging contexts to field participants. Because rules are contested and models disputed, these fields provide less support and guidance to social actors than more highly structured fields. On the other hand, they also impose fewer constraints, allowing more autonomous and innovative behavior on the part of actors.

We see profound institutional change as involving destructuration processes in which previously existing stable organizational fields are destabilized and disrupted, together with restructuration processes in which new types of actors compete and struggle to create a new social order. While we hope to shed light on these fundamental transformations, we are mindful that our study, for all its complexity, provides us with only one case of this phenomenon. Nevertheless, it is an important instance of a more general social trend affecting all modern societies: the ascendance of corporate forms and intrusion of managerial logics into ever more arenas of social life.

Two

THE CASE OF THE
SAN FRANCISCO BAY AREA:
FOCAL POPULATIONS AND
ORGANIZATIONS

OUR INTEREST IS IN UNDERSTANDING the nature and extent of changes that have taken place in healthcare delivery systems during the last half century in the United States. The case we selected to study these changes is the San Francisco Bay Area, a large metropolitan complex situated on the West Coast of the United States. In this chapter, we describe why we chose this particular geographic region, as well as the specific cases of Bay Area organizations and populations of organizations we use to examine and illustrate developments in the healthcare field.

SAN FRANCISCO BAY AREA

The nine-county San Francisco Bay Area is a large metropolitan region in the state of California on the West Coast (fig. 2.1). The commercial and cultural center of the region was and is the city of San Francisco. With the discovery of gold in California in 1849 and the resultant influx of immigrants through its natural harbor and as the western terminus of the transcontinental railroad, San Francisco became the central hub of transportation, immigration, and commerce in the Far West by the 1870s (Bryant 1994; O'Connor 1994). Across the bay, Oakland and the East Bay became and remain the region's major industrial center. To the north, agriculture predominates in Sonoma and Napa counties and, the South Bay, once an agricultural center in its own right, is now best known as the home of the Silicon Valley. This area has developed its own metropolitan focus in San Jose, the largest and most rapidly growing city in the Bay Area.

We chose the Bay Area to study the development of and changes in medical care delivery systems for several reasons. Certainly, data availability and convenience were considerations. It made sense for us to study the region local to us, so we would have relatively easy access to a wide variety

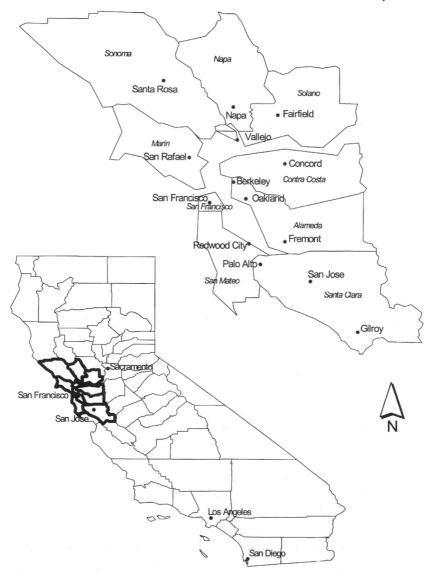

Figure 2.1   San Francisco Bay Area

of both quantitative and qualitative data sources, prior knowledge of the area's history and potential resources, and the ability to discuss our research with local informants knowledgeable about the Bay Area healthcare scene. But we also wanted to select a geographically and demographically diverse region with a history of both traditional and innovative healthcare. We planned to examine the embeddedness of our chosen region in its broader environments—economic, political, cultural—and wanted to study a region that both reacted to and helped shape these environments over time. Thus we sought a distinctive region that has historically been and remains on the cutting edge of developments in healthcare.

Because of its large immigrant population, alternative healthcare approaches, particularly Asian medicine, developed more rapidly and were accepted earlier in the Bay Area than in other parts of the United States. Immigrant communities also formed a variety of fraternal associations that pioneered the development of prepaid medical services. When the associations attempted to open their plans to the public, the California Supreme Court declared them illegal in 1938 (Grant 1988). Following World War II, however, the region hosted Kaiser Permanente, an originally deviant, then innovative, prototype HMO and hospital system. Because of Kaiser Permanente, California and the Bay Area have been leaders in the movement toward managed care. Other examples of more recent innovative healthcare financing arrangements include the development of unusually strong and active business coalitions to purchase health insurance. San Francisco also played a leading role in developing community-based services for AIDS patients.

More so than many other areas of the country, the San Francisco Bay Area has experienced rapid population increases, with the number of residents rising nearly threefold between 1945 and 1990. At the same time the numbers of physicians serving the area has increased even more rapidly, giving the Bay Area one of the highest physician-patient ratios in the country.

While distinctive in these and related ways, the Bay Area includes many traditional healthcare facilities and shares much in common with the rest of the nation. Its provider organizations include a large number of traditional healthcare organizations, such as nonprofit hospitals and independent physicians' practices. The region is also home to two world-renowned academic medical centers, Stanford University and the University of California, San Francisco.

The Bay Area has exhibited both traditional and innovative healthcare systems throughout its history. We chose to focus our study, however, on developments during the latter half of the twentieth century, rather than during the region's entire history, for several reasons. First, data availability and convenience again factored into our decision. We rely on statistical data from government agencies for many of our analyses, and these data are both more accessible and more reliable for the postwar period. Second, and more important, the Bay Area, along with the rest of the nation, underwent substantial transformations during World War II that marked the postwar period as a new era. Mobilization for the war provided the impetus for tremendous economic and demographic expansion in California and the Bay Area. During the early 1940s, California experienced the largest growth of any state, gaining over one million new inhabitants, and the Bay Area had a larger increase in its civilian population than any other metropolitan region in the United States (Abbott 1981). During the war years, more than 10 million servicemen and women were stationed in the West, and many of them returned to this area at the conclusion of the war (Nash 1973).

The federal government had an enormous effect on these developments in the Bay Area. Since the time of the Great Depression and the New Deal, the federal government has provided a disproportionate amount of funding to the West—as much as three times the national average (Nash 1973). In the 1940s, federal expenditures in California totaled more than $35 billion, constituting about 10 percent of all federal spending during World War II (Nash 1973). These expenditures were associated with the expansion of manufacturing, particularly shipbuilding (Abbott 1994). The Bay Area was also home to dozens of military installations. As Abbott observes: "The federal government in 1939 was the leading landlord and largest general contractor in the West. By 1943 and 1944, it was also the dominant employer" (1994: 483).

As the war drew to a close, several developments in the Bay Area marked changes in the healthcare field. Private, employer-based healthcare systems, such as at the Kaiser Industries shipyards, were opened to the public. Significantly, Kaiser's health plan introduced prepaid, capitated medical insurance to the general public. In addition, the end of World War II represented a watershed for hospital foundings and expansion. Aside from the incentives provided by the Hill-Burton act, a federal initiative that subsidized hospital construction and expansion, there was also a great deal of pent-up demand for more hospital beds. Proposed bond issues to build hospitals, left hanging for years during the war, were readily approved once postwar euphoria set in.

The San Francisco Bay Area emerged from the war a large and vigorous metropolitan area. Containing a population of nearly 2.2 million persons, it served as one of the major regional metropolises of the United States at the midpoint of the century. San Francisco was the uncontested financial and insurance capital of the West and functioned as the center of commercial activity for its hinterland, specializing in financial and administrative services, warehousing and wholesale trade functions and transportation services (Duncan et al. 1960). Continued postwar expansion fueled many new developments in the healthcare field. Our history and analysis begins with these midcentury changes.

ORGANIZATIONAL ACTORS IN THE HEALTHCARE FIELD

Of the many ways social actors vary, we emphasize three: types of social actors, functions in the healthcare system, and institutional roles.

Types of Social Actors

Six types of social actors are identified:[1]

1. Individuals. In the course of our study we refer to many talented and unusual individuals who, through their ideas or actions, were able to affect the direction of change in the healthcare sector. We describe the effect of actors both near—such as Henry J. Kaiser—and remote that made a difference in Bay Area healthcare.[2]

2. Associations of individuals. We focus on professional associations, such as the American Medical Association, that allow members with common characteristics to represent themselves as a corporate body that serves their collective interests. Associations are a special class of organization.

3. Populations of individuals. This type of social actor enters our study in chapter 5, where we consider the effects of the sociodemographic characteristics of Bay Area residents on healthcare. We examine various characteristics of residents, including those of patients and physicians.

4. Organizations. We trace the development of several individual organizations—Kaiser Permanente Medical Care Program, Stanford University Medical Center, San Jose Hospital, and Palo Alto Medical Foundation—as one of the primary subjects of our study.

5. Associations of organizations. These corporate bodies are made up of member organizations. We examine the influence of collectivities of major healthcare provider organizations, such as the American Hospital

---

1. Many of these units are nested in the sense that individual persons are members of organizations, populations, and associations; organizations are members of populations and associations.

2. The "new" social history reminds us that we should not overemphasize the role of "great men"— or great women—in affecting the course of events. While there is value in this prescription, the biases of the new institutionalism in organization studies pushes in the opposite direction, tending to provide too "oversocialized" a view of the behavior of social actors (see DiMaggio 1988, Powell 1991). In our study, we attempt to avoid both types of errors.

Association, as well as associations of healthcare purchasers, such as the Pacific Business Group on Health.

6. Populations of organizations. We have chosen five populations of organizations as the primary subject of our investigation: hospitals, HMOs, home health agencies, end-stage renal disease centers, and integrated healthcare systems. We also examine two secondary populations, medical groups and preferred provider organizations (PPOs).

Our study focuses primary attention on organizations and populations of organizations. These are the subjects of our investigation and we describe them in detail in the following sections. The other types of actors are treated primarily as aspects of their environment.

Functions of Social Actors

A second way in which our social actors differ is in the primary functions they perform in healthcare. As briefly noted in chapter 1, we distinguish among four functions in the healthcare field: buying services, supplying services, pooling/bearing financial risk, and oversight or governance. In the simplest case, one type of social actor provides each function. The buyer of services is also the ultimate consumer: the patient. The supplier of services is a single, independent professional provider, such as a physician. Insurance companies spread financial risk across a population of purchasers, and professional associations of practitioners, whose authority is endorsed by state agencies and public health officials, perform oversight functions. In the complex contemporary healthcare field, however, many different social actors serve each of these functions (see fig. 2.2). On the purchaser side, most individuals do not directly pay for the services they receive. Instead, they participate in health plans offered and partially subsidized by their employers or the federal government. On the provider side, individual physicians are increasingly likely to be members of medical groups or physician networks, or to be employees of HMOs or hospitals.

The variety of organizations acting as intermediaries has greatly increased in the last few decades. Commercial insurance companies still offer conventional indemnity insurance coverage, but many also organize, manage, or contract with HMOs or other types of health plans. And among the oversight bodies, professional associations such as the American Medical Association—active at the local, state, and national levels—increasingly share governance functions with a variety of local, state, and federal authorities, and with corporate systems coordinating the services of providers or the demands of clients.

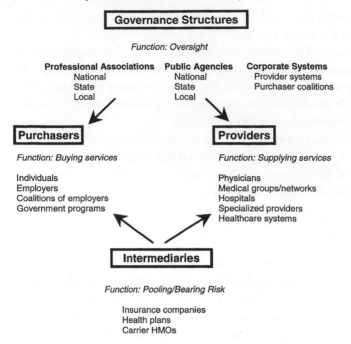

Figure 2.2   The Healthcare Field: Principal Social Actors and Functions

In addition to changes in the composition of actors performing functions, we also observe actors performing more than one function. Medical groups, hospitals, and other organizational forms, for example, provide settings for delivering services but also perform oversight functions, supplementing the internalized and interpersonal controls provided by individual professionals and their associations. For example, hospitals conduct utilization review (to determine if hospital admission and the procedures performed were warranted by the patient's condition) and quality assurance assessments (Somers and Somers 1961; Goss 1963; Roemer and Friedman 1971; Freidson 1975; Flood and Scott 1987). Also, some medical groups now offer their own health plans and so have taken on the risk-pooling and risk-bearing functions associated with insurance carriers.

Purchasers have become more organized and active in attempting to influence the type, cost, and quality of the care they buy. Many employers acting alone or in coalitions have begun to assume some of the functions formerly associated with intermediaries as they, for example, actively participate in the design of benefit packages. At the same time, they are also beginning to share in the oversight function by conducting surveys of employee satisfaction and even utilization reviews of services received (see chaps. 5 and 6).

Intermediaries, in particular, have recently taken on new types of functions in recent years. The new health plans and carrier HMOs not only perform the insurance functions of pooling risks, but actively participate in the management of care, assuming roles formerly performed by providers and governance units. The "arms-length" relation between providers and financial intermediaries has evolved into a much closer and, some would argue, intrusive arrangement. These developments are associated with the rise of managed care systems, which we discuss later in this chapter.

Finally, governance units have also expanded their functions over time. One of the major shifts recorded in our study occurred in 1965 when, with the passage of Medicare and Medicaid legislation, the federal government became a major purchaser of healthcare services. It is largely because of this new responsibility as buyer that the government has been compelled to become more active in its regulatory roles, enlarging on its earlier role as backup for professional controls to become a more active participant in quality assurance and cost-containment functions. We detail these changes in the role of the nation-state and professional bodies in chapter 6.

The variety of ways in which particular types of functions can be performed and, particularly, the many possibilities for combining varying types of functions, provides the seedbed out of which new organizations and new types of organizations emerge. We will be particularly attentive to this process as a major mechanism of field structuration. Our study focuses on provider organizations, but we examine other social actors and the functions they serve in order to fully understand changes in providers.

Institutional Roles of Social Actors

A third major dimension along which social actors vary is in the nature of the role they play in relation to the surrounding social structure. We identify two types of roles: carriers and agents. We view all social actors as institutionally constructed in the sense that their identities—characteristics and capacities—are socially designed. They embody institutionally defined meanings and are both empowered and constrained by the nature of the roles they assume and are assigned. These two roles are embedded in and created by particular social contexts, which are made up of agreed upon norms and meanings that shape and define social reality (Archer 1988; Dietz and Burns 1992).

In our study of organizations embedded in institutional environments, the norms and meanings of primary concern are framed by institutional logics. We define a carrier organization as one that embodies an identifiable institutional logic. For example, if one of the primary logics shaping the healthcare field is that the provision of healthcare is a charitable, not-for-profit service to the community, then nonprofit, eleemosynary hospitals are carriers of that meaning. All social actors act as carriers of their institutional context in the sense that their characteristics and capacities are socially defined, and, by embracing these logics, they reproduce and help to perpetuate them.

Social actors also have, to a variable extent, a capacity for social agency: the ability to shape in a deliberate way the actions of others or the rules governing those actions (Giddens 1979; Sewell 1992). The recognition of social agency is an important safeguard against an overly deterministic view of the influence of social structure. Still, it is essential to recognize that social agency, like all social behaviors, is shaped by social structure. Agency is not evenly and uniformly distributed among social actors but varies substantially by the actor's location in the social structure.

While there is no way to distinguish these roles definitively, we treat our organizational populations primarily as providing evidence concerning the role of organizations as carriers of institutional logics, and we employ the case studies of organizations to help ascertain when and how actors exercise agency. Although we deal with the full range of types of social actors, our primary focus is on those organizations and populations of organizations that provide healthcare services and that serve as carriers of institutional logics.

FOCAL POPULATIONS OF ORGANIZATIONS

Selecting the Populations

The major focus of our investigation is not individuals but organizations, and not single organizations but populations of organizations. We selected five populations for primary study: hospitals, health maintenance organizations, home health agencies, end-stage renal disease centers, and healthcare systems. We chose these five populations to encompass both the more traditional and the more contemporary forms of healthcare organizations, the more general and the more specialized.[3]

3. The five types of organizations singled out for intensive study are not, of course, the only populations of organizations providing health care services. Setting aside those organizations providing

Investigating more than one population has several advantages but also poses conceptual and methodological challenges. One main advantage is the ability to examine the interdependence that exists among these forms. An important feature of any organization's environment is the number and nature of other organizations located in the same area attempting to provide identical or similar services. Such organizations exist in a competitive relation one to another but, at the same time, can also supply mutual benefits to one another. Similar organizations may form temporary alliances allowing them to engage in collective action to improve their position, or they may develop more selective and lasting linkages that allow them to function as a unitary actor for some purposes. Moreover, the growth or decline of populations, relative to competing forms, may be seen, at least in part, as reflecting which logics are in decline and which are in ascendance. Such trends within a field can only be observed if the dynamics of several populations are compared and contrasted.

A primary conceptual problem, however, involves arriving at a clear and serviceable definition of the boundaries of these organizational forms. As Thornton and Tuma point out, "before doing [population-level] research on organizations, scholars need to consider whether a set of organizations truly has a unitary character over time and can be appropriately treated as a distinct population of organizations" (1995: 31). Defining organizational populations presents problems, whether one focuses on similarities of form or structural blueprints (Hannan and Freeman 1977, 1989) or "archetypes" (Greenwood and Hinings 1988), on distinctive competence ("comps") (McKelvey 1982), or similarities in "constitutive information" about how to organize (Suchman forthcoming). We know, for example, that even a well-established, traditional form such as the voluntary hospital subsumes a range of functions and exhibits a considerable variety of forms. Times of rapid change, as in the latter decades of the period of our study, encourage the breakdown of conventional organizational forms and the cobbling together of new and different arrangements. The rise of integrated delivery systems also has increasingly blurred the traditional boundaries of provider organizations, since primary care, specialized care, and extended care have been combined under one organizational canopy (Shortell, Gillies, and Anderson 1994, Shortell et al. 1996). HMOs and preferred provider

---

primarily mental health services or those engaged in long-term care, such as skilled nursing facilities and nursing homes, other provider populations include medical group practices, AIDS service organizations, specialty clinics of various sorts, free-standing centers providing ambulatory, surgical, urgent care, and emergency services, and various types of "alternative" providers, including hospice organizations, home birth centers, acupuncture and herbalist clinics, chiropractic clinics, and holistic health centers.

organizations (PPOs) suffer from similar boundary definition problems because of a pronounced trend toward hybrid combinations of medical plans (Miller and Luft 1994).

These substantive matters are mirrored by methodological concerns. When the boundaries of an organizational population are unclear, omitted members may contribute to selection bias and a consequent misestimation of models (see Berk 1983). We attempt to avoid these potential short-comings by using clear, a priori definitions of organizational forms that can be reasonably maintained over the historical duration of our analysis. We also explicitly consider interdependence among organizations (and organizational forms) that may blur those definitions.

Data Collected on Focal Populations

For each of the five populations we elected to study, we collected observations for all organizations on an annual basis. These observations include eight types of measures: (1) *accreditations and qualifications,* which indicate an organization's standing with oversight agencies and trade organizations; (2) significant organizational *events,* including foundings, mergers, closures, and name changes; (3) *linkages* with other organizations, including contractual arrangements, system memberships, and vertical integration; (4) the organization's *market niche,* (5) *ownership* status, (6) portfolio of *services,* (7) *size,* and (8) *utilization* of services.[4]

The resulting population data sets are structured in an organization-year format to enable us to study change over time. Thus, in the case of hospitals, we have one entry for each hospital that existed in the Bay Area in 1945, one entry for each hospital that existed in 1946, and so on. This kind of data set has a number of theoretical and methodological advantages over simpler cross-sectional, panel, and event-count designs (Tuma and Hannan 1984: chap. 2). Cross-sectional designs, which offer a snapshot of an organizational field at a single point in time, fail to support temporal and causal analyses. Panel data, which isolate features of an organizational field at two or more discrete points in time, are highly dependent on the particular time points chosen and cannot distinguish discontinuous from incremental change. Event-count designs include data from more time points than panel designs but aggregate organizational events to the population level, leaving it unclear whether changes at the population level are due to the entry

---

4. All measures were not available for all years or for all populations, and there is necessarily some variation in the types of measures selected for each population (see table A.2).

of new actors, the demise of old ones, or the transformation of existing organizations.

Given these considerations, we collected continuous-time, organization level data for each of our five focal populations; we also use several event-count data sets for descriptive purposes. The measures we use are described in more detail as appropriate throughout the volume and in Appendix A.

Hospitals

We selected hospitals because, for many decades, they have been "the central workplace of the American health care system" (White 1982: 143). Increasingly, however, these traditionally dominant forms are beleaguered and marginalized. Some are dying; most are undergoing dramatic changes in structure; and all are struggling to survive.

Appearing during the mid-nineteenth century, most hospitals developed as "voluntary institutions" having solid roots in the local community, enjoying support from community elites or ethnic groups, and embracing a strong philanthropic and service ethic. Unlike their European counterparts, U.S. hospitals adopted an open staff model, with community physicians organizing to control admitting privileges among their colleagues (Glaser 1963). During the twentieth century, hospitals have become much more dependent on physicians, who decide what patients are to be admitted and what services they are to receive, and their support base has shifted from donations to the marketing of services.

Until the early 1980s, hospitals were able to charge patients or third-party payors for usual and customary fees. New federal payment schemes, however, have substituted prospective payment for reimbursement, and hospitals receive a fixed amount for most patients determined by diagnosis. Rather than encouraging as much care as justifiable, incentives now reward as little care as required. Confronted with increasing competition for patient dollars, hospitals have begun to embrace conventional business practices, such as marketing, cost-benefit analysis, and strategic planning. Moreover, hospitals that for so long functioned as independent organizations responsive to local community concerns have, since the 1970s, increasingly become components of larger, corporate systems (Burns 1990; Starr 1982; White 1982).

Although established in the previous century, hospitals did not grow rapidly until the early part of the twentieth century. By the 1920s, more than 7000 hospitals existed in this country (Alexander and Amburgey

1987). Their rapid growth was occasioned both by the development of aseptic procedures controlling cross-infection and by the development of more efficacious therapeutic techniques. As a result of these improvements, middle-class patients chose to use hospital facilities in greater numbers (replacing an earlier clientele of poorer patients, who had formerly been forced to use them). The total numbers of hospitals declined during the Depression but recovered following World War II. Aggregate numbers hovered around the 7000 level before beginning a slow but steady decline after 1980.

There are many types of hospitals, so in order to study these orga- nizations, we required a clear delineation of the population boundaries. The *Dictionary of Health Services Management* defines a hospital as "an establishment that provides—through an organized medical staff, perma- nent facilities that include inpatient beds, medical services, and continuous nursing services—diagnosis and treatment (both surgical and nonsurgical) for patients who have a variety of medical conditions" (Timmreck 1982: 296). We narrowed this definition by excluding psychiatric facilities, both because the functions of mental and other hospitals are quite distinct and because very different policy environments have affected the two organizational forms during the last fifty years (Foley and Sharfstein 1983; Scott and Lammers 1985). We also chose to exclude drug and alcohol rehabilitation, geriatric, and chronic-illness hospitals because of overlap with rehabilitation clinics and nursing homes. The latter forms, providing services for chronic or long-term care, utilize technologies quite different from those employed in the acute-care facilities. Our definition includes both general hospitals and specialized facilities. A final definitional concern was how to treat hospitals that were members of larger delivery systems. We decided to explicitly model hospitals at the facility level and treat hospitals and healthcare systems as separate, but interrelated, populations.

The data sources for the hospital population included AHA's *American Hospital Directory* (1945–48), the annual directory issues of the AHA journal *Hospitals* (1949–71), the *AHA Guide to the Health Care Field* (1972–92a), and the annual hospital disclosure reports from California's Office of Statewide Health Planning and Development (OSHPD 1976– 91). Further details regarding sources will be found in Appendix A.

Health Maintenance Organizations

While we selected hospitals because of their historic centrality in the field, we selected HMOs as representatives of the wave of the future—or at least, an important transitional form (Morrison and Luft 1990). HMOs are among the newest, least understood and most controversial of healthcare organizational forms, representing the cutting edge of what has come to be known as *managed care* (Inglehart 1992; Kongstvedt 1996). The goal of managed care is to provide healthcare in as cost efficient a manner as possible, and the responsibility for attaining efficiency is shared by intermediaries that provide insurance or financing, physicians, and service delivery organizations such as hospitals (Miller and Luft 1994). Thus, managed care organizations bring into close association operations that had traditionally been widely separated and segregated because of physicians' fears that financial controls could jeopardize their clinical autonomy (Starr 1982).

Historically, managed care arose in the late 1960s as a solution to escalating costs in the Medicare and Medicaid programs and accusations that U.S. medical care was inefficient (Starr 1982; Gruber, Shadle, and Polich 1988). A handful of organizations that successfully operated with prepaid health plans, preventive care, and/or a group practice of physicians—such as the Ross-Loos Clinic in Los Angeles (founded in 1929), the Kaiser Permanente Medical Care Program (1945), the Health Insurance Plan of Greater New York (1947), and the Group Health Cooperative of Puget Sound (1947)—served as models for managed care plans (Luft 1981). In the early 1970s, Minnesota physician Paul M. Ellwood and colleagues coined the term "health maintenance organization," defined its organizational characteristics, and successfully lobbied the Nixon administration to endorse the HMO as the new national healthcare strategy (Starr 1982; Brown 1983b; Gruber et al. 1988). The HMO Act of 1973 encouraged the formation of HMOs, but because of initially overrestrictive legislation, the major growth in the population did not occur until the early 1980s (Gruber et al. 1988).

An HMO is formally defined as "an organized system of healthcare delivery available to persons in an enrolled group who reside in a specific geographic area. The HMO provides a specific set of [contractually defined] health benefits to its members including the services of physicians and other health care professionals" (Zipperer and Pace 1993: 97). HMOs include several key features that differentiate them from traditional ways of organizing medical care (Luft 1981; HIAA 1996). Members of the enrolled group (or their third-party payors) pay a fixed annual or monthly fee for a designated set of services or conditions. The HMO then gives a similarly fixed amount, called compensation by capitation or a per capita rate, to the selected group of practitioners that serves its population. Because these payments are fixed but patient care responsibilities are open-ended, physicians must assume at least part of the financial risk or gain of providing services. HMO members have financial incentives to use those practitioners and procedures that are covered by the plan, and thus, unlike in indemnity (fee-for-service) plans, have a restricted choice of providers.

Many varieties of managed care plans have emerged, and continuing innovations and combinations of plans make their delineation difficult. Intermediaries vary greatly in the range of functions they perform, which may include contracting with purchasers, determining enrollee eligibility, creating and managing provider networks, and paying providers for services provided. Plans also vary greatly in the extent to which providers are exposed to financial risk. Table 2.1 summarizes the major forms now operating: varieties of HMOs, point-of-service (POS) plans, and preferred provider organizations (PPO). We discuss HMO subtypes and POS plans here (see the section "Other Organizational Populations" for a discussion of PPOs).

The U.S. Department of Health Services classifies HMOs into four models: staff, group, network, and individual practice association (IPA). Other observers have added a "mixed" model. In the staff model, physicians are salaried employees of the HMO. Both the group and network models compensate contracted physicians on a capitated basis. The group model contracts with one group practice, whereas the network model contracts with a variety of groups and/or individual physicians. The most common form, the IPA, is an HMO that contracts with a network of physicians from various settings (solo and group practices), in which the physicians are compensated by capitation and/or fee-for-service plans. An HMO that does not fit neatly into one of the four categories or is a combination of the other models is considered "mixed" (Miller and Luft 1994).

The different types of HMOs vary in the extent to which patients are allowed to exercise free choice of physician. Choice is most restricted in staff and prepaid group practice forms and least restricted in IPAs. In recent years, some HMOs have added a POS option. This allows members to see practitioners that do not have a contractual relationship with the HMO, provided they pay a higher copayment or deductible.

Although, as noted, a distinctive feature of HMOs is to bring together financing and delivery functions, there are differences among various types in how closely the functions are connected. Table 2.1 also shows how types of HMOs are subject to different sets of accreditation and regulatory bodies. Original HMO forms were designed to integrate health plans—combining insurance and marketing functions—with provider organizations. Such forms exist, as exemplified by Kaiser Permanente, but have been joined by

Table 2.1 Types of Managed Care Organizations

Type of Organization	Organization Design	Accreditation Bodies	Regulatory Bodies
Health maintenance organization (HMO) Staff model (practitioners are salaried employees of the HMO)	An organized system of healthcare that provides a comprehensive range of healthcare services to a voluntarily enrolled population in a geographic area on a primarily prepaid and fixed periodic basis	National Committee for Quality Assurance (NCQA) Accreditation Association for Ambulatory Health Care (AAAHC) Utilization Review Accreditation Commission (URAC)	Federal licensing agencies, state insurance commission, state departments of mental health, state departments of public health
Group model (HMO pays a group of practitioners a negotiated, per capita rate, which is then distributed among the individuals)		Joint Commission on Accreditation of Healthcare Organizations (JCAHO)	
Network model (practitioners work out of their own offices under contract with the HMO)			
Individual practice association (IPA) model (practitioners continue individual group practice with compensation by capitation and/or fee-for-service plans)			
Mixed model (combination of two or more of the above)			
Point-of-service (POS)	An organized system of healthcare provided by an HMO model with the option of delivery of services outside the network at a higher copayment or deductible	NCQA JCAHO URAC	State insurance departments
Preferred provider organization (PPO)	A network discount, fee-for-service provider arrangement with incentives to stay inside the network at a decreased copayment and/or deductible; has structured quality and utilization management	NCQA JCAHO URAC	State insurance departments

SOURCE: Adapted from table 2.1 of Edmunds et al. 1997, pp. 43–44.

a modified version, called "carrier" HMOs.[5] These companies sell medical plans, offer management and marketing services, and contract for services with multispeciality group practices, IPAs, or individual physicians (Enthoven and Singer 1996). These "carrier" HMOs may be either network, IPA, or mixed models. Many have attempted to compete by contracting with and offering to their customers access to a broader variety of types of provider systems.

Our data on HMOs include all varieties, and we distinguish between subtypes in some analyses. The primary data source for the HMO population is the National HMO Census, an annual study performed by Interstudy (1976–92) under a contract arrangement with the U.S. Department of Health and Human Services.[6] The National HMO Census provided most of the necessary data for our analyses; however, in some cases, we supplemented or verified Interstudy's data with information from the *Managed Health Care Directory* (AMCRA 1994–95).

Home Health Agencies

We selected our third population, home health agencies, because it is interrelated with both hospitals and managed care. Home health agencies provide in-home care to patients with a variety of short-term and chronic illnesses and injuries. In 1995, the majority of California home healthcare was given to heart disease, stroke, cancer, diabetes, Alzheimer's disease, and AIDS patients (Cohen and King 1996). Much of this care was previously given in hospitals, rather than the patient's home, and thus HHAs represent the "unbundling" of previously combined services provided in one organization (Fennell and Alexander 1993; Scott 1993). Although home health was "unbundled" from mostly nonprofit hospitals, newly forming HHAs are much more likely to be for profit (Gray 1986). Large proportions of HHA patients are elderly, and thus HHAs are strongly affected by— and seek profits from—federal programs. On account of rapid advances in technology, the decreasing costs and increasing portability of many medical treatments makes owning or contracting with HHAs, not surprisingly, very attractive to managed care organizations.

Like hospitals, HHAs originated in the nineteenth century. The predecessors of modern HHAs, nonprofit visiting nurse associations (VNAs),

5. The use of "carrier" here is distinct from our use of "carrier" as an institutional role of a social actor.

6. Douglas R. Wholey kindly made available to us his data set in machine-readable form, compiled from the Interstudy census.

developed during the 1880s to provide nursing and social services to urban and immigrant populations. In the 1890s, there were approximately 35 VNAs in the United States (Waters 1909). In the early decades of the twentieth century, the number of VNAs grew considerably. A national social movement to improve public health, emphasizing sanitation, preventive medicine, and outreach programs, led to the creation of the National Organization for Public Health Nursing in 1913 and brought attention to the work of visiting nurses. VNAs also thrived as a result of perceived imperfections in public health agencies. Around the time of World War I, there were more than 2000 associations in the United States (Buhler-Wilkerson 1989).

While the number of VNAs declined rapidly during the Great Depression, there were more than 400 associations in 1945 (70 percent of all HHAs at the time), and over 600 in 1965 (Ryder, Stitt and Elkin 1969). The character of home health, though, was significantly affected by the passage of Medicare in 1965, and VNAs began to lose their prominence among HHAs in the years that followed. Medicare legislation included a section on the "Conditions of Participation for Home Health Agencies," which required that eligible HHAs offer at least one service, such as physical therapy, in addition to general nursing care. This regulation broadened the traditional mandate of home healthcare with the explicit aim of encouraging the development of more comprehensive services. Medicare requirements also began to redirect the mission of these agencies away from long-term services for the chronically ill to providing short-term care. Many VNAs did not qualify for reimbursement under the new guidelines (Salvatore 1985). In 1990, more that 115 VNAs were still in operation (Buhler-Wilkerson 1991), but many had merged with other HHAs (see Case Illustrations 3.A, 8.C).

Today, a home health agency is defined as a facility that provides "comprehensive health care, including skilled and supportive services, necessary to maintain a person in his or her place of residence" (Timmreck 1982: 291). In 1990, there were approximately 5800 such facilities in the United States (Scalzi et al. 1994). For certification and licensing purposes, however, each state gives a somewhat distinct definition of a home health agency. For instance, in California, a home health agency broadly refers to any agency providing or arranging for the provision of skilled nursing services in the home (Estes, Harrington, and Benjamin 1994). Although conducted under the supervision of a physician, most home care is provided by nurses, other allied health professionals, or by family members.

Bounding any population of HHAs is difficult because of the large number of such facilities that provide nonmedical services (e.g., Meals-on-Wheels) or merely serve as suppliers of medical equipment. We use Medicare certification to aid in bounding our population. HHAs that are not Medicare certified frequently emphasize social over medical services and also exhibit differences from Medicare-certified HHAs in finance patterns, linkage activities, and business strategies (see Estes, Harrington, and Benjamin 1994). We therefore restrict our study population to Medicare-certified HHAs.[7]

Our main data sources for the population of HHAs in the San Francisco Bay Area were annual reports from the California Office of Statewide Health Planning and Development (OSHPD 1978–92). This archive was supplemented by earlier listings from the Social Security Administration, beginning in 1966.

End-Stage Renal Disease Centers

We selected end-stage renal disease centers as our fourth population because they represent the "carving out" of a specialized function (treatment of kidney disease) from a generalized organizational form (hospitals). Like home health agencies, many ESRDCs are independent organizations that provide medical care outside the hospital. Unlike home health agencies, however, they treat just one highly specialized population, provide a narrow range of care, and treat patients in a variety of locations: freestanding facilities, hospitals, and the home. These differences allow us to distinguish between our two specialized provider populations. We also selected ESRDCs because, more so than our other populations, their formation and growth was driven by technological advancements. Renal disease centers also rely more on government funding than our other populations because of federal programs (described below) that reimburse renal disease treatments for all patients, not just the elderly and the poor. Consequently, many ESRDCs are for profit and represent the growth of proprietary forms in the healthcare field.

Such a facility is "specialized to treat outpatients with chronic kidney problems or kidney failure" with dialysis or transplantation (Timmreck 1982). ESRDCs slowly emerged as an organizational form after the first kidney transplant was performed in 1956 and dialysis became available in the early 1960s; previously, only dietary therapies were used to treat chronic renal failure. The initial growth of ESRDCs in hospitals and the Veterans'

---

7. Our population, however, does include those HHAs that have temporarily lost their Medicare certification but had previously been certified.

Administration system, however, was threatened by inadequate facilities, labor shortages, and the high costs of treatment (Schmidt, Blumenkrantz, and Wiegmann 1983). The scarcity of dialysis machines generated a need for patient screening and the creation of hospital selection committees to determine priorities for treatment. Organ procurement was a problem for transplantation, leading to the increased involvement of the Public Health Service, which began funding regional procurement networks in 1965.

In 1967, responding to the exorbitant costs of kidney dialysis, the Bureau of the Budget recommended that a national program be created to help cover the costs of ESRD patients (Kutner 1982). Congress approved legislation (Public Law 92–603) in 1972 extending Medicare coverage to chronically ill patients requiring dialysis or kidney transplantation. In its first (and only) effort to provide universal coverage in one disease category, the federal government assumed responsibility for 80 percent of the treatment costs of eligible patients. Following the enactment of the program, the organizational ranks of ESRD providers, formerly limited to large hospitals, swelled with the founding of independent dialysis facilities and renal disease centers (Kutner 1982). The dialysis market also became highly attractive to investor-owned organizations, which, by 1980, constituted three-quarters of independent facilities throughout the United States. By 1988, there were 1740 ESRDCs in the United States.

Because of the close association between ESRDCs and Medicare funding (and the corresponding certification requirements), the boundaries surrounding this provider population are relatively clear compared with other organizational forms in the healthcare field. The main issue surrounding the population boundaries concerns overlap with other populations, since some hospitals and home health agencies provide dialysis services similar to those available in freestanding ESRDCs. We include all types of organizations that provide ESRD treatment, explicitly acknowledging the overlaps with other organizational forms.

The data sources we used for the ESRDC population include the Health Care Finance Administration's provider directories (1978–92) and the Social Security Administration's listing of Medicare-certified facilities (beginning in 1973).

Multihospital and Integrated Healthcare Systems

We selected multihospital and healthcare systems for our fifth and final population because of their rising importance to the field, both as providers and governance units. Early healthcare systems were nonprofit, primarily religious, organizations made up of horizontal linkages among hospitals (see Case Illustration 8.A for a description of Bay Area healthcare systems that existed in 1945). Most built their own facilities to treat specialized populations or underserved areas, and were relatively small in number so that they had little impact on the field. For-profit multihospital systems were not formed until 1965, when investors saw opportunities for profit from selling management services to hospitals and providing care to Medicare patients. As the turbulence and uncertainty of the healthcare field increased in the early 1970s and the field searched for new ways to organize care, many hospitals joined systems in an attempt to ensure their survival. Prior to 1965 only about 5 percent of nonfederal hospitals belonged to systems; all were exclusively nonprofit at the time. By 1995, more than 270 systems existed incorporating more than 2500 hospitals—approximately 50 percent of all acute-care hospitals in the United States.

Multihospital systems are defined as "religious, investor-owned, or other organizations that own, lease, sponsor, or contract-manage two or more hospitals" (AHA 1983a: B3). Although the term "multihospital system" is still commonly used to describe a simple horizontal linkage of hospitals, the healthcare environment is increasingly witnessing the emergence of newer, vertically integrated forms. In an attempt to weather market conditions and contain costs, these new systems are striving to build a tightly coupled organization that embraces all aspects of pa-tient care, including financial integration (e.g., incorporation of payment mechanisms into the system), physician integration (linking physician groups more formally with the system), and clinical integration (providing services ranging from prevention to hospice care) (Shortell, Gillies, and Anderson 1994). Because this population has changed dramatically since the early 1980s, our population boundaries incorporate both multihos-pital systems and these more integrated healthcare systems. We view these systems as both providing linkages among member organizations of our other populations and constituting a distinctive new population of organizations.

To build our healthcare systems data base, we used the *AHA Guide to the Health Care Field* (AHA 1986–97a) and *Directory of Multihospital Systems* (AHA 1980–85b). We supplemented this information with annual facility reports from OSHPD. Because systems and system-membership data were not regularly collected on a national level until the late 1970s, we used a combination of systems' annual reports, systems and hospi-tal histories, and hospital listings from the AHA guides to the health-care field for the period 1945 to 1979. Finally, we also interviewed and surveyed local hospital administrators to obtain more detailed information on decision-making authority between systems and their component organizations.

OTHER ORGANIZATIONAL POPULATIONS

In addition to the more comprehensive event history data gathered on the five types of organizations that constitute the study's focal populations, we have gathered simple event count data for two other populations in the Bay Area. These two, medical groups and preferred provider organizations, closely interact with our focal populations and have become centrally important in the field. Although both make up populations of provider organizations, we treat them as aspects of our five focal populations' environments.

Medical Groups

A medical group practice is commonly defined as an association of at least three medical practitioners "made up of any combination of licensed physicians, engaged jointly in providing medical services" (Field 1976: 23).[8] Although increasingly prevalent in the current environment, medical groups—particularly those incorporating innovative organizational arrangements, such as prepaid insurance plans, the use of allied health occupations, and preventive medical programs—historically have met with varying degrees of opposition and controversy from the medical establishment.[9] As a consequence, most medical groups are not organized as corporations. Rather, they create "a dual structure involving a clinic organization comprising the medical practitioners and a property corporation that own[s] the plant and equipment" (Starr 1982: 213). The use of this structure, along with the reliance on primarily conventional payment methods and the

---

8. Most definitions employ a minimum number of at least three physicians as a rule-of-thumb to ensure that a group is "formally organized," exhibiting not only economies of scale inherent in the sharing of facilities and services, but also some degree of organizational structure and coordination mechanisms (PHS 1963a: 4, Freidson 1975, Wolinsky and Marder 1985). We use the more conservative criterion of six physicians.

9. Even after the influential Committee on the Costs of Medical Care encouraged medical group practice in its final report of 1932 (MacColl 1966: 11–12), most of organized medicine still considered it to be antithetical to the ideals of physician autonomy and solo practice. In California, changes to the Business and Professions Code in 1937 and a series of court cases in the 1930s and 1940s enforced a ban on the so-called "corporate practice of medicine," leaving group practices to operate in a circumscribed legal netherworld (Grant 1988).

clinical reputation of certain well-established, prestigious group practices,[10] enabled medical groups to avoid for the most part the outright condemnation of organized medicine.

Group practice has grown substantially since the end of World War II and at present enjoys much greater acceptance. Still, by 1991, only between one-fifth and one-third of all active, nonfederal physicians were involved in such arrangements.[11]

We obtained simple counts of medical groups, by facility, involving six or more fulltime equivalent physicians operating in the Bay Area for the period 1946–93. Data covering the early time period come from comprehensive surveys conducted by the U.S. Public Health Service (Hunt 1947; Pomrinse and Goldstein 1960). Data for the later period are from the membership directories of the Medical Group Management Association (MGMA 1961–93, selected years), founded in 1926 and one of the oldest and most representative associations of group practices (Stevens 1976). Information on the Permanente groups was supplemented from the annual reports of the Kaiser Permanente system (KP 1960–1993, selected years).

Preferred Provider Organizations

PPOs are defined as "an entity representing a group of physicians and/or hospitals that contracts with employers, insurance carriers, or third party administrators to provide comprehensive medical services on a discounted fee-for-service basis" (Zipperer 1995: 257). PPOs differ from HMOs in that they are not generally allowed to "pass risk" on to providers—that is, physicians are reimbursed for services rendered rather than given a capitated payment to care for defined groups of patients (see table 2.1). Increasing adoption by PPOs of operating procedures used by HMOs,[12] and cross-sponsorship of plans, have, however, tended to blur the differences between the two forms of delivery systems (Barger, Hillman, and Garland 1985; Trauner 1983).

10. One of the earliest and most famous examples is the Mayo Clinic, organized in Minnesota during the 1880s. In the Bay Area, the Palo Alto Medical Clinic provides an instance of another large and highly regarded group.

11. The AMA survey of medical groups in 1991 reported approximately 33 percent of active, nonfederal physicians in the United States to be in group practice, although this figure may count some physicians more than once if they were members of more than one group (Havlicek, Eiler, and Neblett 1993: 33–37). Current AMA data from surveys of physicians show that approximately 20 percent of all active physicians are in group practice; however substantial numbers of physicians are "not classified" in these surveys (Fennell and Leicht 1998).

12. These procedures include case management, utilization controls, and even limited capitation on providers, as well as restrictions on patients using services outside PPO panels (Barger, Hillman, and Garland 1985: 42).

In California, PPOs were relatively unheard of before the early 1980s. In 1982, reforms in the state Medicaid program that introduced selective contracting (see chap. 5) prompted insurance companies and purchasers to lobby for companion legislation lifting restrictions in the California Insurance Code. Specifically, they wanted insurance carriers to have the legal right to obtain alternate payment rates (discounted or competitive in other ways) from hospitals (Bergthold 1990; Barger, Hillman, and Garland 1985; Trauner 1983). Following the passage of this legislation, PPOs have been formed by insurance brokers and third-party administrative firms, provider-sponsored organizations reacting to HMO growth, and purchaser-sponsored health insurance plans (AMCRA 1990: ix).

To obtain a quantitative indicator of the growing importance of PPOs in the trend toward managed care, we gathered data on the numbers of PPO plans existing for each year from 1983 to 1995 with service areas in the San Francisco Bay Area. The sources for these data were Trauner's (1983) report on early PPO development in California, the American Managed Care and Review Association's directories of PPOs (AMCRA 1985–91, selected years) and *Managed Health Care Directory* (1994–95).

In addition to these data on healthcare provider organizations, we also collected information on other types of organizations, including business and community coalitions of healthcare buyers and professional associations. We describe these data and their sources as appropriate in later chapters.

FOCAL ORGANIZATIONAL CASE STUDIES

While our study design focuses primary attention on populations of organizations, we also examined four organizations in the Bay Area: the Kaiser Permanente Medical Care Program (Northern California Region), the Palo Alto Medical Clinic, Stanford University Hospital, and San Jose Hospital. We selected these four organizations as subjects for case studies based on the different roles each played in the development and delivery of healthcare, both regionally and nationally.

Kaiser Permanente Medical Care Program

The Kaiser Permanente Medical Care Program is one of the nation's oldest and largest health maintenance organizations. Founded in the 1930s at Kaiser Industries projects at the Colorado River and Grand Coulee Dam and brought to the San Francisco Bay Area shipyards during World War II,

Table 2.2 Organizations: Four Case Studies

Organization	Population(s)	Founding Date(s)	Primary Role
Kaiser Permanente Medical Care Program (KP)	Hospitals HMOs HHAs ESRDCs Healthcare systems	1933 for Kaiser workers 1945 opened to public	Prototype HMO
Palo Alto Medical Clinic (PAMC)	Medical groups	1931	Prototype group practice
Stanford University Hospital (SUH)	Hospitals	1912 San Francisco 1959 Stanford campus	Traditional academic medical center
San Jose Hospital (SJH)	Hospitals Healthcare systems	1923	Traditional community hospital

Kaiser Permanente (KP) opened to the public in 1945 (Smillie 1991; Hendricks 1993). Its unique combination of healthcare service delivery and financing includes two legally separate but functionally intertwined organizations: the nonprofit Kaiser Foundation Health Plans and Hospitals (one national organization with regional subsidiaries), which enrolls members in prepaid health plans and owns and operates KP facilities; and the for-profit Permanente Medical Groups (one in each region), that hire staff physicians to practice in groups and provide preventive and comprehensive care exclusively to Kaiser health plan members. Although located primarily on the West Coast in the 1940s, KP offered health plans in twelve regions (including Ohio, North Carolina, and Texas) by 1994, with a total enrollment of 6.6 million members (KP 1994). In the Bay Area, KP owned thirty-one facilities (including fifteen hospitals), enrolled 2.4 million patients, and employed 3600 fulltime physicians.

We chose to study Kaiser Permanente primarily because of its role as a prototype health maintenance organization, its substantial Bay Area market share, and its representation in all of our focal populations (it owns hospitals, HHAs, and ESRDCs, and is both an HMO and a healthcare system). We also chose KP because of its changing degree of congruence with the healthcare field (see chap. 1), which influenced its treatment and behavior in different eras. In the 1940s and 1950s, local medical societies opposed and persecuted KP because of the many ways it deviated from normative medical practice (Hendricks 1991, 1993). But in the late 1960s, as medical costs escalated, health policy experts and government officials held up KP as a model of future healthcare (Williams 1971; Somers 1971a, 1971b). In the 1980s and 1990s, KP faced increasing competition from other, looser forms of HMOs and began to react to change rather than instigate it. In sum, the case of Kaiser Permanente allows us to study an organization that was both a carrier and an agent in the healthcare field.

Palo Alto Medical Clinic

The Palo Alto Medical Clinic (PAMC) was founded by Dr. Russell Lee in 1931 and represents an early and continuing example of an innovative medical group. PAMC, like KP, was a pioneer in numerous aspects of medical care (see Fortney 1980; Casalino 1997, for descriptions of its history). As an early multispecialty group practice, it provided a model for other clinics. PAMC was also an early provider of prepaid healthcare, developing its first such plan in 1946 for Stanford University students. When Stanford faculty members later joined the plan and were perceived as overutilizing its services, PAMC added a copayment provision. This practice was adopted by the designers of Medicare and Medicaid plans, to whom Dr. Lee served as a consultant.

In 1980, PAMC formed the Palo Alto Medical Foundation, a nonprofit organization containing three divisions: (1) the Health Care Division, including PAMC and clinics in Fremont (founded in 1984) and Los Altos (1994); (2) the Education Division, founded in 1981; and (3) the Research Institute, founded in 1950. The Health Care Division has strong ties to local hospitals, particularly Stanford University Hospital, but operates under the goal of "outpatient everything." To further its efforts, the Palo Alto Medical Foundation became an affiliate of Sutter Health, a healthcare system headquartered in Sacramento, in 1992 (Miller and Cochrane 1994). In 1995, PAMC served over 130,000 patients and employed approximately 160 physicians.

Stanford University Hospital

We selected the Stanford University Hospital (SUH), a component of Stanford University Medical Center, because of its role as an influential referral center and provider of tertiary care for the greater Bay Area. Representative of traditional academic medical centers, Stanford's medical school opened in 1908 and its first hospital, located in San Francisco, opened in 1917 (Cutting 1955). The medical school and hospital continued to grow during succeeding decades and, in 1959, the medical center moved into a newly constructed facility on the main campus at Stanford. Throughout most of the period of our study, the medical center flourished as a leading center of academic research and medical innovation—a model of a research-oriented medical school (Knox 1979).

Heavily dependent on federal research support and on referrals from community physicians, SUH has experienced difficulty in sustaining both vital flows in recent years, as federal support for research has dwindled and community physicians have referred fewer of their patients to the teaching hospital. Confronting the reality of diminished resources and faced with ever increasing competition for dollars and patients, SUH effected a merger in 1997 with its longtime rival academic hospital, the University of California Medical Center in San Francisco. Stanford Hospital's 611 licensed beds and 100 specialty areas are now part of UCSF–Stanford Health Care, a healthcare system with four hospitals, 1350 beds, 12,000 employees, and 2000 fulltime physicians.

San Jose Hospital

The choice of San Jose Hospital (SJH) reflects our interest in including among our cases one representative community hospital. Unlike the other cases selected, SJH was less often considered a central player or an innovative change agent and more often behaved as a follower or reactor to environmental changes. It acted primarily as a carrier of traditional logics rather than as a social agent effecting change. Founded in downtown San Jose in 1923 as a for-profit corporation under the leadership of a group of physicians, the hospital was converted to nonprofit status in 1937 (Visions 1984). SJH attempted to secure an adequate flow of patients during the Great Depression by instituting a hospitalization insurance plan that quickly became connected with regional Blue Cross plans developing in California at that time. When demand for services increased at the end of World War II, SJH grew as San Jose expanded.

During its early years SJH benefited from being located in a rapidly growing urban center. By the 1970s, however, it found itself in a deteriorating area that was rapidly losing its middle-class residents. It attempted to secure a flow of patients by contracting with an experimental HMO and later with a preferred provider group of physicians. Beginning in 1986, SJH was acquired by the parent organization Health Dimensions, later renamed the Good Samaritan Health System, which was sold in 1995 to Columbia/HCA, the nation's largest for-profit hospital system. This system is currently refuting rumors that it will close the 300-bed SJH but, as Good Samaritan CEO Michael Guthrie stated in 1994, "what goes on at that location will be dramatically different in the next six to eight years" (Alvarado 1994b).

Data Sources

Each case study involved somewhat different data collection activities, but in general we employed the following sources: (1) archival materials obtained from the organization, including memos, annual reports, catalogs and brochures, and histories written by organizational participants; (2) periodicals, including local and national newspapers, magazines, and journals; (3) historical accounts written by nonparticipants; and (4) interviews with former and current organizational leaders and informants.

Contribution of Case Studies to Larger Project

While the population-level data described earlier are employed to trace the historical trends characterizing the evolution of medical care organizations in the Bay Area, the four case studies allow us to investigate the response of particular organizations to these trends and other events occurring throughout this period. We employ the case studies to determine how specific organizations did and did not react to various developments and how specific organizations did and did not attempt to influence them. By allowing us to observe occasions of leadership and influence on the part of these organizations and their members, as well as their absence, the case studies focus attention on the varying capacity for social agency, thus helping to balance the structural emphasis present in the population-level analysis (see Caronna, Pollack, and Scott 1997).

The case study materials inform all our analyses, but are employed to provide the basis for a series of case illustrations that appear throughout this volume. We use the cases to exemplify, amplify (and sometimes to contest or challenge) results from our quantitative, more macro-level analyses. These case illustrations rely primarily on the four case studies, but are not restricted to these materials.

CONCLUSION: DIVERSE DATA, MULTIPLE LEVELS

Just as we attempt to combine and integrate a number of theoretical arguments, we also employ a variety of types of data and data-gathering techniques in order to illuminate changes in the organization of healthcare services. Among the types of data gathered are: census data on individual providers, particularly physicians and consumers of medical care; archival data on the characteristics of selected organizational providers; historical information on the four organization cases; survey data on the characteristics of hospital systems; and archival and historical information on changes in the political, economic, and regulatory context of these actors (the latter are described in chap. 6). These data cover developments occurring in or affecting the San Francisco Bay Area's healthcare delivery system over a 50-year period, from the end of World War II to the present.

While attention is focused on the geographically bounded San Francisco Bay Area, we recognize the internal diversity of this metropolitan community by attending to county-level variations in both demographic characteristics and the nature and distribution of organizational providers (detailed in chap. 5). And while we restrict attention to provider systems and consumers operating in this region, we take account of the effect on these actors of activities occurring outside the area and of relations linking local actors to distant events and parties at both the state and national levels. Because organizations are open systems, it is important to recognize the extent to which nonlocal environmental influences—some of them at great distances from the units affected—impact local organizations. And because organizations are cultural systems, it is important to recognize the extent to which noncontemporary events and long-established beliefs and practices affect today's happenings.

The focus on multiple types of actors—individuals, organizations, associations—as well as the use of multiple types and levels of data connect our case study of the Bay Area to wider currents and broader influences. The approach emphasizes that all social activities are situated in historical time and institutional space (see Scott and Christensen 1995). The use of diverse types of data also takes into account the recognition that any specific observation is subject to distortion and bias but that observations from diverse sources and of varied types may, in combination, provide a more accurate rendering of the events they purport to depict.

Three

CHANGING HEALTHCARE
DELIVERY SYSTEMS

HAVING INTRODUCED SOME OF THE individuals and organizations that are major players in the regional field of healthcare services, we now turn to changes over time in the focal organizational populations. The broad subject of our study is historical change in healthcare institutions. Detailing changes in the types, numbers, and connections among organizational providers offers insight into the fundamental ways in which the healthcare system has been transformed. The aim of this chapter is to provide a descriptive overview of the changes occurring in medical care organizations in the San Francisco Bay Area during the 50-year period since World War II. We focus primarily on four of the five populations of organizations on which we have gathered systematic data—hospitals, home health agencies, health maintenance organizations, and end-stage renal disease centers—although we also report changes in the numbers of two other organizational populations: preferred provider organizations and medical groups. The fifth population, hospital systems, is discussed in chapter 8, where we consider the development of more integrated forms of healthcare delivery.

Before presenting an overview of changes occurring in the numbers and types of organizations providing healthcare services in the Bay Area, we place these developments in perspective first, by briefly summarizing major trends in the U.S. healthcare field as a whole, and second, by describing theories of organizational change. In considering these topics, we begin the task of spelling out the ways and the extent to which we are presented with an instance of profound institutional change.

MAJOR TRENDS IN U.S. HEALTHCARE DELIVERY SYSTEMS

A number of major trends affecting the organization of medical services in the U.S. have been identified by researchers (Scott 1993; Fennell and

Alexander 1993). We focus on six significant trends, all of which are reflected in developments in the Bay Area. This discussion identifies some of the more general dimensions along which change in provider systems can be observed. We also note inconsistencies and complexities when we review these processes at closer range and in greater depth for the Bay Area. First, however, we outline the general tendencies.

Increased Concentration

During the past fifty years, medical resources engaged in the delivery of health services have become more concentrated. This trend is evident among both individuals and organizations.

• Individual providers, such as physicians, are less likely today to operate as independent practitioners and more likely to practice in an organizational setting, including group practices, HMOs, and hospitals.

• Healthcare organizations, such as hospitals or urgent care centers, are more likely to operate as component units of larger systems. About half of all U.S. hospitals now operate as members of some type of larger administrative system.

A shift in the concentration of and connections among individuals and organizations, that is, *relations among actors,* is one of the ways in which profound institutional change is evidenced.

Increased Specialization

Both individual providers, such as physicians and nurses, and healthcare organizations have become more specialized.

• The number of recognized medical specialties (certified by specialty boards) has greatly increased, particularly during the second half of this century.

• In a similar fashion, nurses exhibit increased specialization, although these developments are more closely related to locus of practice (e.g., surgery) than to differences in training. And a host of specialized parapro-fessional occupations have emerged (e.g., inhalation therapist, radiology technician) that are certified to provide highly specialized services.

• A wide variety of specialized organizational forms has developed in recent years, such as neighborhood health centers, renal disease units, freestanding surgery centers, urgent care centers, and home health agencies. A number of these are viewed as reflecting the practice of service "unbundling," whereby a cluster of services once performed in a generalized organization, such as a hospital, is disaggregated and re-formed as separate units.

Specialization is one of the processes that produces *new types of social actors,* an indicator of profound change. Note also that both the trend toward increasing concentration and increasing specialization are observed to occur at *multiple levels* (the examples point to changes at both the individual and the organizational level).

Increased Integration and Diversification

While many service units move in the direction of increased specialization, other organizational units tend toward increased horizontal and vertical integration and increased diversification. Horizontal integration—the combining of similar organizations—changes the *scale* on which services are delivered, a process described above as increased concentration. Vertical integration increases the *scope* of services, involving a broadening of the organization's domain (Chandler 1990). A vertically integrated organization "links the stages of production and distribution of its product into a chain" that incorporates earlier or later stages (Clement 1988: 100).

• Many hospitals have chosen to integrate vertically, adding services that involve patients at stages earlier or later than those requiring acute care, the core service domain of traditional hospitals. Thus, hospitals may integrate "forward" into ambulatory services by opening outpatient clinics or urgent care centers; or they can integrate "backward" by including extended care facilities or home health agencies.

Diversification involves the decision to produce goods or services unrelated to the organization's conventional domain.

• Healthcare organizations are also increasingly engaged in carrying out services unrelated to their primary domain. These types of services involve a different type of "final consumable output" than that ordinarily produced by healthcare units and so requires these organizations to develop new skills or to deal with different consumer groups (Clement 1988: 106). Among the types of nonrelated services currently being offered by hospital systems are office building management, real estate development, and the operation of retirement communities (Ermann and Gabel 1984).

Vertical integration offers yet another way in which *new types of social actors* are appearing in the healthcare field, and diversification is a process that challenges and changes conventional *field boundaries.*

Increased Linkages among Healthcare Organizations

In addition to the emergence of multihospital chains and vertically integrated healthcare systems, which represent relatively stronger and more tightly coupled connections among organizations, healthcare organizations have increased their involvement in other types of linkages entailing somewhat looser and more flexible connections.

• A growing number of hospitals and other types of healthcare units are managed under contract, with management systems providing both general and specialized administrative services to "independent" units (Morrisey and Alexander 1987).

• A large number of healthcare organizations are linked by "strategic alliances." The concept of alliance "refers to a voluntary, loosely coupled interorganizational relationship between two or more organizations that are linked in ways that preserve the legal identity and autonomy of each, as well as most of their functional autonomies" (Christianson, Moscovice, and Wellever 1995: 99–100; see also, Longest 1990; Kaluzny, Zuckerman, and Ricketts 1995). Although the variety of modes of linkage is great, they most often take the form of long-term contracts.

• A variety of confederations, consortia, and associations have developed among various parties in the healthcare arena. Such connections among multiple individuals or organizations are formed to serve interests that the members share in common.

All of these types of connections among individuals and organizations signify some of the additional ways in which *relations among actors* in the healthcare sector are currently changing.

Increased Privatization

The American healthcare sector has long been composed of a mix of public and private—both nonprofit and for-profit—forms. In the last few decades, however, the proportion of private forms has markedly increased, in particular, the number of for-profit providers (see next section). This development may reflect, at least in part, a broader effort during the past two decades to reduce the role of government and the size of the welfare state generally (Offe 1984), although whether this is in fact happening is much in dispute (Brown 1988; Ruggie 1996). What is less controversial is the observation that public organizations are currently less involved in the direct provision of services (Osborne and Gaebler 1992). Even when public funds are involved, service provision is increasingly contracted out to private organizations. In 1988, "nearly half of all government spending on goods and services" by the U.S. federal government went to outside, private organizations (Donahue 1989: 8). This implies that the role of public sector organizations is increasingly changing from providing goods and services to overseeing their production.

• Fewer new public organizations for delivering health services have been created in recent years. There has been a long-term decline in the portion of healthcare services provided by public organizations as compared to private forms.

Shifts between public and various types of private ownership arrangements is one of the important ways in which the *types of social actors* in an organizational field undergo change. Their roles and relations to one another are also changing. Today, public actors are more likely to fund and to police a general set of rules or guidelines for service provision rather than to provide the service themselves.

Increased Market Orientation

Numerous indicators suggest that an earlier conception of healthcare delivery as being immune from market forces is rapidly being transformed. These changes are reflected both in ownership arrangements and in the behavior of healthcare organizations.

• There has been a substantial increase in the number of for-profit forms offering healthcare services, especially among more specialized organizational providers (Gray 1986).

• While nonprofit forms remain the dominant type in some organizational populations such as hospitals, they have largely shifted from a "donative" to a "commercial" character (Hansmann 1987). The former receive their income primarily in the form of donations from "patrons"; income for the latter comes chiefly from the sale of goods and services. Clearly, organizations whose income depends more on the number and nature of services provided will be more sensitive to market considerations than will organizations whose income derives primarily from philanthropic sources.

• There is a "blurring" of the distinction between for-profit and nonprofit forms and behaviors. Many non-profit organizations operate for-profit components and vice versa. And most nonprofit organizations have embraced the competitive orientation and strategies of for-profit providers (Fennell and Alexander 1993).

In addition to reflecting changes in the *type of social actors* in the field, a shift from professional service norms and models to more commercial and market-oriented approaches signals an important change in the *meanings* associated with given activities within the field and in the *institutional logics* that direct, motivate, and legitimate the behavior of field actors.

In short, across several critical dimensions, such as new types of social actors, changing relations among actors, new logics governing action, and shifting boundaries, the field of organizations providing healthcare is in transition—a transition of such a nature as to suggest that we are observing an instance of profound institutional change.

THEORIES OF ORGANIZATIONAL CHANGE

A General Typology

In a comprehensive review of the many theories that have been proposed to account for the ways in which organizations—or indeed, any types of social unit—change, Van de Ven and Poole (1995) construct a typology of developmental theories that, they believe, encompasses the main arguments that have appeared over the years. Four types of argument are identified:

Life-cycle theories embrace the metaphor of organic growth and attempt to identify stages in the development of the entity from its initiation to its termination. Change is viewed as immanent: the developing entity contains within it an underlying logic or program that regulates the process of change. For example, Kimberly (1980) has applied this model to examining changes occurring in the development of a medical school, and D'Aunno and Zuckerman (1987) describe how hospital federations may be viewed as following a life-cycle model of development.

Teleological theories assume that the entity is purposeful and adaptive, directed toward some goal or desired end state. Development is viewed as an iterative process of goal setting, implementation, evaluation, and goal modification. Most strategic management theories assume this perspective, focusing on managers as intendedly rational decision makers. This perspective has only recently been embraced by healthcare managers as the image of the administrator has changed from that of "caretaker" to "risktaker" (Shortell, Morrison, and Robbins 1985: 220).

Dialectical theories assume that the entity exists in a pluralistic world of conflicting forces that compete with each other for domination and control. Stability and change are explained by alterations in the balance of power among opposing entities. Many conflict theories addressing the emergence of and competing claims among professional occupations have embraced this perspective (e.g., Larson 1977; Abbott 1988). Begun and Lippincott (1993) provide a useful characterization of the ways in which professionals in the healthcare arena compete and cooperate to achieve and maintain legitimacy and market power.

Evolutionary theories assume that change occurs through a continuous cycle of variation, selection, and retention. New elements (rules, roles, organizations) arise through random change; selection occurs primarily through the competition for scarce resources; and retention preserves some elements, either because they improve fitness or because of inertia. The study by Van de Ven and Grazman (1994) of the genealogy of healthcare systems in Minnesota (described below) illustrates this perspective.

It seems unnecessary—indeed, inappropriate—to choose among these views, since we can observe instances of all four types of change in our study. This is particularly so if we recognize that the changes may take place at various levels of analysis. Thus, not only may individual persons and organizations be observed to exhibit some relatively predictable changes through their life cycle (Kimberly and Miles 1980), but so may organizational fields or industries, which often become more stable or "mature" over time. Most of the types of actors with which we deal regard themselves as "rational" and capable of pursuing goals that themselves may change over time. At the same time, different actors in this sector often seek conflicting goals. We observe various types of actors—governmental agencies, healthcare providers, professional associations—engaged in dialectical processes as they carry on contests of power and control. Finally, changes in the mix of organizations at the population and field levels need not occur primarily by one type of organization transforming itself into a different type, but may result from environmental selection processes, as some organizations and organizational forms die out and different ones are created.

Underlying Van de Ven and Poole's (1995) typology are two sets of distinctions that identify contrasting assumptions about the source and the nature of change. We discuss these distinctions and then add a third which is important to our study.

Internal versus External Sources of Change

Whereas the first two "motors" of organizational change in Van de Ven and Poole's typology emphasize factors internal to organizations, the latter two stress external causes. In his general typology of organization theories, Pfeffer (1982) also identifies this distinction as a principal dimension helping to differentiate among organization theories. In general, theories such as resource dependence, population ecology, and institutional theory emphasize external sources of change, while strategic management and transaction cost approaches stress internal actors and processes.

Van de Ven and Grazman (1994) employ the internal-external distinction in their study examining the genealogies (i.e., social histories) of the development of four major healthcare systems in the Minneapolis–St. Paul area over a period of 150 years. They classified organizational events into "internal" and "external" forms of change or growth, based upon whether "the previous organizational units or resources that were combined to create the new organizational form existed solely within the parent organization alone or came, in whole or part, from two or more organizations" (1994: 9). Events classified as "internal" included foundings, openings, expansions, renovations, and closings of the organization or its subsidiary units. "External" events included mergers, acquisitions, and affiliations with other organizations. Van de Ven and Grazman report that during the period 1845 to 1963, changes in healthcare organizations occurred largely by means of combining or recombining units internal to the organizations, whereas after 1963 changes were more likely to occur as a result of external recombinations and mergers. The researchers view the period around 1963, during which there was increasing evidence of changes in governmental policy regarding healthcare, as "an important breaking point in the time series of genealogical events for the Twin Cities populations of health care organizations" (1994: 21). As noted, we also view this period as one involving significant change, although we target the critical date as 1965 rather than 1963 (see chaps. 1 and 6).

The internal-external distinction may appear at first to be both obvious and useful, but it is in fact difficult to apply and may be quite misleading when one is studying "open systems," such as organizations (see Katz and Kahn 1978; Scott 1998). "External" or environmental factors not only constrain and influence organizations and their participants; they also infiltrate, construct, and empower them. On the other hand, organizations and participants are not the passive pawns of external events, allowing external forces to freely reshape them, but take steps to control, modify, and challenge these forces. When dealing with organizations and environments, we need to recognize the extent to which "internal" actors—both individual and collective—affect and manage "external" contexts and, at the same time, the ways in which "external" contexts construct actors and constrain and empower action (Caronna, Pollack and Scott 1997).

The distinction between internal and external is even more difficult to apply when one is studying an organizational field. The field itself contains many of the actors and forces that constitute a significant part of the environment for any given actor. For example, the numbers and types of hospitals operating in a region is a salient aspect of the environment for the other types of healthcare organizations. Thus, at the field level, many "environmental" elements are endogenous to the field of study (Scott, Mendel, and Pollack 2000).

Intentional versus Unintentional Change

A second important distinction underlying the typology is that of intentional versus unintentional change, with teleological and dialectical theories falling in the former camp and life-cycle and evolutionary theories falling in the latter. Fennell and Alexander stress this dimension in their review of recent transformations in the healthcare field. They identify *strategic change* models as those in which "the organization (or the healthcare system) actively chooses one course of action over another" (1993: 97). This approach is exemplified by strategic management perspectives, as pioneered by Porter (1980), and applied to the healthcare field by Shortell and colleagues (Shortell, Morrison, and Robbins 1985; Shortell and Zajac 1990; see also Topping and Hernandez 1991). The strategic management perspective has been widely embraced by managers of healthcare systems during the last two decades, in part because it treats managerial action and decision-making as pivotal to organizational outcomes. In addition, it is compatible with the increased market orientation of the sector.

Other perspectives for studying organizational change can also be accommodated under the intentional change umbrella. Prominent examples include resource dependence theory as developed by Pfeffer and Salancik (1978). Even though this approach stresses the importance of external, environmental factors affecting organizations, it also emphasizes that managers can take an active role in "managing their environments" by developing appropriate linkages with vital exchange partners. Transaction cost economics, as elaborated by Williamson (1975, 1985), even more strongly views the role of managers as designing their organizations and developing linkages with the environment in such a way as to reduce the costs associated with developing and monitoring exchanges. Applications of these arguments to healthcare systems include those by Mick (1990a) and Hurley and Fennell (1990).

In contrast to these "active" and purposive perspectives on organizational change, other theories embrace a more "passive" conception, emphasizing the role of market selection processes or blind environmental forces.

Principal exemplars of this type of theorizing are the ecological models first developed by Hannan and Freeman (1977) and Aldrich (1979) and subsequently applied to a number of healthcare organization populations—including HMOs (Christianson et al. 1991; Wholey and Burns 1993; and Strang 1995), rural primary care centers (Ricketts et al. 1987), and home health agencies (Estes et al. 1992).

In their early work, ecological theorists stressed the constraints on organizational adaptation: organizational structures were viewed as inertial, especially when considered in relation to the environments in which they were located (Hannan and Freeman 1977). But more recent versions soften this stance. In 1984, Hannan and Freeman refined their views on inertia, recognizing that some aspects of organizations (e.g., marketing strategies) are more adaptable than others (e.g., goals).[1] Subsequent empirical studies have supported the view that inertia is not a ubiquitous feature of organizations, but one that sets in with senescence, as organizations gradually "lock-in" to particular administrative and technical procedures (Hannan, Burton, and Baron 1996). Contemporary ecological analysts are therefore more likely to view organizational passivity as a variable than as an a priori assumption.

Parallel shifts have occurred in institutional theory frameworks, which began by employing a passive conception of organizational actors. Early versions of institutional approaches, for example, stressed the extent to which organizations conform to cultural frameworks, independent of efficiency considerations (Meyer and Rowan 1977; DiMaggio and Powell 1983).[2] Later analysts—as well as later works by many of the same analysts—acknowledged that these theories presented an "overly socialized" view of organizations, understating their capacity for agency and for strategic action (Perrow 1986; DiMaggio 1988). More recent versions of institutional theory emphasize that many if not most organizations operate in environments characterized by conflicting logics and rules and recognize that conformity is only one of a range of organizational responses to institutional demands, with others including manipulation, defiance, avoidance, and compromise (Oliver 1991; Scott 1995).

---

1. We employ Hannan and Freeman's "hierarchical" conception of organizational elements in chapter 4, when we contrast ecological with adaptive sources of change in hospitals.

2. The sense in which organizational actors are "passive" is quite different in classic organizational ecology and institutional formulations. Ecologists equate passivity with the relatively slow rate with which organizations react to environmental threats and opportunities. For institutionalists, passivity refers to the tendency of organizations to adopt unreflectively current fads and fashions, becoming marionettes to their institutional environments.

Thus, to a large extent, the theoretical distinction between active and passive organizational actors has begun to fade or at least soften. At the same time that strategic choice theorists have come to recognize barriers to directed change, ecological and institutional theorists increasingly recognize that organizations can evolve and exert influence, even if under constraints. Changes in an organizational field will reflect some combination of selection and adaptation, some admixture of organizational inertia, organizational learning, and dumb luck.

Even more to the point, ecologists increasingly have come to recognize that "variation" and "selection" processes are not disembodied events but the products of human action. Organizations do not simply die of old age; owners and managers decide to sell or dismantle them. And new organizations do not magically appear on the landscape: someone must assemble the resources and personnel and assume the risks of starting a new enterprise. Ecologists have given much more attention of late to these entrepreneurial activities and their implications for population dynamics (Romanelli 1991; Aldrich and Fiol 1994).

For these reasons, the *ecological* and *adaptive* components of organizational change (i.e., the extent to which long-term historical change in populations of organizations can be attributed to differing rates of organization founding and dissolution or to the transformation of existing organizations) should not be conflated with debates over organizational intentionality. Rather, the importance of this distinction is to acknowledge both potential modes of change in organizational populations and not blind oneself to one or the other. For us, the important questions—which we explore in depth in chap. 4—concern the comparative influence of each component and the relative role of inertia, the dimensions along and the degree to which existing organizations are (or are not) capable of change.

Incremental versus Discontinuous Change

Organizational researchers have come to recognize the importance of another aspect of change: the magnitude or scale of changes that are observed. This third distinction is not reflected in Van de Ven and Poole's typology but is important to our research. Students of evolutionary change have observed that change may occur in an episodic rather than a gradual tempo. Abrupt upheavals produce a "stepwise rather than a continuous pattern of change" (Astley 1985: 230). This common pattern has been labeled by population biologists as one of "punctuated equilibrium" (Eldrege and Gould 1972). Periods of gradual change are "punctuated" by periods of turbulence. Thus, the distinction is made between *incremental* change, smaller changes that occur during periods of equilibrium, and *discontinuous* change, which occurs during periods of major disruption in the normal order of things (see Nadler and Tushman 1995).

As with all dimensions of change, this distinction can be utilized at multiple levels of analysis. For our present purposes, the most important distinction is that between the organizational and field levels. Meyer, Brooks, and Goes (1990) develop a typology that cross-classifies magnitude of change with level of analysis (see table 3.1). Incremental change at the organization level is termed "adaptation," while discontinuous changes for organizations represent "metamorphosis." At the industry or field level, incremental changes are labeled "evolutionary," while discontinuous changes are "revolutionary." We consider all four types of change in our examination of events in the Bay Area.

While it is clear that the two levels of change are likely to be connected so that, for example, periods of revolutionary change at the field level are likely to be associated with significant transformation at the organizational level, we also need to recognize the possibility of "loose coupling" between environments and organizations. Environments and organizations within them are connected but not in a tight or deterministic manner. Our organizational case studies reveal instances of what appear to be revolutionary changes at the field level that profoundly affect some types of organizations but are of little or no consequence to others (see Case Illustration 6.B).

Meyer and colleagues (1990, 1993) developed their model of revolutionary change by observing conditions in the San Francisco Bay Area (limited to four counties) affecting 30 medical-surgical hospitals. The hospitals were studied intensively during the period 1987–89, but more general information was gathered to characterize conditions from 1960 to 1989. They selected this field and time period because they were interested in how individual organizations adapt to rapidly changing environments. However, the study population was changing so rapidly that the researchers were forced to shift their focus from individual organizations to field-level processes and to elevate their theoretical models from studying adaptive changes to studying revolutionary changes. In important respects, this study served as a touchstone for our own research.

Van de Ven and Grazman (1994), in their study of healthcare organizations in the Twin Cities, also noted the importance of the pace of change. Employing their distinction regarding the source of change, whether managerial or environmental, they report that "managerial actions have their greatest effect on changes in organizational forms during benign

Table 3.1 Types and Levels of Change

	INCREMENTAL	DISCONTINUOUS
Organizational level	**Adaptation**	**Metamorphosis**
	Focus: Incremental change within organizations	Focus: Frame-breaking change within organizations
	Mechanisms: Strategic choice, resource dependence	Mechanisms: Life cycles, Strategic reorientations
	Illustrative analyses: Child 1972, Pfeffer & Salancik 1978	Illustrative analyses: Greenwood & Hinings 1988, Tushman & Romanelli 1985
Organizational field level	**Evolution**	**Revolution**
	Focus: Incremental change within established fields	Focus: Emergence, transformation, and decline of fields
	Mechanisms: Natural selection, institutional isomorphism	Mechanisms: Quantum speciation, environmental partitioning
	Illustrative analyses: Hannan & Freeman 1989, Meyer & Rowan 1977	Illustrative analyses: Astley 1985, Schumpeter 1947

SOURCE: Adapted from fig. 1 of Meyer, Brooks, and Goes (1990).

Copyright John Wiley & Sons Limited. Reproduced with permission.

environmental periods, while environmental events exert the greatest influence on changes in organizational growth and evolution during more turbulent and competitive periods" (1994: 1).

CHANGES IN POPULATIONS OF HEALTHCARE ORGANIZATIONS

We present a descriptive overview of changes occurring within several populations of healthcare organizations in the Bay Area during the period 1945 to 1992. We will describe trends observed for four of the five focal populations and present simple count data for two other organizational populations: medical groups and preferred provider organizations (PPOs).[3] Definitions of these populations and discussions of data sources are provided in chapter 2 and appendix A.

3. As already noted, the fifth population, hospital systems, represents a special category of organization to be discussed in chapter 8, which deals with the increasing integration of healthcare systems.

Trends in Focal Organizational Populations

Hospitals

At the beginning of our study period, a large number of hospitals were already in existence in the Bay Area, some of them dating well back into the nineteenth century. We lack data on the formative period that witnessed the emergence of this population during the decades after the 1850s and its growth during the first century of its existence. More so than for the other organizational populations studied the data set compiled on hospitals is "left-censored": we lack observations recording the timing of early entries into and exits from this population and are only able to examine its later development and what appears to be the onset of its decline.

When our systematic data set begins, in 1945, 83 hospitals were operating in the Bay Area. Throughout the study period, up to 1992, 67 hospitals entered the population, involving 65 foundings of new organizations and 2 equal-status mergers.[4] Entries of new hospitals occurred primarily during the 1950s and, especially, the 1960s, with relatively few organizations entering after 1970 (fig. 3.1).

While entries into the hospital population were clustered by time period, exits have been more evenly distributed—though more occurred during the latter half of the study period, after 1965 (see fig. 3.2). In total, 81 exits were observed, 53 because of the demise of the organization, 11 because of "transformation" into a different form (for example, a skilled nursing facility), and 17 as a result of a merger or acquisition.

The combined effects of entries and exits produce the density plot exhibited in figure 3.3, which also contrasts density of generalist hospitals with generalist and specialist forms combined. It is apparent from this graph that the hospital population increased in size slowly between 1945 and 1960, then rapidly between 1960 and 1970, only to decline steadily after that date. More recent data reveal that the Bay Area hospital population has contracted another 10 percent after 1992, dropping to 76 facilities in 1997. The proportion of generalist to specialists hospitals has increased throughout the period of study. Note that while the general trends in the healthcare sector, described earlier in this chapter, favor an increase in the number of specialist organizations, this is not true for hospitals.

---

4. Entries are counted as equal-status mergers when two organizations stop submitting separate facility reports to OSHPD or AHA, but instead submit these reports as a "new" combined organizational entity. Note that this administrative definition of "equal-status" mergers does not exhaust all possible types of mergers, which are counted in our data as either foundings or acquisitions.

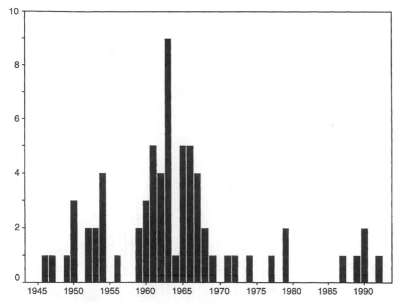

Figure 3.1   Bay Area Hospital Entries, 1945–92

Specialist hospitals—such as tuberculosis or eye, ear, nose, and throat facilities—represent a shrinking proportion of the hospital population in 1992 compared with 1945.

At first viewing, it may appear that, although they have experienced ups and downs, hospitals in the Bay Area have managed to hold their own throughout the study period since roughly the same number of hospitals existed in 1992 as there were in 1945. However, such a conclusion ignores two other important considerations: first, during this period, the population of the Bay Area increased nearly threefold (see chaps. 2 and 5), so that the relative number of hospitals has greatly declined. Second, although the number of hospitals remained about the same and their capacity (average numbers of hospital beds) has remained fairly constant (following the closing of the large military hospitals at the end of World War II), their capacity utilization—ratio of occupied beds to total beds—has declined after 1980 (see fig. 3.4).

Taken together, these descriptive data indicate that (1) there are significantly fewer hospitals per capita in the Bay Area in 1992 than there were in 1945–1.36 per 100,000 compared with 3.78; and (2) there was an even more dramatic decline in occupied hospital beds per capita in the Bay Area in this period: from 14.68 per 1,000 in 1945 to 3.04 in 1992. The care of

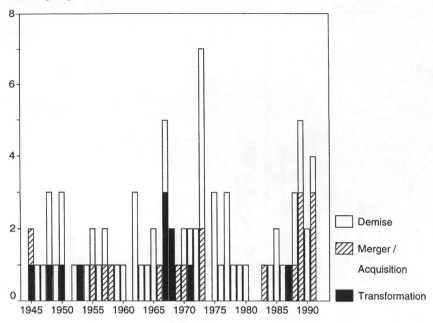

Figure 3.2   Bay Area Hospital Exits, 1945–91

patients has increasingly moved outside of hospitals into ambulatory and more specialized types of facilities.[5]

Ownership trends in the Bay Area reveal that the proportion of government-owned hospitals (federal, state, county, district, and city facilities) has declined from about 40 percent in 1945 to approximately 25 percent in 1992 (see fig. 3.5). By contrast, nonprofit forms have increased their proportion from 40 percent in 1945 to over 60 percent in 1992. For-profit forms have declined slightly from 20 percent in 1945 to approximately 15 percent in 1992. Whereas Bay Area hospitals have become more privatized during the period of study, the dominant trend has been from public to nonprofit forms rather than toward for-profit forms.

Comparing the trends for Bay Area hospitals to trends for U.S. hospitals as a whole, one can note some fundamental similarities (see Alexander and Amburgey 1987). Hospitals in both the Bay Area and in the country have declined in density since the late 1960s and early 1970s. Although capacity

5. Taking note of the declining occupancy trends in combination with hospitals' heavy expenditure for technologies and continuing high staffing levels, Herzlinger (1997: 221) observes: "The American hospital system, with 1995 occupancy of only 59.7 percent is like a lavishly outfitted jumbo jet that flies only two-thirds full on its average trip."

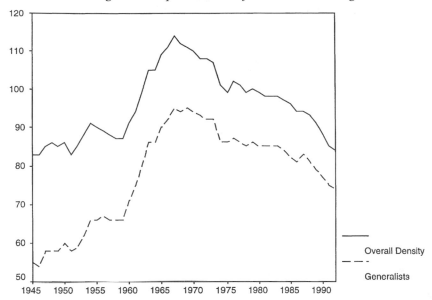

Figure 3.3 Bay Area Hospitals, 1945–92

utilization in the Bay Area has tended to be lower than that for the entire U.S., the trend over time has also been roughly parallel, particularly in the dramatic fall in bed occupancy after 1980. In addition, local and national ownership patterns have converged, primarily as a result of the significant reduction in the proportion of government-owned hospitals in the Bay region since the 1940s. With matching declines in the fraction of for-profit facilities, the voluntary nonprofit form is now the most prevalent ownership status in both hospital populations. In terms of facility size, however, the mean number of beds per hospital in the U.S. declined to a little over 190 by 1985 from around 240 in the early 1960s, while the mean bed number at the local level has remained relatively steady. This deviation may reflect the presence of several large urban and teaching hospitals as well as more intense facility consolidation in the Bay Area.

While our data reveal substantially fewer hospitals per capita in the Bay Area in the closing decade of the twentieth century than at midcentury, it is important to recognize that, while beleaguered, this population exhibits great resilience. Although half-empty and driven from their position of centrality in the field, many hospitals continue to survive. That so many have been able to do so is testimony to their strong roots in the communities they serve.

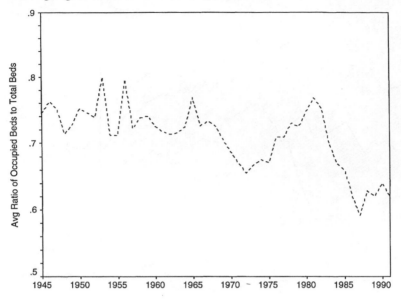

Figure 3.4   Bay Area Hospital Capacity Utilization, 1945–91

Most of these surviving hospitals have been obliged to make substantial changes in their structure and operation as a cost of continuing to do business. Many of them have become parts of larger systems, and all of them have taken steps to develop alliances with other similar and different organizations. We discuss these types of adaptations in chapter 8.

Health Maintenance Organizations

Unlike hospitals, which were an invention of the nineteenth century and existed in large numbers at the outset of the study period, HMOs represent a relatively new organizational form (see chap. 2). While this form did not generally become prominent until the late 1970s, in 1945 Kaiser Permanente (KP), an important pioneer model of the HMO form, opened to the public in the Bay Area (Case Illustration 3.A describes the development of various components in the KP system).

Figure 3.6 depicts the annual entries and exits of organizations in and out of the HMO population. The figure graphically illustrates the extent to which KP was an "outlier" (or pioneer) when it appeared in 1945. The next entry into this population did not occur until 1965, and it was only following federal legislation in 1973 that significant numbers of entries

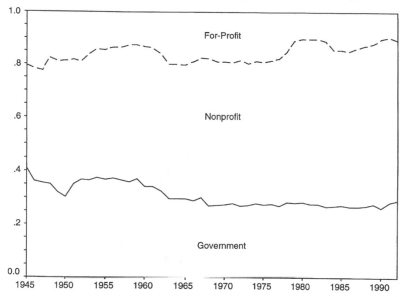

Figure 3.5   Proportion of Bay Area Hospitals by Ownership Type, 1954–92

occurred. Most of the 36 entries into the Bay Area population occurred after the mid-1970s, and there is evidence of a decline in foundings during the latter part of the study period. During the same period, we recorded a total of 16 HMO exits, 8 by dissolution and 8 by merger. Taken together, the entries and exits yield a pattern of rapid growth in the organizational population during the 1970s and early 1980s, followed by some decline in the 1990s (see fig. 3.7). Other sources reveal that this decline was reversed after 1992, when our systematic data ends. In 1997, for instance, 31 HMOs included the Bay region in their service area (AAHP 1997), compared with 24 in 1992.

Enrollments in HMOs have increased steadily since 1980 and, by 1992, averaged more than 170,000 patients per HMO in the Bay Area.[6] In California as a whole, more than 12 million people were enrolled in HMOs by 1994, representing about 35 percent of the residents of the state, compared with 20 percent in other states (Interstudy 1994). HMO market penetration in the Bay Area (measured as covered lives divided by total population) has been even more substantial, rising from a mere 0.5 percent of the population in 1945 to 48 percent in 1990 (fig. 3.8). Not surprisingly,

6. Kaiser Permanente (KP) is excluded from this calculation since its large size would necessarily skew the enrollment average.

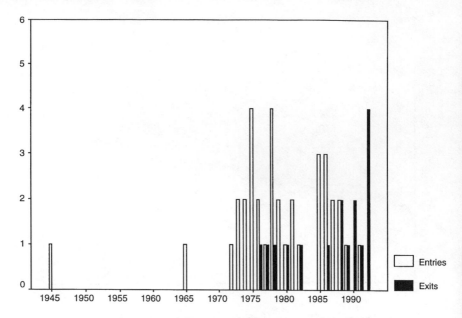

Figure 3.6 Bay Area HMO Entries and Exits, 1945–92

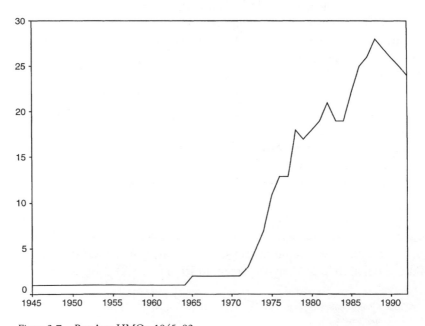

Figure 3.7 Bay Area HMOs, 1945–92

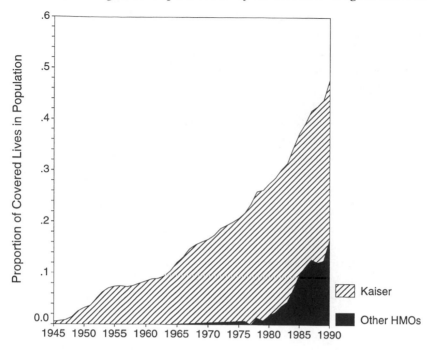

Figure 3.8   Bay Area HMO Market Penetration, 1945–90

Kaiser Permanente's share completely dominated the market until the early 1980s; even in 1990, KP enrollments in the region outnumbered those of all other HMOs combined by a nearly 2:1 ratio.

Average hospital stays for Bay Area HMO patients declined from approximately 550 days per thousand patients in 1977 to roughly 400 days in 1985. As Luft (1981) was the first to show, HMOs achieve most of their savings by reductions in the hospitalization of their patients, both in terms of admissions and length of stay. HMO practice contributed significantly to decreases in hospital utilization during the 1980s.[7]

As previously described (see chap. 2, esp. table 2.1), HMOs come in a variety of types—group, staff, network, and independent practice associations, although these categories have become less distinct over time. In recent years, differences among the various types of HMOs—as well as between HMOs and other arrangements such as PPOs—have become increasingly blurred, so they constitute "more of a continuum rather than separate

7. In the United States as a whole, national data reveal that this trend has continued into the 1990s; for instance, average hospitals days per 1000 non-Medicare members dropped from around 297 in 1993 to 277 in 1994 (Hoechst Marion Roussel 1995).

categories" (Morrison and Luft 1990: 82). Nevertheless, broad differences between staff and more individualized physician models are still discernible.

Staff and group models were the most prevalent types of HMOs prior to 1980, but since that time, IPAs have become the most rapidly growing type (fig. 3.9). The IPA contracts with individual physicians in diverse settings, including physicians in independent and group practice, to provide care, typically on a discounted fee-for-service basis. As Strang (1995) points out, the IPA form of HMO is most consistent with physician's normative beliefs and preferred mode of practice.[8] This model also offers patients a greater range of choice of physician. Over half of the HMOs serving the Bay Area in 1992 were of the IPA type.

Early forms of HMOs were primarily nonprofit in status, but for-profit forms have come to dominate the field. The development of the latter was encouraged by revisions in the HMO Act in 1976 making for-profit as well as nonprofit forms eligible for federal loan guarantees for start-up costs. The phase out of federal support during the early 1980s further encouraged the growth of for-profits that could raise capital for start-up and expansion from equity markets (Christianson et al. 1991). In the Bay Area, for-profit organizations overtook nonprofits during the latter half of the 1980s and constituted about 65 percent of the HMO population in 1994.

In summary, with the exception of Kaiser Permanente, HMOs did not become prevalent as an organizational form until federal legislation in the early 1970s furnished both resources and legitimacy. Following a slow gestation period during their first decade, this form has grown relatively steadily, both in numbers, up to 1990, and in enrollments up to the present time. IPAs and for-profit forms now constitute the dominant mode of HMO, in both the Bay Area and the nation.

A comparison of the Bay Area's HMO population with that of the country at large proves instructive in revealing that our region was a leader in the "HMO movement." In the late 1970s, when HMO market penetration in the San Francisco Bay Area was already over 25 percent, market penetration at a national level was a mere 3 percent. While the bulk of Bay Area entries occurred between the mid-1970s and mid-1980s, entries at the national level did not peak until 1986–87 (Christianson et al. 1991: fig. 3). The "first-mover" status of the Bay Area is also reflected in comparisons of density statistics—the number of HMOs active in the

---

8. IPAs, like PPOs, operate in such a loosely-coupled fashion that some observers argue that they exist at some point about halfway on the continuum between pure market relations and an organizational form (Robinson 1998).

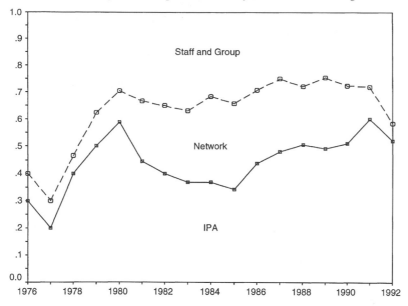

Figure 3.9   Proportion of Bay Area HMO Subtypes, 1976–92

nine-county region in 1979 represented approximately 9 percent of all health maintenance organizations in the entire United States. Although that percentage later dropped to around 5 percent in the late 1980s, the historical presence of HMOs in our study area can hardly be taken to be typical of other metropolitan regions.

Home Health Agencies

The pioneer models for home health agencies were visiting nurse associations that developed during the 1880s to assist persons with healthcare needs in their homes, particularly in urban areas (see chap. 2). The impetus for these associations was to enable persons requiring regular nursing services and nonmedical services such as hot meals to receive these in their own homes, preserving their independence for as long as possible. VNAs, both public and private, reached an early peak in the first two decades of this century and then entered a long period of decline. These forms have recently been renewed and, in the case of the subset we focus on, revised to incorporate medical services. Such arrangements can prevent or shorten hospitalization and other more expensive alternatives and so are increasingly viewed as a method of reducing healthcare costs. In 1961,

HHAs became eligible for federal support through the Community Health Services and Facilities Act and, in 1965, received a major boost when Medicare authorized funding for certified agencies.

Our data set is restricted to HHAs certified to receive Medicare funding, since these are the principal providers of healthcare services. Since our data series begins in 1966, it includes information on the vital rates for this population during its major recent growth period. In 1966, 21 HHAs were in existence in the Bay Area, of which about one-third were VNAs. Most of the growth of HHAs did not take place until the late 1970s, which witnessed a substantial increase in the founding rate (fig. 3.10). The increase in foundings coincides with the liberalization of federal policies regarding HHAs: in 1978, end-stage renal disease patients became eligible for Medicare funding for home dialysis, and in 1980, for-profit organizations were no longer excluded from reimbursement under Medicare (see Estes et al. 1992). Annual exits remained relatively low until the mid-1980s.

The combination of foundings and exits indicates a relatively steady increase in the number of both hospital-based and autonomous HHAs throughout the study period, with surges in the mid-1980s and early 1990s (fig. 3.11).[9] Early on, the hospital-based subtype represents a very small proportion of the organizational population (10 percent in 1966), expands to almost 40 percent of the population by the mid-1970s, and then hovers between 30 and 40 percent through the end of the study period. Clearly, the initial wave of new integrated HHAs between 1966 and 1975 represented a recognition on the part of hospitals that they needed to expand their service niches beyond traditional acute care.

Nonprofit forms dominated the HHA population during the 1960s and 1970s, but for-profit forms began their increase in 1980 and now account for more than 60 percent of the market. Meanwhile, the more traditional VNAs have declined steadily throughout the study period, from a high of 30 percent of all autonomous HHAs in 1966 to a low of 10 percent in 1992. Many of the HHAs in the Bay Area are affiliated with other forms—both hospitals and HMOs (see chap. 8).

Considering national figures, the size of the Medicare-certified HHA population has grown in a fashion similar to the Bay Area population, including a steady increase since the 1960s and a major wave in the first half of the 1980s (Estes et al. 1992; Scalzi et al. 1994b). With regard to ownership patterns, the nation in general also experienced a relative

9. Growth in the Bay Area HHA population has continued to be strong in the 1990s, with some fifty agencies being added to the HHA census between 1992 and 1994 (OSHPD 1994).

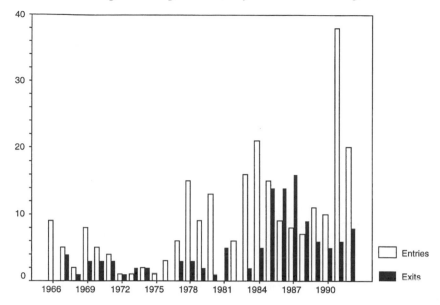

Figure 3.10   Bay Area HHA Entries and Exits, 1966–92

decline in VNAs, with most increases in the number of HHAs coming from proprietary forms, especially after 1980 (Spohn, Bergthold, and Estes 1988). However, for-profits still only comprised 15 percent of HHAs nationally by 1990 (Scalzi et al. 1994b: 13), well below the percentage reported above for the Bay Area (which reflects the tendency among the western and southwestern regions of the United States toward proprietary HHAs [Estes et al. 1992]). The HCFA administrative region containing the San Francisco area has also been one of the most volatile markets in terms of agency entries, exits, and clientele changes (Scalzi et al. 1994b: 12–13).

In summary, following a long period of decline (prior to 1945), HHAs became newly popular during the 1960s and, with the help of Medicare funding, have experienced substantial growth in recent decades. While early organizations were either nonprofit (typically VNAs) or public (typically state and municipal programs), for-profit forms now dominate the population of providers in the Bay Area.

End-Stage Renal Disease Centers

End-stage renal disease centers are the joint product of recent developments in technology and changes in funding policies at the federal level. Prior to the development of kidney transplantation and dialysis procedures in the 1950s, no such facilities existed. Prior to the extension in 1972

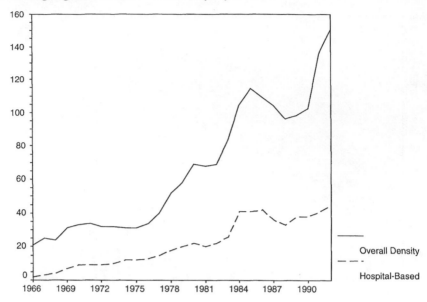

Figure 3.11   Total and Hospital-Based Bay Area HHAs, 1966–92

of Medicare coverage to chronically ill patients, the only facilities that existed were located in major hospitals. It is only with the combination of these two factors that independent ESRDCs began to emerge (Rettig and Levinsky 1991).

The ecological dynamics of ESRDC units in the Bay Area are summarized in figure 3.12, including a total of 48 entries and 13 exits during the period of analysis. As anticipated by our historical discussion (chap. 2), an initial wave of ESRDC foundings emerged in the wake of the 1972 Medicare amendment, with further entries encouraged by the market reforms of the 1980s. Organizational exits are more sporadic, only occurring in a consistent fashion after the mid-1980s.

Figure 3.13 shows the corresponding ESRDC densities and numbers of hospital-based facilities. In 1969, only 10 ESRD providers existed in the San Francisco Bay Area and all of them were hospital-based. By 1991, the total number of units had grown to 45 and only one-third of them were hospital-based. During the twenty-three year period shown in the figure, all but twelve ESRDC entries involved autonomous units.[10]

10. As in the case of the HMO and HHA populations, the ESRDC population continued to grow in the years following our systematic data collection. Between 1992 and 1997, nine facilities were added in the Bay region, representing a 20 percent increase in provider numbers (HCFA 1997).

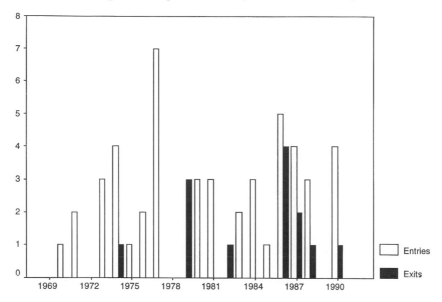

Figure 3.12 Bay Area ESRDC Entries and Exits, 1969–91

Like vertical integration, ESRDC ownership patterns have changed dramatically over the past few decades. Government-owned units have declined noticeably, from around 27 percent of the Bay Area population in 1980 to less than 15 percent in 1991. At the same time, the proportion of for-profits has increased from 30 percent to almost 50 percent. The proportion of nonprofit centers has fluctuated around 40 percent during the period.

Treatment modalities have also continued to evolve since the 1960s, leading to service differentiation among ESRD providers. One important dimension of differentiation involves the availability of transplantation and/or dialysis outpatient services. In this respect, three basic "types" of providers can be identified: (1) *generalists* include those units that are "approved to furnish the full spectrum of diagnostic, therapeutic, and reha-bilitative services required for the care of ESRD dialysis patients (including inpatient dialysis furnished directly or under arrangement)" (HCFA 1990: 61); these providers do not perform transplantation; (2) *low-end specialists* include those units that perform either in-patient or outpatient dialysis, but not both; and (3) *high-end specialists* include units that emphasize transplantation (but may offer dialysis treatment as well). Between 1980 and 1991, the subpopulation of low-end specialists in the Bay region

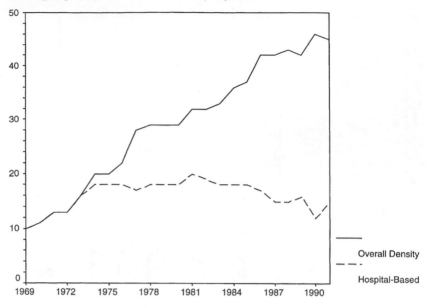

Figure 3.13   Total and Hospital-Based Bay Area ESRDCs, 1969–91

grew dramatically, expanding from about 40 to 70 percent of all ES-RDCs. Generalists in the population have experienced a concomitant decline, from a little over 50 percent of the population to a mere 20 percent.[11]

Again, it is useful to compare the Bay Area trends in the ESRDC population with national developments. In the first comprehensive census of ESRD providers, Katz and Proctor (1969) identified 111 centers nationwide. At the time, around 9 percent of these centers were in the Bay Area, which—as in the case of HMOs—was clearly ahead of the curve in introducing these new organizational forms. By 1990, the national numbers had grown to almost two thousand ESRD providers, with the Bay Area's share shrinking to a little over 2 percent of the total (HCFA 1990), consistent with its representative share of the nationwide patient population. A cross-sectional analysis of ESRD providers in 1990 reveals that the structural characteristics in the Bay Area had also become representative of those

11. ESRDC providers continue to display a responsiveness to technological innovations. Earlier procedures required that patients be treated approximately three times a week on an in-patient basis. More recently, "home hemodialysis" techniques have allowed dialyzers to be employed on an out-patient basis, and alternative procedures, such as peritoneal dialysis (which is also available on an out-treatment basis), have become important supplements to original dialysis methods.

of providers in the country as a whole—about a third of providers were hospital-based, both locally and nationally, and about half were for-profits, again in both instances.

Before turning to two other healthcare populations, we call attention to the broad representation of Kaiser Permanente (KP) in each of our focal populations. Kaiser Permanente is unique among our organizational cases and other Bay Area healthcare providers in many ways. Its complex, interconnected organizational structure is distinctive: members enroll in prepaid health plans and are given preventive and comprehensive medical treatments by a salaried, group practice of physicians in KP-owned and operated facilities. Because of its size, age, and general significance to the Bay Area healthcare field, we describe KP's development in Case Illustration 3.A.

Case Illustration 3.A   Kaiser Permanente's Representation in Focal Populations

In our study of the population of Bay Area systems, we pay particular attention to Kaiser Permanente because it is and has been the largest healthcare system in the region since the 1950s (as determined by number of facilities and market share). We also take into account KP's representation in our focal populations, its influence on those populations, and its distinctiveness (or lack thereof) compared to general population trends.

KP leaders formed what we would today consider an integrated healthcare system (see chap. 8). It combines a full range of facilities and services, provided by its own staff of physicians, with comprehensive health plans. The tight coupling of these components (e.g., KP members see only Permanente physicians at KP facilities; Permanente physicians treat only KP members at KP facilities) stems from KP's necessary self-reliance in its formative years and makes KP distinct from more loosely coupled systems that developed later.

In the 1940s and 1950s, local medical societies refused to grant Permanente physicians privileges in community hospital. KP had to build or acquire its own hospitals to treat its members, beginning with the purchase and renovation of a 54-bed hospital in Oakland in 1942. KP's expansion of its hospital facilities peaked as membership grew in the 1950s and 1960s (Smillie 1991; see Case Illustration 5.A), at the same time that the overall Bay Area hospital population experienced its most entries. By 1995, KP owned thirteen general hospitals and 30 medical offices in the Bay Area, with either one or two hospitals in each of the nine Bay Area counties (except Napa, where it has medical offices but no hospital). Some of the hospitals offer specialized treatments: the Oakland hospital is one of seven in the Bay Area with a renal transplant facility and is KP's only Bay Area ESRDC.

At the same time that KP was building hospitals, its leaders recognized the need to reduce hospital utilization to cut costs. Although home health services were a cost-effective solution to excessive hospitalization, KP did not introduce home health care until Medicare provided reimbursement for these services in 1965 (KP 1966). Initially such care was restricted to the elderly, but in time the service was offered to all members. The first services were provided by the Hayward hospital through a contract with a VNA. By 1992, KP was operating 8 HHAs, all affiliated with Kaiser hospitals. Between 1978 and 1992, KP's proportion of the Bay Area HHAs declined from 15 to 5 percent (OSHPD 1978–92).

Because of its success at treating patients for reduced costs, KP was considered a model for policy makers and researchers seeking solutions to rising healthcare costs in the late 1960s (Williams 1971; Somers 1971a, 1971b). Minnesota physician Paul Ellwood labeled KP and similar providers "health maintenance organizations" and lobbied the federal government to support the formation of HMOs. Most early HMOs, including KP, fit the group/staff model, but later models were more flexible. To compete with these forms, KP has recently changed some aspects of its program. For example, it added point-of-service plans, in which members may receive medical care from outside doctors for higher co-payments (Kramon 1989; Winslow 1994). Physician members of the Permanente Medical Group, however, remain the primary providers of care.

In sum, KP's influence on the Bay Area healthcare field was and is far-reaching. Because of the circumstances surrounding its early history as well as its commitment to comprehensive care, KP's healthcare system bridges many populations of principal players in the field (see fig. 2.2). As a provider, it operates hospitals, HHAs, and an ESRDC, as well as other types of facilities and programs. As an intermediary between purchasers and providers, it offers health plans to individuals and employers. In light of the scope and magnitude of KP's involvement in the Bay Area, we are careful to consider KP's multiple roles and considerable influence throughout our study.

Trends in Two Other Populations

In addition to the four preceding organizational populations on which we have collected annual data on numbers and selected characteristics, we also counted the numbers of two other forms: medical groups and preferred provider organizations.

Medical Groups

Medical groups represent a long-standing, although historically marginalized, model of practice enabling groups of physicians, usually specialists, to share facilities and some services. As medical groups organize an increasing proportion of all physicians, they not only constitute new units that directly compete with individual practitioners for the delivery of medical care but also comprise basic building blocks for other types of healthcare systems.

The prevalence of group practice contributes to the formation and growth of HMO and PPO networks (Christianson et al. 1991; Barger, Hillman, and Garland 1985), and contracts with HMOs, PPOs, and hospitals now constitute a substantial component of medical group operations.[12] This overlap with other provider populations is even more pronounced for group model HMOs, such as the Kaiser Permanente system, in which Permanente medical groups exclusively serve patients enrolled in the Kaiser health plans. Thus, the count data reported in figure 3.14 overlaps somewhat with the data on numbers of HMOs reported in figure 3.7. We define groups at the facility level and count only those groups that include six or more physicians.

From only ten medical groups existing in 1946, by 1993 the Bay Area had become home to 79 such facilities, including Permanente Groups (fig. 3.14).[13] The number of these groups in the KP system has, until near the end of the study period, increased steadily and comprised the largest share of the group practice population in the region. Nevertheless, its relative numbers have declined from over 60 percent in the early 1960s to 37 percent in 1993.

Preferred Provider Organizations

PPOs function as intermediaries between insurance companies or employers and providers, whether groups of physicians, individual physicians or hospitals. They contract with these providers not on a capitation basis, as do HMOs, but on a discounted fee-for-service basis. Thus, although these organizations swell the wave of "managed care," they represent the response of the more traditionalist or conservative faction of providers and insurers to the challenges posed by HMOs.

Following the passage of enabling legislation in California in 1982, PPOs developed rapidly, initially focused in the San Francisco Bay and Los Angeles metropolitan areas (Trauner 1983; White and Arstein-Kerslake 1983). Only two PPOs operated in the San Francisco Bay Area in 1983,

---

12. Fifty-four percent of medical groups in the United States in 1991 contracted with one or more HMOs, two-thirds (64 percent) contracted with one or more PPOs, and a relatively substantial share of their revenue was derived from these sources—approximately 15 percent from each. Over 17 percent reported a relationship with a hospital involving joint ownership or shared fiscal accountability (Havlicek, Eiler, and Neblett 1993).

13. Although we treat KP as one HMO organization and formally all its Bay Area physicians belong to the Permanente Medical Group of Northern California, each clinical medical office of the KP system is counted as a separate "medical group" in our study to make the Permanente data consistent with data on other medical groups.

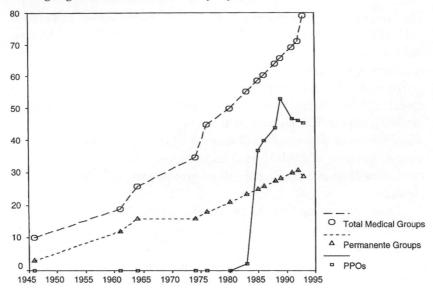

Figure 3.14   Bay Area Medical Groups and PPOs, 1945–93

but the number rose rapidly to a peak of 53 in 1989, before dropping slightly to 45 in 1994 (see fig. 3.14). The proportion of these plans with statewide, as opposed to more limited regional coverage, also showed a substantial increase throughout the period.

Comparing Population Trends

Having reviewed the development of four populations of healthcare providers and described some of the changes in their characteristics, we find it instructive to compare the relative density of each type in the Bay Area over time (see fig. 3.15). Note that we have complete trends throughout this period for only two of the four focal populations: hospitals and HMOs. We were unable to obtain complete information for the earliest HHAs and ESRDCs. This is not only, or even primarily, a data problem, however, but a substantive and theoretical issue, which we discuss below.

Although the data set is not complete, it allows us to discern the contours of the major trends in these populations during the past half century. Hospitals were unchallenged and dominant until the mid-1960s, when other different and more specialized types of providers began to emerge. From that point to the present, the numbers and influence of hospitals have declined while the numbers and relative prevalence of

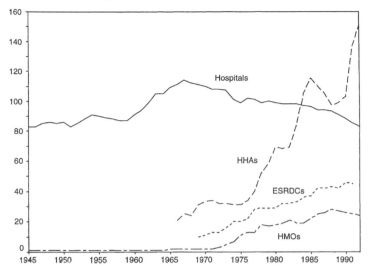

Figure 3.15   Bay Area Organizational Populations, 1945–92

the newer types of providers have grown. The steepest and most impressive growth rates are exhibited by HHAs, whose numbers continue to rise rapidly up to the end of the study period. The other populations have grown less quickly, but still steadily through the late 1980s, when HMOs exhibit a slight decline in numbers (of organizations, not of enrollments).

If we add to this picture the density data depicted in figure 3.14 for the other two populations—medical groups and PPOs—we have further evidence of the ascendance of the newer forms. Medical groups existed in very small numbers prior to the early 1960s, when they began to show a steady rate of increase. PPOs did not exist as a recognized form of healthcare provider in California until 1982, but grew rapidly throughout the 1980s, tailing off a bit at the end of the study period.

These density plots provide a graphic portrait of one of the most important ways the field of healthcare organizations has changed during the past half century. Carroll and Hannan (1989) have argued that organizational density can be employed as an important indicator of the legitimacy of an organizational population. As we will discuss in more detail in chapter 7, legitimacy is a complex and multifaceted concept. In their usage, Carroll and Hannan emphasize the cognitive aspects of legitimacy—the "taken-for-grantedness" of the organizational form in the sense that "relevant actors regard it as the 'natural' way to achieve some collective goal" (1989: 525).

They argue that the higher the density, the greater the prevalence of a given organizational form, the stronger the sense that it represents the legitimate way to organize (up to a point where "further proliferation is unlikely to have much effect on its taken-for-grantedness"). We embrace this insight and add that, in organizational fields in which competing forms exist, *relative* prevalence provides a useful gauge of how varying organizational forms are faring in the competition for support from the institutional environment. From this perspective, in the fifty years since World War II, hospitals have been losing their monopoly position as the primary model or organizational archetype for delivering medical care services, and are increasingly being challenged by the emergence and expanding numbers of more specialized rivals.

Another way to describe these trends is to examine the changing profile of organizations located in or providing services for a given county at the beginning, middle, and end of the study period. These data are presented in table 3.2 for two Bay Area counties: San Mateo, the median county in terms of population size (of individuals), and Santa Clara County, the largest county in the area. The first four rows of the table present data on the numbers of hospitals, HHAs, HMOs, and kidney disease centers for 1945, 1972, and 1992. We note that in the first period (1945) for both counties, hospitals stand virtually alone as an organizational provider of healthcare services. In the middle period (1972) hospitals retain their numerical and, no doubt, normative and behavioral dominance in both counties, although we begin to see the emergence of new provider forms. The number of hospitals doubled in Santa Clara County between 1945 and 1972, but the resident population of this county had increased more than four times during this period. There was no increase in the number of hospitals in San Mateo County even though its resident population had more than doubled.

By the end of the study period (1992), hospitals had not grown further in numbers whereas the other organizational populations continued to increase. The number of ESRDCs and HHAs more than doubled during the two decades since 1972, and the numbers of HMO exploded.

The other important change, recorded in the last row of table 3.2 is the transition of hospitals from being independent and freestanding facilities to becoming members of multihospital systems. In 1945, none of the hospitals in the two counties belonged to these corporate entities; by 1972 about a third of the hospitals had made such connections, and by 1992, all of San Mateo's hospitals and two-thirds of Santa Clara's hospitals were system members.

Table 3.2 Organizational Populations in San Mateo and Santa Clara Counties

Organizational Population	San Mateo			Santa Clara		
	1945	1972	1992	1945	1972	1992
Hospitals	7	7	7	8	16	15
HMOs[a]	1	1	19	1	2	17
HHAs[b]	n/a	2	15	n/a	4	33
ESRDCs	0	1	3	0	2	8
Multihospital system members	0	2	7	0	3	10

NOTES: a. Number of HMOs with enrollees in these counties.

b. Excludes HHAs which are not Medicare-certified.

Blurred and Shifting Boundaries

An important criterion of profound institutional change is whether new types of social actors—such as new organizational forms—are being created and whether organizational populations and fields are experiencing changes in their boundaries. This chapter has already provided substantial evidence regarding the development of new kinds of healthcare organizations during the past half century. For example, organizations like HMOs and ESRDCs did not exist at all in midcentury and now are present in substantial numbers.

What about boundary changes? We have alluded to such processes on occasion, but it is time to collect the evidence we have. It is considerable. We just noted that hospitals are increasingly becoming component units of larger, more integrated systems. The extent and types of such integration vary, as does the extent to which a hospital member retains its independence and original identity. The fact that more than two-thirds of the hospitals in the Bay Area are now members of such systems represents one important instance of boundary change. Moreover, these systems connect to and combine with a diverse set of organizational forms.

The newer types of organizations also give evidence of changing and blurring boundaries. We have noted that HMOs come in many varieties and that these subtypes are evolving, with various hybrid and difficult-to-classify subforms (Morrison and Luft 1990). Even Kaiser Permanente, historically a closed group/staff HMO, has recently blurred its boundaries with other types of HMOs. It is also becoming increasingly difficult to

Table 3.3   Blending of Medical Groups with Other Delivery Forms in the Bay Area, 1993

Medical Groups involved in:	Excluding KP Medical Groups	Including KP Medical Groups[e]
HMO network[a]	52%	70%
PPO network[b]	70%	44%
Home health services[c]	10%	43%
Hospital connection[d]	12%	44%

NOTES: Figures for local medical groups excluding the Permanente medical group facilities of the Kaiser Permanente (KP) system are comparable to national statistics gathered by the AMA in 1991: HMO network (61%), PPO network (64%), and close connection with hospital (17%) (Havlicek, Eiler, and Neblett 1993).

a. Includes medical groups that are staff HMOs, are organized to provide services to an HMO, or have contracts with one or more HMOs.

b. Includes medical groups that have contracts with one or more PPO.

c. Includes medical groups offering home health services.

d. Includes medical groups that are jointly owned by or share fiscal responsibility with at least one hospital.

e. For purpose of these comparisons, each Permanente medical group facility of the Kaiser Permanente system is counted as a separate medical group (29 in the Bay area in 1993).

SOURCES: MGMA (1961–93), KP (1960–94).

distinguish HMOs from alternative provider models such as preferred provider organizations (PPOs), as we have reported.

We indicated above in our discussion of medical groups the sense in which they constitute important building blocks, participating in and linking with broader healthcare systems. To illustrate the extent of such linkages as well as the special role that the KP system plays in the Bay Area, we assembled data on selected linkages for medical groups in the Bay Area for 1993 (see table 3.3). As indicated, more than half of these groups were associated with an HMO (of the IPA type), and 70 percent were involved in one or more PPO plans. A small proportion, around 10 percent, were involved in providing home health services or had a close affiliation with a hospital. As indicated, the latter types of connections were much more characteristic of KP groups. If data for the KP system are excluded, Bay Area figures for medical group linkages are quite comparable with national level data (see table 3.3 note). While these types of affiliations and linkages can be viewed as providing information on the increasing number of horizontal and vertical connections among healthcare forms (see chap. 8), they can also be seen as evidence for the increased extent of blending of organizational forms and blurring of traditional boundaries between forms. Case Illustration 3.B describes this blending and blurring for one particular medical group, the Palo Alto Medical Clinic.

Case Illustration 3.B **Blurred Boundaries of the Palo Alto Medical Clinic**

The Palo Alto Medical Clinic's history of linkages with other organizations includes close affiliations with other clinics, HMOs, and PPOs. In many cases, these linkages blurred and/or expanded what were considered the boundaries of the medical group. Because of its pioneering influence on other medical groups, PAMC's linkages affected not just its own boundaries, but the expectations for the boundaries of medical groups in general.

PAMC formed the United Medical Clinics in 1965 with three other local medical groups. Over the next ten years, the number of the United Medical Clinics' patients enrolled in prepaid plans grew. After the 1976 California Knox-Keene act required all prepaid health plans to be administered by HMOs, the United Medical Clinics and Blue Cross jointly created TakeCare, a nonprofit HMO, to accommodate its patients (Casalino 1997). Owned by Blue Cross, TakeCare only contracted with multispecialty medical groups, which encouraged a close bond between the clinic and the HMO. Unlike other, looser linkages, "there was a good deal of HMO–medical group interaction and cooperation . . . the medical groups helped create TakeCare's medical policies and promoted the HMO to their patients" (Casalino 1997: 111).

The United Medical Clinics' involvement in the administration and marketing of TakeCare expanded and blurred PAMC's medical group boundaries. In 1988, the clinics attempted to buy TakeCare when Blue Cross offered the HMO for sale, which would have created further blurring. Blue Cross chose another buyer, but the clinics and the HMO retained their tight linkage. In 1990, nearly all of the clinics' HMO patients were enrolled in TakeCare, and, in 1991, the Palo Alto Medical Clinic became a part owner of TakeCare by buying stock in the HMO, which it later sold at a substantial profit (Casalino 1997). Nevertheless, after several years of close coordination, PAMC ended its nearly exclusive relationship with TakeCare in 1994 and contracted with more than ten different HMOs.

In addition to linkages with other medical groups and HMOs, PAMC's boundaries were blurred and expanded by its relationships with Stanford Hospital and two local surgicenters. Since Stanford Hospital's founding in 1959, it has maintained close ties with community physicians (see Case Illustration 7.A). Members of PAMC were and are extensively involved at Stanford Hospital. As the closest hospital to the clinic, most PAMC patients are treated at Stanford, and many PAMC physicians are faculty members at the medical school. With these two institutional affiliations, PAMC physicians bridge the hospital and group practice and blur the boundary between the two organizations.

PAMC's involvement in freestanding surgicenters began in 1974 when an Arizona-based organization founded one in Palo Alto (Casalino 1997). The clinic immediately took advantage of this new surgical option, using it extensively, and bought a majority interest in it in 1990. In 1992, PAMC became involved with a second surgicenter when it joined with Helian Health to build a Recovery Inn in Menlo Park, the city north of Palo Alto. This upscale surgicenter, designed for private patients, has two operating rooms and seven patient suites.

In sum, PAMC's linkages with other healthcare organizations have expanded considerably over the last thirty years. In the process of affiliating and working with other clinics, insurers, and provider organizations, the boundaries of the clinic have become more porous, less clear, and more expansive.

As for HHAs, and ESRDCs, our lack of data on the earliest period for these forms is not simply an absence of information but poses a substantive and theoretical problem—one closely connected to issues of definition and boundaries of organizational forms. Let us consider each type. HHAs have been in existence since the 1880s. From the earliest period, they have tended to cluster into two broad types: those that perform medical and skilled nursing services and those that primarily provide assistance with living, including meal preparation and physical rehabilitation. The conventional and most convenient way to distinguish between these types of providers is to employ the criterion of whether or not they are certified by Medicare, since only those providing healthcare services are eligible for this type of reimbursement. Thus, in the case of this population, certification by a federal agency provides a relatively clear criterion of the boundaries between these two subtypes (Estes et al. 1992). The difficulty this standard poses for an historical study such as our own is that it cannot be employed prior to 1965, when the Medicare program was created.

Turning to ESRDCs, this specialized facility could not exist until the development of science and technology gave rise to new therapeutic equipment and procedures. During its formative period, such "centers" existed only as innovative equipment owned by hospitals engaged in highly specialized treatment programs. ESRD services often did not exist during the early 1960s, even as distinct organizational units within hospitals. Only gradually were these services differentiated into specialized units within hospitals, then as freestanding centers. The fact that our AHA data set picks up on this class of services in 1969 largely reflects growing federal support (e.g., kidney procurement programs) that allowed ESRD provision to gain heightened recognition. Again, we find that federal policies and guidelines with respect to who can be reimbursed for services plays an important role in the creation of a distinct population of provider forms. As technology continues to develop in this area, we are witnessing a blurring of the boundaries between HHAs and ESRDCs as the former increasingly perform functions previously reserved for the latter.

CONCLUSION

While a number of general trends affecting healthcare organizations were described in the opening section of this chapter, our review of changes in healthcare organizations in the Bay Area has thus far provided evidence regarding only a subset of these: concentration, specialization, and privatization/market orientation. Later chapters will deal with other trends as they have affected the Bay Area. Increasing concentration is intimated by the growing density of a number of providers, including HHAs, HMOs, and ESRDCs. Evidence was also provided regarding the rapid growth of medical groups and PPOs in recent decades. More detailed indications of concentration—focusing on the interrelationships of some of these organizational populations—will be offered in chapter 8.

Increased specialization is witnessed in the numbers of new, specialized provider forms—for example, HHAs, and ESRDCs. At the same time, it is noteworthy that specialization within forms has decreased in a number of cases; hospitals, for instance, are far less likely to thrive in specialist niches than they were fifty years ago and there are trends away from specialism among HMOs as well. The complexity of institutional change in healthcare is such that dynamics of change at one level (e.g., specialization *among* forms in the organizational field) may run counter to the dynamics at another level (reduced specialization *within* organizational forms).

The trend toward privatization is evident in three of the organizational populations reviewed. Hospitals, HHAs, and ESRDCs are now less likely to be organized as public facilities than they were formerly. HMOs have never operated as public systems, and the numbers of public (state and county) hospital systems has also declined. With the exception of hospitals, all of our organizational populations are more likely to be operated as for-profit than as nonprofit institutions today than was the case a few decades ago. Hospitals, the most traditional and conservative form of healthcare delivery organization, is the only population in which the proportion of nonprofit units increased during the period of our study.

Four

PROCESSES SHAPING ORGANIZATIONAL POPULATIONS: ECOLOGICAL AND ADAPTIVE CHANGE

IN THEIR REVIEW OF HISTORICAL trends among U.S. hospitals, Alexander and Amburgey (1987) call attention to a neglected distinction in organization theory that empirically separates population-level changes resulting from differential numbers of organizational entries and exits from those produced by modifications in existing organizations (cf. Aldrich and Pfeffer 1976). Here, we attempt to decompose change processes into these two broad categories, which in chapter 3 we termed *ecological*—involving the effects of differential foundings and dissolutions of organizations—and *adaptive*—involving the transformation of existing organizations.[1]

As this chapter demonstrates, similar levels of aggregate change may be comprised of very different underlying dynamics and relative mixes of these two modes of change, often varying across populations and types of organizations. We also examine the degree to which adaptive and ecological dynamics interact with a second dimension of change introduced in chapter 3—that distinguishing *incremental* and *discontinuous* transitions in organizational environments.

In subsequent chapters, we offer a more detailed examination of environmental factors—in particular those relating to the material-resource and institutional environments—which have contributed to these changes. It is clear that both modes of change interact with and reflect transformations in demographic, regulatory, and funding environments of organizational populations. For example, some legislative initiatives will both encourage

---

1. This distinction is often confounded with debates over *intentional* versus *unintentional* sources of change (see chap. 3). For example, adaptive change is frequently referred to as "strategic," implying intentionality, but this seems inappropriate. Both types of change may be viewed as instances of strategic choice: in the case of ecological change, some actor(s) must decide whether to found and invest in a new organization or, conversely, whether the time has come to terminate the existence of the organization in its present form. In the case of adaptive change, actors take steps to modify existing organizations in the hopes of making them more viable. The difference resides primarily in what type of strategic decision is being made.

new organizations and support existing ones (such as the Hill-Burton program, which allocated funds to build new hospitals as well as enlarge current facilities) and other programs will favor one type of change over another (such as the HMO Act, which focused primarily on incentives for the creation of this new organizational form). We describe these connections when they appear most relevant in the following inquiry.

CHANGES IN HOSPITAL CHARACTERISTICS

With an approach developed by Ruef (1997), it is possible to use longitudinal data to disaggregate net rates of population-level change, viewed as fluctuations in the total or mean level of some characteristic (e.g., hospital bed capacity). The *ecological* component of these changes is the amount of fluctuation that would have occurred if all of the existing organizations in the population were assumed to be structurally inert—incapable of internal change—so that population-level changes could only occur through differential rates of entries and exits. The *adaptive* component is represented by the difference between the observed net rates of change and those engendered by ecological processes.[2] We illustrate this decomposition with a concrete example of annual bed capacity changes in Bay area hospitals.

Hospital Size

Bed Capacity Levels

Bed capacity is a common measure of hospital size since it assesses the ability of facilities to handle patient loads. Size has long been of interest to students of organizations because of its strong association with a number of important organizational characteristics—differentiation and formalization (Blau 1970; Kimberly 1976), economies of scale (Stigler 1958), and power stemming from political influence or dominance in the market (Perrow 1991). The latter two concerns are most relevant given our interest

2. Gauging the relative degree of change taking place in both components can be important from an individual organization's perspective, as well. Even an organization that remains relatively inert may find its strategic position within an industry or market greatly altered depending on entries and exits by similar or different organizations—a process that Ruef (1997) has termed *ecological drift*. In effect, instead of an actor moving across a stage, the background scenery changes. This is similar to the experience of the Kaiser Permanente system as it went from "extreme nonconformist" in the 1950s to a "model program" in the early 1970s, all the while fundamentally maintaining the same organizational form (see Case Illustration 6.B).

in organizational survival. In the following discussion, however, we will not limit ourselves to the size dynamics of individual hospitals but, rather, examine shifts in the bed capacity of our hospital population as a whole.

Historically, the total bed capacity for all nonfederal hospitals in the San Francisco region increased from approximately 12,000 in the immediate post–World War II years to 19,000 around the passage of the Medicare and Medicaid acts in 1965. This was followed by a period of stability up to 1970, and then some declines thereafter.[3] Figure 4.1a plots the annual changes in total bed capacity as smoothed trends. To what extent are these changes driven by expansions or contractions in existing hospitals— by adaptation—as compared with the ecological dynamics of hospital entry and exit? Figure 4.1b shows a decomposition of the bed capacity fluctuations into adaptive and ecological components. To illustrate how these components are derived, consider the adaptive and ecological activity for two time points during the study period. In 1950, for instance, we find that the total bed capacity in the nine-county region had grown by 456 beds from the previous year.[4] Adaptive changes (e.g., new hospital wings) on the part of facilities that existed in both 1949 and 1950 accounted for 185 beds of the total expansion. The remaining addition of 271 beds resulted from three new hospitals that entered the population in 1950, minus the bed capacity of one hospital that exited by the end of 1949. These dynamics are represented in the ecological component of change.

While the adaptive and ecological dynamics are oriented in the same direction in 1950, this does not necessarily have to be the case. For example, in 1989 the total bed capacity contracted by 26 beds from the previous year. Adaptive changes actually contributed to an expansion, with 183 beds being added by existing Bay area hospitals. But this expansion was counteracted by ecological changes, with five exiting facilities and only one entry, which resulted in an elimination of 209 hospital beds.

Reviewing the overall trends in figure 4.1b, we observe that adaptive change on the part of these hospitals consistently increased bed capacity in the region between 1945 and 1970. Not surprisingly, this set of changes largely coincided with the period of Hill-Burton funding, which provided financial aid for hospital expansion programs. During the following twelve

3. The total bed capacity levels for the Bay Area translate into an average hospital size ranging from 180 beds in 1950 to nearly 240 beds in 1990. It is also noteworthy that nonfederal and federal hospitals in the region have converged to the same mean bed capacity over time, overcoming significant disparities observed during the immediate postwar period (when federal hospitals averaged over 350 beds).

4. Because figures 4.1a and 4.1b are based on smoothed rather than raw data trends, all numbers used in the examples will also reflect the smoothed estimates.

years (1970–82), adaptive trajectories were more likely to involve contractions, as indicated by negative bed capacity growth rates. This trend was reversed in the early 1980s, when market-reform measures, such as selective contracting and prospective payments for Medicare patients, were introduced.

While the adaptive changes before 1982 seem to correspond to broader historical patterns, the trend reversal during the most recent era is unexpected. Why did existing hospitals add beds in the period of heightened market competition? A detailed examination of individual hospitals reveals that much of this "adaptive" activity was due to acquisitions. When one hospital acquires another, we treat this event as comprising both ecological and adaptive components. Ecologically, it represents the exit of one existing organization. But it also denotes an adaptive change in the acquiring hospital, which has thereby increased its capacity for service. The increase in number of hospital beds during the late 1980s and early 1990s seems to be primarily the result of such consolidation activities.

The ecological component displays a trend that is different from its adaptive counterpart. Following the two years of "ecological downsizing" that occurred immediately after 1945 (reflecting the closure of some facilities during the demobilization activities following the end of World War II),

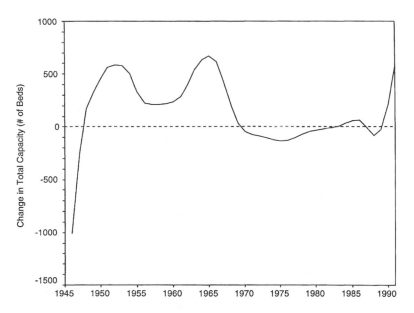

Figure 4.1a   Net Change in Total Bed Capacity of Bay Area Hospitals, 1946–91

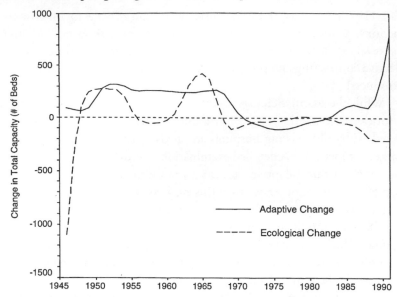

Figure 4.1b   Adaptive and Ecological Components of Change in Total Bed Capacity of Bay Area Hospitals, 1946–91

NOTES: All time trends have been smoothed.

Changes are reported as differences in bed capacity from previous year.

the impact of the Hill-Burton legislation appears to have produced net ecological increases in bed capacity, as hospital entries in the region were encouraged. These were also years of substantial growth in the resident population of the Bay area (see chap. 5). Unlike the adaptive component of these changes, the ecological dynamic reversed itself in the mid-1950s—a time when some specialist facilities, such as tuberculosis hospitals, were closed as a result of medical advances and changes in treatment philosophy. It resumed its positive trajectory in the early 1960s, only to end, once and for all for our study period, with the implementation of the Medicare and Medicaid programs. Between the late 1960s and the present, ecological dynamics favored exits over entries; moreover these exits involved not just more, but also somewhat larger facilities than those leaving the population during the earlier period.

The history of capacity expansion and contraction of one Bay area facility, San Jose Hospital (SJH), demonstrates the abundant variations of decisions and events that comprise both ecological and adaptive change (see Case Illustration 4.A). Moreover, it accentuates the complexity of certain commonly assumed theoretical distinctions of organizational change, as discussed in chapter 3: adaptive changes that are not necessarily "intentional" (e.g., aging and obsolescence of facilities), unintended changes resulting from initially "intentional" decisions (frequently interpreted as "failures"), and types of changes producing both ecological and adaptive consequences (e.g., mergers and acquisitions). The chronology of SJH's experiences also reflects the adaptive and ecological trends for the population of Bay area hospitals as a whole, which we later relate to periods of incremental versus discontinuous change.

Case Illustration 4.A **Facility Expansion and Contraction: San Jose Hospital**

San Jose Hospital (SJH) was founded in 1923 by local physicians to fill a need for hospital services among San Jose's growing middle class.[1] The original hospital began with 84 beds, adding a 33-room wing in 1925. Subsequent major expansions in the 1940s and 1950s were undertaken as SJH grew with the community. In 1946 at the conclusion of World War II, the hospital purchased and relocated four surplus barracks from the San Bruno Naval Base, which provided an additional 38 ward beds. With the help of federal Hill-Burton funds, a 65-bed extension was constructed in 1953, after which time the naval barracks were phased out.

In 1957, SJH expanded both internally, by building a 126-bed surgical wing, and externally, by acquiring Alum Rock Hospital. Alum Rock, a 67-bed tuberculosis facility, was intended for use as a satellite of the main hospital, but many physicians refused to admit patients there because of its remote location. In time, Alum Rock was converted to a nursing home and eventually eliminated by the extended care section of a new 252-bed wing in 1968.

In the early 1970s, SJH merged with Doctors Hospital, a 121-bed facility, later renamed Park Alameda. This event marked the last major expansion of SJH, as the rest of the decade saw a reversal of fortunes for the once prosperous hospital. Locally, SJH faced shifting patient demographics and a diminishing resource base. At the time of its founding in the 1920s, SJH's surrounding neighborhood was a desirable residential area with many professional and mercantile families. Beginning in the late 1960s and throughout the 1970s, the neighborhood experienced an influx of persons on fixed or low incomes and a flight of former residents and businesses to the suburbs. Meanwhile, changes in federal and state health policies, such as Medicaid rates and Health Systems Agency controls, further contributed to the hospital's struggles. In 1972, SJH operated at a loss for the first time, and in 1974 its board decided to decrease bed capacity by selling Park Alameda to Santa Clara County.

During the turbulence and increased competition of the 1980s, a series of failed strategies to improve aging facilities and reposition itself in the local market led SJH to merge with several other local hospitals in order to maintain its viability. But severe financial problems persisted in the 1990s (see Case Illustrations 8.C and

8.D). In 1994, rumors circulated that its parent system would close SJH or convert its beds to non-hospital uses (Alvarado 1995b). Although this did not occur, SJH, like other Bay Area hospitals, has reduced its bed capacity in an attempt to forestall closing entirely.

1. We rely on Visions and Progress (1984), a commemorative history of SJH, for the events surrounding the hospital's early development.

Bed Capacity Distributions

Just as overall rates of change may be comprised of widely varying combinations of ecological and adaptive alterations, changes in the total or mean level of an attribute (such as bed capacity) may result from very different patterns of distribution within an organizational population. Organizational ecologists have identified three types of distributional transformations—stabilizing, directional, and disruptive (Amburgey, Dacin, and Kelly 1994).[5] *Stabilizing* transformations describe a reduction in the dispersion of some organizational characteristic because of strong pressures on both tails of the population distribution. For example, if there were an optimal size for hospitals, then overly small or large hospitals would be eliminated, reducing the size dispersion among the remaining members. *Directional* transformations refer to a shift in the mean of some organizational attribute, either up or down, because of pressures on one tail of the population. It could be the case that hospitals need to attain a certain size in order to be viable, but there are no survival problems associated with being large. *Disruptive* processes involve pressures on the members near the mean of a population such that a polarized or bimodal distribution results. For instance, midsized hospitals might find themselves under particular disadvantage in having to compete with both small and large providers.

In order to examine the patterns typifying the Bay area population of hospitals, we compared changes in their size distribution for four periods. Figure 4.2 shows sequential snapshots of aggregated hospital logged-size distributions during the 1950s, 1960s, 1970s, and 1980s. The pattern of change revealed is most consistent with the operation of *stabilizing* processes over this time period. From the successive changes in the shape of

5. Ecologists have referred to such patternings of change as stabilizing "selection," directional "selection," and disruptive "selection," emphasizing ecological influences (e.g., the termination or continuance of either smaller or larger organizations) on an attribute. Both adaptive and ecological processes can, however, contribute to such distributional shifts in the characteristics of organizational populations.

the distribution, it is clear that the upper and lower tails are disappearing, reflecting decreases in the numbers of smaller- and larger-sized hospitals. In the first decade, the standard deviation of the logged-size distribution (assessing the amount of dispersion in size among hospitals) is 1.04; by the 1980s, the measure has dropped to .86. This evolution is consistent with suggestions by health economists that economies of scale accruing to hospital bed capacities are curvilinear, increasing up to an optimal size range and decreasing thereafter (cf. Feldstein 1988). An institutional perspective might also predict such a stabilizing tendency but interpret it as a product of mimetic, normative, or regulatory pressures (DiMaggio and Powell 1983) to conform to an "acceptable" facility size.

At the same time, there is evidence of a *directional* process at work, since the average size of hospitals in the Bay area increased over the four decades. Again, this can be attributed to either technical or institutional demands. Hospitals may have become larger because the mean of the initial distribution was below that of optimal scale economies or because of institutional pressures toward hospital expansion. Although we do not further explore this particular issue,[6] in later chapters we examine material and institutional influences on the general dynamics of hospital and other provider populations.

Hospital Attributes

Size is, of course, only one of many important features of hospital organizations. Hannan and Freeman (1984) have proposed a hierarchy of organizational attributes—goals, formal structure, technology, and marketing strategy—that are rank-ordered in terms of structural inertia (i.e., resistance to change). Their argument amplifies Scott's (1981) identification of core versus peripheral features of organizational structure and his suggestion that the former are less easily modified than the latter. The pursuit of new and different goals is more likely to be accomplished by selection—when a new organization replaces an existing one—than by adaptive change. By contrast, altering service portfolios or developing connections to other organizations are types of adaptive modifications that are more readily implemented.

We will compare a number of hospital characteristics to evaluate this hierarchy of inertia in organizational attributes. For our analysis,

---

6. We also refrain from decomposing these distributional transformations into their ecological and adaptive components.

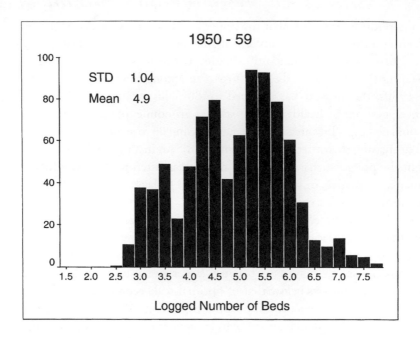

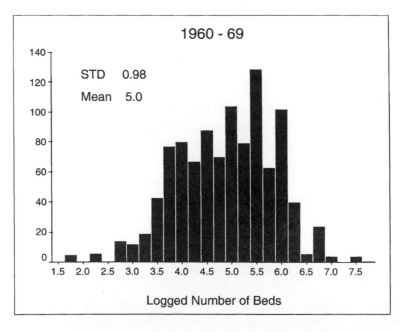

Figure 4.2   Distributional Change in Bed Capacity of Bay Area Hospitals, 1950–90

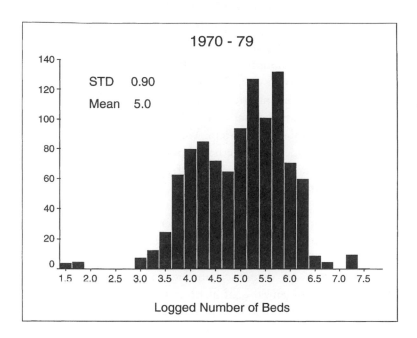

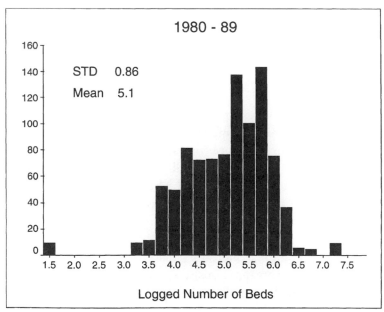

Figure 4.2 continued

NOTES: All distributions are aggregated by decade.

Log transformation was applied to hospital bed capacities in order to eliminate positive skew in distributions.

we index goals broadly through ownership type: for-profit hospitals are oriented toward different types of goals—in particular, maximizing returns to stockholders—than are nonprofit or public forms, which tend to give more weight to community service. Our indicators of formal structure are hospital size, since larger organizations tend to be more highly formalized and bureaucratized (Blau and Schoenherr 1971), and whether a given facility is a member of a multihospital system. We capture technology with the numbers of services provided and whether a hospital operates an outpatient service. Lacking the data to assess market strategy, we instead examine the extent to which hospitals have developed various linkages to their institutional environment, focusing, in particular, on the number of technical and managerial accreditations obtained.[7] Like market strategies, these linkages must be highly responsive to changing environmental conditions and are therefore likely to exhibit relatively low levels of structural inertia.

Despite the significant theoretical implications associated with the proposed hierarchy of organizational attributes, it has more often been assumed in empirical studies than investigated. The reason for this neglect may be methodological. While the argument of differential inertia in organizational features appears straightforward, the direct comparison of raw rates of change in components is not. First, one's conclusions may vary according to the choice of (often qualitatively different) indicators. For example, is formal structure to be measured by organizational size, centralization, or hierarchical complexity? Second, high net rates of change may be evident even in a truly inertial attribute, but can result from the replacement of older with newer organizations rather than by modifications in existing ones. These problems may be avoided when structural inertia is conceptualized in terms of the *relative* rates of adaptive and ecological change across indicators of the several attributes. With this approach, an attribute is considered to be more inertial when a higher proportion of change in that feature is due to ecological processes and a lower proportion is due to adaptation.[8]

Table 4.1 reports the overall proportion of population-level change in the means of our hospital indicators that is explained by adaptive transformations (of extant organizations) as opposed to ecological dynamics (entries and exits from the population). We find empirical support for

7. A more detailed analysis of the determinants and effects of hospital accreditations is reported in chapter 7 and Ruef and Scott (1998).

8. The proportion of change due to adaptation is simply 1 minus the proportion accounted for by ecological processes, and vice versa. This holds regardless of the net rates of change, which, as discussed above, are likely not to be comparable across indicators and attributes.

Table 4.1 Proportion of Change in Bay Area Hospital Attributes Accounted for by Adaptation, 1946–91.

	Overall (1946–91)	Professional Dominance (1946–65)	Federal Involvement (1966–82)	Market Orientation (1983–91)
Goal orientation				
Ownership type[a]	0.398	0.369	0.393	0.461
Formal structure				
Size (bed capacity)	0.515	0.465	0.508	0.640
System membership[b]	0.529	—	—	—
Technology				
Service portfolio	0.586	0.556	0.628	0.566
Outpatient services	0.823	0.796	0.889	0.759
Institutional linkages				
Accreditations	0.774	0.725	0.772	0.899
AHA membership	0.673	0.617	0.660	0.811

a. Proportion averaged over all ownership categories (for-profit, nonprofit, government).

b. Lack of system membership changes during the first period (1946–65), and to a lesser extent during the second, does not make temporal comparisons meaningful for this attribute.

the existence of an inertial hierarchy of organizational attributes. Only 40 percent of the change in ownership status is accounted for by adaptive dynamics while 82 percent of the change in outpatient services and 77 percent in accreditation portfolios is explained in this manner. While there is some variation across the specific indicators, the rank ordering of the four types of organizational attributes coincide with that predicted by the structural inertia theory of Hannan and Freeman (1984).

Appendix B includes a more formal statistical test of the hierarchical ranking using an analysis of variance procedure. To summarize the results, we find that population-level changes in institutional linkages (e.g., accreditations) and technology (service portfolios) are significantly less likely to be generated by ecological dynamics than are changes in formal structure and goals (ownership). The evidence supports the argument that organizational features exhibit an order that makes some "core" characteristics more resistant to change than others. These core characteristics are more likely to be modified by ecological than by adaptive processes.

Table 4.1 further disaggregates these overall proportions into the three major eras in U.S. healthcare introduced in chapter 1, in order to see whether these temporal variations are related to periods of either incremental or discontinuous change. As mentioned in the previous chapter, discussions of organizational evolution (McKelvey 1994; Meyer, Goes, and Brooks 1993) have called attention to important contextual differences between unpunctuated, placid environments and punctuated, turbulent environments. Under the former conditions, social ecologists have theorized that the development of organizational populations will be dictated overwhelmingly by ecological processes and that adaptive change will be minimized (Hannan and Freeman 1984, 1989). Under the latter conditions, however, the parameters controlling ecological dynamics tend to be in rapid flux, permitting a greater role for adaptation during periods of turbulence.[9]

This speculation generally dovetails with conceptions of organizational change offered in neoclassical economics, which point to the capacity of firms for rapid, adaptive responses under the turbulent conditions of market emergence. Neoinstitutional scholars are likely to be more skeptical, pointing out that the publicly observable "rituals" that organizations undertake in response to changing environments may mask underlying rigidity in core technical routines (Meyer and Rowan 1977).

Our typology of institutional eras (cf. chap. 1) allows us to deduce some preliminary hypotheses with respect to the preponderance of ecological and adaptive change. During the period of professional dominance (1945–65), the environment of healthcare organizations in the United States was fairly placid; during the era of federal involvement (1966–82), it evidenced a mixed state, as characterized by Alford's (1975) phrase "dynamics without change"; more recently with the advent of a managerial and market orientation (1983–present), the environment of the sector has been subject to "hyperturbulence" (Meyer, Goes, and Brooks 1993). Consequently, we would expect that the adaptive component of change should experience a continuing rise in preponderance in American healthcare over the past five decades.

The exploratory analysis in table 4.1 suggests that this trend generally holds for Bay area hospitals. Population-level changes in ownership, formal structure, and institutional linkages have increasingly come to be influenced by adaptive transformation. Prior to the passage of the Medicare and Medicaid acts in 1965, adaptive factors accounted for 37 percent of ownership changes in our hospital population, for 47 percent of size changes, and for 73 percent of changes in accreditations. During the more tumultuous period of market reforms (1983–91), these percentages have been 46, 64, and 90, respectively. At least in this regard, the dynamics of change in

---

9. Organization researchers have distinguished between two principal parameters in this regard: *carrying capacity*, which indicates the (nonzero) density at which no entries or exits are likely to occur in an organizational population, and the *intrinsic growth rate*, the rate with which the population density adjusts itself toward the carrying capacity (Hannan and Freeman 1989).

organizational populations appear to be influenced by the general tempo of environmental transformation. Organizations respond to conditions of turbulence by overcoming inertial constraints and undertaking a greater degree of adaptive changes in their goals, formal structure, and institutional linkages.

A noteworthy exception to this tendency has been in the core technology of these hospital facilities, where the impact of adaptive dynamics has hovered around the same range throughout the study period—for example, accounting for approximately 60 percent of all organizational change in service portfolios. This finding implies, as institutional scholars have argued, that features of organizations that are not easily buffered from external change (e.g., goals, size, linkages) will be responsive to environmental contingencies. The technical core, on the other hand, which is ostensibly sealed off from most such disturbances (see Thompson 1967; Scott 1998), will display a more constant level of structural inertia. Note also that the buffering mechanisms that hospitals deploy do not affect the absolute level of inertia exhibited by their core activities per se but rather the extent to which that level of inertia is affected by environmental demands.

CHANGES IN ORGANIZATIONAL OWNERSHIP

Ownership status frequently signifies important differences in organizational goals, in the expectations and evaluations placed on organizations, and in the identity and behavior displayed by these collective actors. The ownership of healthcare providers can be categorized in terms of three broad classifications:

- for-profit facilities, including corporate and other proprietary forms
- nonprofit facilities, including religious and other eleemosynary forms
- government-owned organizations, subsuming municipal, county, district, state, and federal facilities[10]

As described in our discussion of general trends in chapter 3, there has been a broad movement in recent decades toward reduced numbers of governmental as compared with private organizations, and, in some cases, toward reduced numbers of nonprofit forms compared with for-profit

---

10. As throughout the analyses in this study, we exclude federal hospitals—primarily military and Veterans Administration facilities—since they represent distinctive subpopulations.

organizations.[11] In the following analyses, we explore these trends of privatization and corporatization in the Bay area and examine the extent to which they have been the result of ecological or adaptive processes for three of our organizational populations: hospitals, home health agencies, and end-stage renal disease centers.

We examine transition rates between the various ownership forms for existing organizations (table 4.2) and also tabulate organizational entries into and exits from each population. We then juxtapose these data to allow comparison across provider populations (table 4.3).

Trend toward Proprietary Forms

We first examine evidence regarding the transition between nonprofit and for-profit organizational forms. We calculate basic transition rates, reflecting adaptive change in existing organizations, by dividing the number of changes in ownership status by all possible transitions that could have occurred. The formulation thus adjusts the actual number of transitions by a *risk set*—that is, the number of organizations that were "at risk" of experiencing a certain ownership transformation during a time interval.

From table 4.2, we note that ownership changes for provider facilities tend to be fairly rare in general: the overall rate for hospitals is 85 in 4165 or 0.020 transitions per annum, while the rate is quite similar for home health agencies, 35 in 1360 or 0.026 per annum, and even lower for end-stage renal disease centers at 0.016 per annum. Focusing first on the transitions between nonprofit and for-profit forms, a somewhat unexpected result is observed: hospitals undergoing a transition of ownership from for-profit to nonprofit forms (35 transitions) outnumbered those converting from nonprofit to for-profit status (21 transitions). These figures become even more dramatic when we adjust them for their respective risk sets. Considering hospitals that were for-profit at the beginning of any given year, for instance, we find that 746 facilities were included in the risk set of possible conversions to nonprofit status and that 35 facilities actually did convert. The effective transition rate for these facilities from for-profit to nonprofit status is therefore 35 in 746 or 0.047 per annum. By comparison, the transition rate of hospitals from nonprofit to for-profit status is only 0.009 (21 in 2451) per annum. Ownership transition rates for hospitals

---

11. It should be noted that these categories, although traditionally maintained as distinct, need not be exclusive. In recent years, some complex corporate systems of organizations have developed that contain both for-profit and nonprofit units (see Gray 1986: 42–43, also chap. 8).

Table 4.2 Adaptive Change in Ownership: Transition Rates of Bay Area Hospitals, HHAs, and ESRDCs

Population and Period	All Transitions	For-Profit → Nonprofit	Nonprofit → For-Profit	Private → Public	Public → Private
Hospitals (1946–92)	0.020	0.047	0.009	0.004	0.018
Hospitals (1979–92)	0.018	0.038	0.009	0.004	0.019
HHAs (1979–92)	0.026	0.021	0.022	0.003	0.024
ESRDCs (1979–92)	0.016	0.023	0.015	0.000	0.000

clearly favored movement in the direction of nonprofit status rather than toward for-profit status.

Within the HHA population, we find that rates of adaptive change between for-profit and nonprofit ownership tended to be approximately equal, at least during the 1979–92 period for which we have data. In order to provide more comparable statistics for hospitals, we computed their ownership transition rates for the equivalent time frame as well. The ratio of hospital conversions to nonprofit status as opposed to for-profit status between 1979 and 1992 (circa 4:1) is roughly equal to that evidenced from 1946 to 1992. Thus, while hospital conversions favored conversions to nonprofit over for-profit status, HHA conversions were balanced between the two forms.

Table 4.3 adds information on ecological sources of change for hospitals and HHAs and allows us to compare the effects of births and dissolutions on ownership with changes resulting from adaptive processes. First, we note that ecological processes had a limited effect on the distribution of ownership forms for the population of hospitals. Entries and exits tended to balance each other, and there was little net change during the period 1946–92. By contrast, ecological processes generated large effects on the ownership distribution of HHAs, with the net increase in for-profit forms outweighing the increase in nonprofit forms.

Comparable data are available for the period 1979–92 for ESRDCs but, as noted above, involve relatively few transition events of any type, and so must be interpreted with caution. Only 8 transitions in ownership occurred for this population in the Bay area, yielding a rate of 0.016 for ESRDCs. Of these, 5 involved shifts from for-profit to nonprofit status (conversion rate of 0.023) and 3 involved transitions from nonprofit to for-profit status (conversion rate of 0.015). Thus, while the number of events is quite small, adaptive processes again favored conversion to nonprofit status. But ecological dynamics strongly favored for-profit forms as they

Table 4.3 Adaptive and Ecological Components of Change in Ownership: Bay Area Hospitals, HHAs, and ESRDCs

	Private		Public
	For Profit	**Nonprofit**	**Government**
Hospitals, 1946–92			
Organizational entries	22	33	8
Organizational exits	25	34	8
Net ecological change	**−3**	**−1**	**0**
Net adaptive change	**−12**	**+17**	**−5**
Home health agencies, 1979–92			
Organizational entries	126	44	8
Organizational exits	59	25	5
Net ecological change	**+67**	**+19**	**+3**
Net adaptive change	**+5**	**−7**	**+2**
End-Stage Renal Disease Centers, 1979–92			
Organizational entries	17	11	0
Organizational exits	5	6	1
Net ecological change	**+12**	**+5**	**−1**
Net adaptive change	**−2**	**+2**	**0**

Notes: Net ecological change = organizational entries − organizational exits.

Net adaptive change derived from separate analyses of ownership conversions.

had for HHAs. Of the 28 new ESRDCs created during this period, 17 (61 percent) were for-profit forms; after exits were taken into account, the net ecological effects favored for-profits by a ratio of over 2:1 (see table 4.3).

Data from these three populations call attention to the complexities involved in generalizing about the widely discussed "trend toward for-profit" forms among healthcare organizations in recent decades. In all three populations, transformations involving a change in ownership status were rare. Of existing organizations undergoing ownership changes, however, substantially more were likely to convert from for-profit to nonprofit status rather than from nonprofit to for-profit for two of the populations: hospitals and ESRDCs. In our data, adaptive processes—the transformation of existing organizations—do not account for the increasingly for-profit orientation of the healthcare sector. That trend is due primarily to the operation of ecological processes.

Drawing these observations together, what can we conclude about population trends in the Bay area regarding the development of proprietary forms of ownership? First, we do observe increasing numbers of such forms in our populations of healthcare organizations, but only in the newer forms, not in the most traditional population.[12] Hospitals were much less likely to assume for-profit forms than HHAs or ESRDCs. We believe that this reflects the fact that older organizations and forms of organizations exhibit substantial inertia: existing legitimated patterns of doing business that have long been utilized are not quickly or easily discarded. Novel archetypes and logics of organizing are more likely to be appropriated by new kinds of organizations.

Second, among two of our three populations—hospitals and ESRDCs—we observed that, while ownership transitions were rare, adaptive processes favored more traditional nonprofit over for-profit forms. For the third population, HHAs, adaptive processes were as likely to favor for-profit as nonprofit forms. Thus, the trend toward increasing numbers of for-profit organizations is largely due to the creation of new organizations of this type, not to the conversion of existing organizations. This finding reflects the power of inertial forces: it is difficult to change existing structures.

It has been observed that much of the advantage of for-profit status for organizations in the healthcare sector is in providing access to capital markets of a type not available to nonprofit forms (see Gray 1986). Generally speaking, organizations that are just being founded have greater need for capital than do organizations already in operation. We also note that public policies changed during the period under review so that for-profit entrepreneurs were able, for the first time, to tap governmental funds supporting new start-up HHAs and ESRDCs. Thus, for-profits enjoyed access to both private as well as public sources of funding, and this may account for their high prevalence among recent organizational foundings in nontraditional forms.

More generally, how, if at all, does the ownership status of an organization affect its behavior, in particular, its delivery of healthcare services? While we do not have empirical data from our project that directly shed light on this subject, it is too important to ignore. Results from previous studies, unfortunately, are not very informative. Literature surveys by DiMaggio and Anheier (1990) and by Sloan (1988) conclude either that there are few or no differences or that the studies are inconclusive. This determination seems inexplicable, since as Schlesinger (1998) points out, there are at least

12. This observation holds as well for the United States in general: for-profit hospitals have not increased proportionally, representing 11 percent of American hospitals in both 1980 and 1994 (AHA 1994; see also chap. 3).

three important ways in which ownership status could affect organizational behavior: (1) by influencing the incentives for administrators and employees; (2) by affecting the expectations and perceptions of those who deal with the organization, including the general public; and (3) by affecting the way in which the organization is treated by regulatory agencies. All of these seem plausible and applicable to healthcare organizations.

Schlesinger (1998) argues that previous examinations of this question are critically flawed because investigators have studied only the direct effects of ownership and have neglected its interactive influence: the ways in which ownership status changes the effects associated with other organizational or environmental characteristics. In his own research on psychiatric hospitals, for example, Schlesinger found that hospitals subjected to higher levels of competitive pressure showed smaller differences between nonprofit and for-profit hospitals in service behaviors (for example, providing treatments for government-sponsored patients or additional chronic care), whereas service differences between nonprofit and for-profit hospitals were larger when these facilities were subjected to greater pressures from community groups, medical professionals, and state regulators. In short, the effect of ownership status on behavior must take into account the wider environmental context in which an organization operates.

Our discussion of the rareness with which existing organizations alter their ownership forms implies that this type of transition event would occur only under extreme circumstances and would present significant challenges to organizations. Two specific instances of ownership change in Bay area hospitals examined in Case Illustration 4.B demonstrate both the profound forces and practical concerns motivating such transitions, as well as their implications for the organizations involved.

Case Illustration 4.B   Causes and Consequences of Ownership Change: San Jose Hospital and Stanford Medical Center

In the 1990s, two of our organizational cases experienced major transformations in ownership status. The nonprofit San Jose Hospital (SJH) was sold along with its parent organization to a for-profit system, and the nonprofit Stanford Medical Center merged with the public University of California, San Francisco Medical Center (UCSF) into a new private, nonprofit entity. Although the first reflects the trend among healthcare systems toward proprietary organizational forms and the second the trend toward privatization, both events represent a response to the contingencies of a market-oriented era. Both also evoked similar types of controversy, indicating the contentiousness of many changes engendered in the current period in the health-care field.

The Sale of San Jose Hospital to Columbia/HCA

Although founded as a for-profit corporation, SJH had converted shortly thereafter to nonprofit status in 1937, motivated by benefits of tax exemption and enhanced public acceptance and fundraising potential within the local community (Visions 1984). Nearly sixty years later, SJH reverted back to for-profit ownership when its parent healthcare system, Good Samaritan, was purchased by Columbia/HCA, the nation's largest commercial healthcare system.

Case Illustration 4.A briefly described the decline of SJH that motivated its de-cision to join in the formation of the local, nonprofit Health Dimensions system, later renamed Good Samaritan. That system performed well for several years but struggled against intensified competition for patients in the 1990s. The loss of a 35-year-old exclusive contractual relation with the San Jose Medical Group (Ansley 1991), a series of restructuring and downsizing measures (Lapin 1991), and financial problems reflected in a $43 million budgetary shortfall in 1994 (Alvarado 1995a; Puzzanghera 1997) eventually inspired a strategy to be rescued by a larger, more financially stable healthcare system.

Although maintaining a nonprofit status was preferred, a more crucial criterion for selecting a buyer was the ability to cover Good Samaritan's debt and inject funds into the failing system. Because of its financial resources, Columbia/HCA emerged as the front runner and acquired Good Samaritan for $165 million in January 1996 (Alvarado 1995b). The resulting conversion of SJH and the Good Samaritan system from nonprofit to for-profit ownership raised a host of concerns. Columbia/HCA had a reputation for hard-nosed deal making, hospital closure, charity case dumping, and national executives out of touch with local community needs, which physicians and residents worried would lead to a reduction in the quality of care at the hospitals (Shiller 1995; Puzzanghera 1997b). California watchdog organizations, such as Consumers' Union, argued that Good Samaritan's immediate financial crisis was unduly prompting the local system to settle for "fire-sale" prices, which would provide only a modest trust fund endowment (required by California law when a nonprofit entity is privatized) for indigent care (Alvarado 1995c, 1995d, 1996).

Several of these fears were realized. In the aftermath of the sale, 342 administrative and corporate employees and 274 hospital employees within the system lost their jobs. Although Columbia/HCA's widely publicized Medicare fraud scandals in 1997 did not directly involve the Good Samaritan hospitals, articles in local newspapers repeatedly linked the cutbacks in staffing to declining quality of care (Puzzanghera 1997a). Nonetheless, the persistent financial woes brought about by both particular demographic shifts in the local area and general movements toward lower hospi-tal utilization and higher competition (see Case Illustrations 4.A and 8.C) impelled SJH and Good Samaritan into the expansive arms and deep pockets of a for-profit "white knight."

The Merger of the Stanford and UCSF Medical Centers

The merger of the Bay Area's two major, and nationally prestigious, academic medical centers in 1997 provides a stunning example of profound and previously unimaginable change. It reflects both the entrance of a facility into a multihospital system (for the Stanford Medical Center) as well as a large-scale and highly contentious transition toward private ownership (for UCSF). This event, which involved several years of lively and frequently acrimonious debate, arose in the context of diminished federal funding for academic medical centers, heightened competition with community hospitals, and decreased numbers of referrals from community physicians (Puzzanghera 1995a). In this constrained environment, the Stanford Medical Center began a cost-cutting program in 1989 that eliminated a thousand jobs over a six-year period (Puzzanghera 1995b). In 1994, Stanford formed Stanford Health Services (SHS) to integrate its hospital and clinical operations. Between 1991 and 1996, SHS eliminated $100 million from its operating budget (Frabotta 1996). During the same period, UCSF Medical Center lost $42 million (Beyers 1997).

Faced with these dire financial circumstances, and even worse prospects, Stanford and UCSF began discussing the possibility of consolidating their medical centers in 1995. Proponents argued that the combination of facilities would alleviate the pressing financial problems, as well as offer economies of scale, leverage in negotiating with managed care companies, and a broader base of patients requiring specialized services (Frabotta 1996; Cisneros 1997; Traugott 1996). Peter Van Etten, CEO of Stanford Medical Center and designated CEO of the merged system, also claimed that it would create a "distinct brand identity" for academic medicine in the Bay Area (Frabotta 1996). UCSF Chancellor Haile Debas called the merger "a vision that would revolutionize health care and create the nation's foremost academic health care center" (Koury 1997a).

Many others, including individual citizens, advocates, organizations, and associations, opposed the plan. Labor union members (mostly employed at UCSF) feared both the possibility that quality of care would diminish in an enterprise of vastly increased scale and the likelihood of layoffs. Unions rallied at several meetings of University of California regents, who, they alleged, were subordinating academic medicine to "purely commercial interests" and "defrauding the taxpaying citizen" (Levander 1996). Other critics, such as UCSF faculty (Carter 1996), voiced concerns that the merger would alter the mission of academic medicine, resulting in substandard training for new physicians and other healthcare professionals and a deemphasis on research and indigent care.

But the strongest controversy involved the legality and efficacy of privatizing the public UCSF facility, in effect transferring $480 million in public assets to a private, nonprofit entity. The UC regents and state legislators heatedly debated privatization. Senator John Burton (D-San Francisco), chair of the Senate Judiciary Committee, referred to the merger as "a giveaway of public property" and led other legislators in protest (Martin, Debas, and Schroffel 1997). In May 1997, Burton and allies passed bills in the California Assembly and Senate to create public oversight of the new corporation, enforce meeting rules, and apply the state Open Records Act for Public

Institutions to University of California Stanford Health Care (Levander 1997), which were signed by Governor Pete Wilson in October 1997 (*San Jose Mercury News* October 15, 1997). Several UC regents also opposed the merger, including Lt. Governor Gray Davis, who termed it a "leap of faith" (Koury 1997b).

Despite these vocal public outcries and reviews by a gauntlet of regulators, including the California Attorney General, the Federal Trade Commission, and the U.S. Department of Justice, the merger was eventually approved by the UC regents and Stanford University trustees in September 1997. The newly created $879 million non-profit corporation is expected to serve one million patients a year (Koury 1997a). The arrangement required compromises between public and private modes of governance and operation, such as modified compliance with open meeting and public record laws and the leasing of former UCSF employees to allow retention and accrual of public-system retirement benefits.

For a time, the merger seemed to be proceeding smoothly; administrative costs had been cut 38 percent and patient stays were up 6 percent. But sixteen months into the merger, UCSF Stanford was confronting a first-quarter operating loss of $11 million and a projected deficit of $66 million by the end of 1999 (Chui 1999). Some regents have begun to call for a breakup, noting that state funds are at risk (Krieger 1999). The administration, however, has insisted that the financial problems can be averted by stringent cost-cutting measures, and it has instituted programs to eliminate one out of six jobs—about 2000 positions—in the network of hospitals and clinics. In addition, difficult and contentious decisions remain as the two hospital systems determine how duplicated services are to be combined.

Clearly, difficult challenges continue to confront university-based and teaching hospitals, even those that are engaged in draconian cost-cutting programs. Faced with the expansion of managed care, reduced patient census, and federal cutbacks in Medicare spending, the ability of teaching hospitals to fulfil their special missions—"to handle the sickest patients, to act as incubators for new cures, to treat poor people and to training budding doctors"—is being threatened (Goldberg 1999).

Summary

Although the transformations of San Jose Hospital to for-profit status and of Stanford and UCSF Medical Centers into a private, nonprofit entity comprise ownership changes of varying scales and natures, they reveal common underlying concerns: the conversion of public resources, a potential neglect of medical training and indigent care, and a general fear of the incursion and power of corporations. In the current struggles and transformations of healthcare systems, critics correctly perceive a fundamental movement away from a community-oriented, charitable system toward a market-oriented, increasingly commercial model of healthcare. The transitions described in these cases also demonstrate the strength of current trends in loosening, if not wholly overcoming, the perennial resistance and inertia that impede any extensive adaptive or ecological changes in such large, complex, visible, and embedded organizations.

Trend toward Privatization

Recall that another major trend in healthcare described in chapter 3 was that toward increased privatization of healthcare organizations. By *privatization* we mean the tendency to rely less on governmental organizations and to utilize private forms, whether nonprofit or for-profit. This type of transition is illustrated in the conversion of the University of California–San Francisco Medical Center (UCSF) from a publicly owned facility to a private, nonprofit corporation (see Case Illustration 4.B).

Considering hospitals first, we note from table 4.2 that while all types of ownership transitions were rare, governmental hospitals were much more likely to convert into private forms than the reverse: conversion of nonfederal public hospitals to private—both for-profit and nonprofit—facilities has proceeded at about four times the rate of private to public conversions (rates of 0.018 and 0.004, respectively). Examining ecological processes, we see that public hospitals held their own during the period of our study, accounting for 13 percent of the new entries and for 12 percent of the exits (see table 4.3). Thus, for hospitals, there is evidence of a trend toward privatization among nonfederal hospitals from 1946 to 1992, and it was produced primarily by adaptive processes involving the conversion of public into private hospitals.

Like hospitals, HHAs revealed low transition rates, but those that underwent any type of ownership change were more than seven times more likely to convert from public to private forms than the reverse. And, in the case of this population, ecological processes were pressing hard in the same direction: 97 percent of the net ecological change occurring between 1979 and 1992 involved the addition of private forms.

As for the renal disease centers, no ownership transitions by adaptation were observed in the ESRDC population involving governmental forms (see table 4.3). And no additions to this population occurred during the study period involving governmental units: all the additions to this rapidly growing population involved private forms. One dissolution of a public unit was recorded. As a consequence of these processes, the proportion of governmental units within this population declined from 27 percent in 1980 to just over 10 percent in 1991.

Thus, more so than the trend toward proprietary forms in the Bay area, the trends toward privatization involved a combination of both adaptive and ecological processes. The hospital population moved in the direction of increased privatization (see fig. 3.5) as a result of the conversion of existing governmental units to private auspices. The HHA population moved in the same direction, but its transformation was fueled by a combination of both adaptive and ecological processes. And the ESRDC population also moved toward increased privatization, but the processes at work were exclusively ecological. Of most importance, all three populations of healthcare organizations exhibited a lower proportion of public compared with private facilities at the end of the study period than at the beginning.

Why did adaptation play a greater role in the conversion of ownership from public to private forms in contrast to the conversion of nonprofit to for-profit forms? It seems likely that some government organizations (e.g., state hospitals) are less deeply embedded in local community structures than are private, especially nonprofit, forms; in addition, the decision processes that determine their fate tend to be more centralized and, often, are physically separated from the operating unit. In a time when the privatization currents run strong and when public funding for community services is being reduced, we would expect few new governmental units to be created and some existing units to be sold off. Still other governmental facilities are contracted out to private companies, but these changes are not captured by our data.

CHANGES IN ORGANIZATIONAL SUBTYPES

While ownership changes constitute one form of fundamental reorganization in the healthcare sector, other significant types of transformation involve shifts in the breadth of medical service provision (e.g., niche generalism vs. specialism) or in the mode of physician organization. We briefly consider evidence regarding the former type of change for hospitals and the latter type of change for health maintenance organizations.

Generalist versus Specialist Hospitals

Transformations of generalist into specialist hospitals (and vice versa) are even more rare than ownership changes. Only 18 of these transformations took place among all Bay area hospitals during the full period of our study, translating into an overall transition rate of 0.004. Disaggregating this by the direction of change, we find that the number of facilities changing from generalist to specialist forms was equal to that changing from specialist to generalist forms—nine in each direction. Because of the varying risk sets in the two cases, however, the effective rate of specialist to generalist transformation (0.021) was 10 times higher than that of generalist to specialist (0.002) form. Moreover, ecological dynamics have also favored generalists heavily, with 60 of the nonfederal hospital entries during the five decades after World War II being generalist compared with only 3 specialist entries. These dynamics in combination explain the marked decline of specialist hospitals during the period of our study, as described in chapter 3.

We therefore reiterate that the general trend toward greater specialization of organizational forms in the healthcare sector does not involve an increase of specialist versus general hospitals. Rather, the proportion of generalist hospitals has substantially increased during the last half century. The widely observed trend toward specialization involves the creation and rapid proliferation of new types of specialist organizations, competing with, but differing from hospitals.

Forms of Physician Organization among HMOs

Our previous discussion of health maintenance organizations (chaps. 2 and 3) noted that there are several subtypes of this organizational form that exhibit a good deal of boundary blurring among them. Our data on HMOs in the Bay area bear out these observations (Kaiser Permanente is excluded from this analysis).

HMOs with enrollees in the Bay area have experienced high rates of adaptive change among different model types (group, staff, IPA, network, and mixed forms). Overall, 29 conversions between various models have occurred between 1976 and 1992, representing an average transition rate of 0.048, or one conversion per organization every 20.7 years. Table 4.4 displays the breakdown of origin and destination model types. Given the preponderance of destinations that are of mixed form (28 percent) and the relatively low number of initial models in this class, it appears that hybridization constitutes the strongest adaptive tendency among these organizations. All other subtypes exhibit relative decline with the exception of the staff model, which grew modestly.

Ecological processes favored loosely coupled HMO forms, in particular, IPA and network forms. During the period between 1976 and 1992, IPA forms experienced a net increase of 10 (19 entries and 9 exits) and networks a net increase of 5 (7 entries and 2 exits). Group models exhibited a net increase of 4 (8 entries and 4 exits), staff models no net change (2 entries and 2 exits) and mixed forms a small net decrease (0 entries and 2 exits).

How are we to characterize this process as a motor of change? Haveman and Rao (1998) view the creation of hybrid organizations as involving the blending of two or more elements from (formerly) distinct forms of

Table 4.4 Adaptive Change in Organizational Subtypes: Initial and Adopted Models of HMO Form Conversions, 1976–92

Type	Initial Model		Adopted Model	
	Number	Percent	Number	Percent
Group	8	28%	5	17%
Staff	0	0%	2	7%
IPA	9	31%	7	24%
Network	11	38%	7	24%
Mixed/other	1	3%	8	28%
TOTAL	29 (100%)			

organizations. When this process is widespread, it promotes incremental, as opposed to radical or discontinuous, evolution of institutions and organizations. Hybrids can be formed as an existing organization elects to borrow and attach a component from a different form or they can be formed by entrepreneurs who construct new organizational forms by combining elements from two or more existing forms, through a process known as "bricolage"—the recombination of existing stock repertories of structure (Douglas 1986).

In the case of HMO structures, hybridization involves not only the so-called mixed/other forms but also, the network and IPA versions. All of these forms combine varying elements into new combinations. For example, the IPA combines the managed care plan with either individual or group practice arrangements. Since these forms involve combinations of existing elements, they are not only easier for entrepreneurs to construct but also more familiar and, hence, more acceptable to their participants. IPAs allow physicians to remain in private practice while cooperating in an organization that has the scale and power to negotiate more favorable contracts (Robinson 1998). Throughout the entire period of our study, the less restrictive HMO models—IPA, mixed, networks—grew more rapidly than the more tightly organized forms—group and staff models. This generalization also applied to HMO forms nationwide (Christianson et al. 1991).

CONCLUSION

We have reviewed a variety of types of data to examine the ways in which two modes of change have affected several populations of healthcare delivery organizations in the Bay area. Adaptive processes entail changes in the structural features of existing organizations; ecological processes entail the differential rates at which organizations are formed or dissolved. Our data and analyses have revealed the complexity entailed in the operation of these two change processes. They have been observed to vary over time in their relative importance for a given type of organization and to vary in the contributions they make to changes occurring across diverse populations of providers. They also have been shown to work sometimes at cross-purposes, adaptive processes inducing change in one direction, ecological processes, in the opposite. Finally, they appear to produce various effects on different organizational attributes, such as goals, formal structure, and institutional linkages.

These patterns result from the features of organizations and organizational populations, the characteristics of their environments, and the interaction across these levels. With respect to organization and population characteristics, we have observed less fundamental change among hospitals, an older and more traditional model of healthcare delivery, than among the newer, more specialized forms such as HHAs and ESRDCs. These findings suggest the possibility that inertial processes operate not only at the level of the individual organization—older organizations being more resistant to change—but also at the level of the population or organizational form— more highly institutionalized forms also being more resistant to change.

Environmental elements affecting such changes include public policies providing support for an extant organizational form (e.g., Hill-Burton funds for hospitals) or for the creation of new forms (e.g., early federal HMO legislation), which, as we describe and examine in depth in later chapters, are rooted in broader fieldwide transformations of governance structures and institutional logics. In this chapter, the interaction of organizational and environmental factors was illustrated by our observation that inertial forms such as hospitals are more likely to undergo adaptive change in more unsettled and turbulent environments.

Turning to a few of our specific results, we observe that hospitals have gradually increased bed capacity during the period of study while simultaneously reducing their occupancy rates (see fig. 3.4). These trends more clearly represent incremental than revolutionary change and result from both adaptive and ecological processes. Ownership changes among hospitals exhibited the expected inclination toward privatization (declining public ownership of hospitals) but no increase in commercial forms. Indeed, the observed pattern of adaptive change favored nonprofit over for-profit forms. Again, the few hospitals undergoing ownership change were more likely to revert to the conventional nonprofit form rather than to adopt the newer, for-profit model.

By contrast, substantial change was exhibited by the newer and more specialized organizational populations, in particular, home health agencies and renal disease centers. Both populations experienced dramatic growth during the period of study and exhibited pronounced trends in the direction of privatization and for-profit forms. In both cases, these tendencies were largely fueled by ecological processes: a surplus of entries of new organizations into the population. Among health maintenance organizations, adaptive and ecological processes contributed toward the growing predominance of the more loosely coupled network and IPA forms over the earlier staff and group models.

Evidence of profound change at the population level is more readily apparent among the newer than the older organizational forms. And these more dramatic changes appear to be differentially borne by ecological than by adaptive change patterns. Change among the newer populations is driven more by differential birth and death processes than by the transformation of existing organizations. On the other hand, there is also evidence of incremental change at work among these forms, as witnessed by the hybridization processes that are fueling the growth of a wide and confusing variety of HMO subtype organizations. Change occurs in manifold ways and encompasses multiple mechanisms. In order to understand the transformations experienced by organizations and organizational populations, it is important to study the processes, as well as the overall level or direction, of change.

Five

RESOURCE ENVIRONMENTS AND ORGANIZATIONAL DYNAMICS

SINCE THE EMERGENCE OF OPEN systems theory in the early 1960s, no serious study of organizations can afford to neglect the wider context within which organizations live and operate. Although early studies of organizations' environments were fairly simplistic, theoretical conceptions of environmental factors and forces have become increasingly elaborated.

In our attempts to understand how and why healthcare delivery systems are changing in the Bay Area, we attend closely to their surrounding environments. As briefly noted in chapter 1, we distinguish broadly between two facets of environments: material-resource and institutional. In this chapter, we focus on the material-resource environment, but also examine how it is affected by institutional forces.

PERSPECTIVES ON MATERIAL-RESOURCE ENVIRONMENTS

The *material-resource environment* includes the tangible resources that organizations—viewed as technical, production systems—use to transform inputs into outputs. It includes factors affecting demand for products or services, the supply of products or services, technologies utilized in transforming inputs into outputs, and the structure of the industry.

In the healthcare field, the principal factors shaping demand for medical services are the sociodemographic characteristics of the human population in the area served, the nature and extent of funding for medical services, and local economic conditions. Factors affecting supply include the number of physicians and other healthcare professionals and public and private funding for medical services. Both demand and supply are affected by the state of technology, including the specialized knowledge, tools, and equipment used to produce medicines and provide therapeutic treatments, as well as the information processing technologies that facilitate diagnosis and support complex financing and billing arrangements. Industry structure involves the extent of concentration and degree of coordination among both buyers and sellers of healthcare.[1]

To examine the material-resource environment of Bay Area healthcare organizations, we draw from several theoretical perspectives. In chapter 4, we relied primarily on two theoretical frameworks—organizational ecology and strategic management—to examine how ecological and adaptive processes interact to produce the observed dynamics of population change. Here we introduce two additional perspectives, health economics and industrial organization economics, to help us account for some additional components of change. We also employ selected arguments from institutional theory. These perspectives do not displace our interest in ecological processes shaping organizational populations, but add additional factors affecting the life chances of healthcare organizations.

Health Economics

Historically, economists did not rush to apply their developing theories and models to the medical care arena. They recognized that market transactions in this sector did not conform closely to conventional economic assumptions and that several characteristics, somewhat peculiar to the healthcare sector, impede the efficiency of market operations. The fact that quality of care is difficult to assess, particularly by the consumer, has a profound effect on market transactions. As Arrow (1963: 951) points out: "Uncertainty as to the quality of the product is perhaps more intense here [in healthcare] than in any other important commodity." Professional providers and analysts continue to disagree about what criteria and indicators of quality are appropriate to employ (Donabedian 1980–85; Flood, Shortell, and Scott 1997). Moreover, much of the demand for care is not directly determined by patients' needs or choices. Rather, physicians act as intermediate agents, exerting substantial influence on medical care services, the choice of institutional setting for the receipt of care, and the amount of care consumed affecting, in particular, the level of physician-initiated visits (Rossiter and Wilensky 1983).

While price is always a central factor considered by economists in evaluating demand, it plays a reduced role in healthcare decisions for two

---

1. Industry structure is also affected by governance arrangements, including regulatory policies. These factors are examined as part of the institutional environment in chapter 6.

reasons. First, demand for most health services is relatively inelastic. That is, it is not particularly sensitive to price differences. Second, and related to this lack of responsiveness, an increasing proportion of care throughout the period after World War II has been covered by "third-party" payors: commercial insurers, employers, and governmental programs. As a result, consumers often do not pay directly for the medical care they consume. And, for their part, only in the most recent decades have these institutional payors begun to take steps to curtail medical care costs by negotiating with providers over the price of services covered.

With respect to the supply side of medical care services, the number of physicians and other specialized medical personnel are restricted by many conditions, including licensure requirements, the high cost and lengthy duration of medical education, and, for many years, the restrictive admissions policies of medical schools (Arrow 1963). Physician density is the factor that has been most widely considered in studies of utilization. Under fee-for-service and/or indemnity arrangements, physician providers have been guided by incentives that encourage them to dispense more rather than fewer services. Not only do they stand to benefit financially by providing more—and more expensive—services, but such actions were believed to be associated with quality care (Fuchs 1968). Thus, up to the advent of managed care arrangements, higher concentrations of physicians have been found to be associated with higher levels of utilization (Hulka and Wheat 1985). Similarly, until the development of prospective payment mechanisms for hospitals and other care facilities, which establish a preset reimbursement determined by patient diagnosis regardless of the amount of service delivered (see chap. 6), the supply of additional beds was found to be related to increasing demand for those beds (Roemer 1961).

Despite the many ways healthcare deviates from conventional economic assumptions, the discipline of health economics began to grow in the 1960s (e.g., Department of Economics 1964; Klarman 1965; Feldstein 1966), and by the 1980s, there existed a substantial body of both theoretical and empirical work (Joskow 1981; Sloan and Steinwald 1980). Economists focused primary attention on factors affecting costs which, from the 1950s forward began to escalate faster than the general rate of inflation. They also examined issues of organizational founding in their exploration of various types of barriers to entry—a body of work we draw on in this and subsequent chapters. Economists often discuss barriers to entry by asking whether some types of organizations operate as "natural monopolies"— monopolies resulting from the inherent characteristics of the enterprise rather than from collusion or regulative controls (Pauly 1974). Economies of scale and geographic localization are particularly prominent in creating natural monopolies.

If the minimum organizational size required to achieve efficient production costs is excessively high, then the number of competitors in a population will diminish, and oligopolistic or monopolistic markets may result. Empirical evidence on such *economies of scale* in the hospital population has proven difficult to evaluate because of the multiproduct nature of these organizations (often involving differences in patient mix and types of services provided). A general conclusion drawn from empirical studies suggests that costs tend to be minimized for hospitals having between 200 and 300 beds (Starkweather 1981; Feldstein 1988), but also that the cost curve is shallow—that is, the diseconomies experienced by smaller or larger hospitals are not substantial. Recall that in chapter 4, we presented evidence to suggest that hospitals in the Bay Area were, over time, becoming more homogeneous in size and tending to converge around a mean of 240 beds.

A second, probably more significant factor in the creation of natural monopolies, is the *localization* of services. Numerous empirical studies have indicated the importance of spatial considerations in defining hospital markets (Folland 1983; Garnick et al. 1987; Luft et al. 1990; Duffy 1992). When emergency care is required, distance to medical facilities is obviously important, but even the choice of less urgent care is subject to powerful constraints on patient travel time, transit costs, and access to transportation (Garnick et al. 1987; Long and Feldstein 1967). In rural areas, such factors clearly lead to cases where hospitals do enjoy a "natural" monopoly. In more urban regions, the service areas of hospitals are more likely to overlap, providing some choice. However, the spatial density of hospitals remains a significant factor in accounting for the extent to which hospitals operate under competitive pressures.

The studies of health economists offer valuable lessons, but leave important areas unexplored. The detailed ways in which healthcare is not a conventional industry remind us of the many institutional factors at work in the field, and the emphasis on the development of natural monopolies reinforces our previous findings and indicates directions for analysis. However, little attention has been paid to the recent, rapid development of diverse organizational providers associated with different mixes of services, types of professionals, and modes of management. We wonder if and how variables that predict utilization of medical care services vary depending on the setting or type of organization providing the care. Our comparative analyses of hospital, home health agencies (HHAs), and end-stage renal disease centers (ESRDCs), reported later in this chapter, are aimed at exploring this question.

Industrial Organization Economics

Since the medical arena does not match the ideal-type of a competitive marketplace, industrial organization economics, which focuses on the relationship between economic performance and market structure, offers a useful complementary perspective. The industrial organization approach recognizes the need to go beyond models that simply deal with aggregate supply and demand considerations to examine the structure of the industry—that is, to take into account the numbers and types of buyers and sellers and the ways in which they are related to one another. Early research in this area involved detailed case studies of particular industries. This work was superseded in the 1950s by comparative studies pioneered by Bain (1951, 1956), who used cross-sectional data from a number of industries. As it developed, this approach gave rise to the "structure-conduct-performance" paradigm, which held sway well into the 1980s.

"Structure" refers to the relatively stable industry configurations comprised of degree of buyer and seller concentration and extent of product differentiation. Such formations are presumed to result primarily from the nature of the products or services being produced and the state of available technologies. Other elements of market structure are also recognized, such as conditions of entry into the market, thought to be shaped by factors such as governmental policies, distribution and scarcity of resources, or accidents of history. "Conduct" pertains to the "behavioral rules" followed by participants in the field, in particular, their business strategies. "Performance" serves as the dependent variable, assessed by comparing outcomes such as productivity or profitability with an ideal model or to other selected industries (Schmalensee 1989).

This model was refined and amplified by Porter (1980), who defined structure as those key features of an industry that determine the nature and type of competitive forces present. Porter emphasized the importance of five features: rivalry among current competitors, bargaining power of buyers, threat of entry, bargaining power of suppliers, and the threat of substitution of other goods or services. For the concept of conduct, Porter substituted a focus on organizational strategy, identifying three generic strategies that an organization might pursue to achieve competitive advantage: overall cost leadership, based on cost minimization and exploiting the experience curve; differentiation, based on creating a product or service widely viewed as unique; and focus, targeting a specialized product group or market segment. LaMont and colleagues (LaMont, Marlin, and Hoffman 1993) have examined the extent to which hospitals have improved their performance based on the use of these strategies. And Luke and Begun (1994) investigate how the strategic conduct of provider organizations varies with the structure of healthcare markets, including degree of buyer and seller concentration, degree of product differentiation, and conditions of entry into the market.

More so than earlier analysts, Porter emphasized the value of *intra*industry analysis—the identification of subsets of organizations within the industry following the same or similar strategies. He argued that to the extent that such differentiation occurs within an industry, competition occurs within rather than between these groups. Two important insights are associated with Porter's approach: (1) within a given industry, "there are many different kinds of potentially profitable strategies"; and (2) "formulating competitive strategy in an industry can be viewed as the choice of which strategic group to compete in" (Porter 1980: 144, 149). In our own approach, we pursue these insights by examining the ways in which different kinds of organizations (e.g., organizational populations), associated with different types of strategies (e.g., specialist vs. generalist), compete in healthcare markets.

The rigorously comparative approach remained dominant until the mid-1980s, when cross-sectional studies began to be challenged by researchers advocating the advantages of using time series or longitudinal data from one or a few related industries. This more recent work criticized the cross-sectional, comparative tradition on several counts, including the difficulty of inferring price-cost margins from accounting data and the reliance on a small number of measures to assess industry structure. In particular, these analysts insisted that all industries are characterized by important idiosyncrasies, and that such "institutional detail" has important effects on firms' conduct that should be taken into account in attempting to measure both structure and performance (see Bresnahan 1989). This shift to focus more closely on the details of particular industries has been accompanied by the increasing use of game theory methodologies to model the strategic behavior of interacting firms under given sets of market conditions (see, e.g., Sutton 1991; McMillan 1992). The theoretical import of these new methodologies is to emphasize that the structure of a given industry is not necessarily determined by factors independent of the conduct and behavior of industry members. Rather, as Norman and La Manna (1992: 2) comment:

Developments in the new industrial economics suggest that most of the factors that enter into market structure, conduct and performance are endogenous. They are derived from the basic economic conditions that characterize the markets under investigation and the strategic interaction of the players in those markets. As a consequence, many of the factors that enter into the various parts of the structure-conduct-performance paradigm are simultaneously determined.

The importance of strategic behavior on the part of organizational participants in shaping the contours of industrial structure has also been recognized by students of the healthcare field (see Starkweather and Carman 1987; Luke and Begun 1994).

Thus, in deciding to focus attention on a single field (or industry), in adopting a longitudinal approach, and in emphasizing the importance of endogenous sources of change and structuration, our own approach appears to be quite compatible with the new thrust in industrial organization economics.

TRENDS IN MATERIAL-RESOURCE ENVIRONMENTS IN THE BAY AREA AND BEYOND

Important changes have occurred in the San Francisco Bay Area's material-resource environment during the past fifty years. While the entire Bay Area has experienced substantial change, there is significant variation across the nine counties included in our study. Thus, we examine both temporal variation and cross-sectional differences of the material-resource environment. We begin by describing some of the more significant changes in the Bay Area and wider economic environment and then proceed to link these developments to changes in the healthcare delivery system.

Changes in Characteristics Affecting Demand

Characteristics of Area Residents

The numbers and types of Bay Area residents constitute the most basic determinant of demand for healthcare services. (For a map depicting the Bay Area, showing the location of major cities and county boundaries, see fig. 2.1.)

Density and urbanization. Overall, the population of the Bay Area has increased threefold between 1945 and 1990, from 2.2 to a little over

6.0 million persons. Whereas the Bay-bounded, peninsular county of San Francisco showed relatively little population growth during this period, increasing from 698,000 in 1945 to 724,000 in 1990, other counties experienced dramatic increases. Six of the nine counties underwent their highest growth rates between 1950 and 1960: Contra Costa, Marin, Napa, San Mateo, Santa Clara, and Sonoma. Among these, the growth rates for Marin, San Mateo, and Santa Clara were the highest, ranging from 42 to 55 percent. Three counties—Santa Clara, Solano, and Sonoma—have continued to exhibit relatively high growth rates on through 1990. By 1990, San Francisco County was exceeded in size of population by three other counties: Alameda (1.3 million), Contra Costa (.8 million), and Santa Clara (1.5 million).

While the Bay Area is generally highly urbanized,[2] there remains substantial variation within the region and even more so over time (see fig. 5.1). In 1945 only 30 percent of Napa and 33 percent of Sonoma County's population was urbanized; and even in 1990 only 72 percent of the latter's population was urban. Still, by 1970, seven of the nine area counties reported over 90 percent of their populations as residing in urban areas.

Minority populations. Whereas only a small racial minority population (defined as nonwhite) existed at the beginning of the period of study, by 1990, over 31 percent of the population in the Bay Area was nonwhite (see fig. 5.1). There exists greater variance in numbers of minorities across the nine counties than over time. San Francisco County has the largest percentage of minority residents, with 46 percent in 1990, up from 8 percent in 1945. Alameda County, which includes the city of Oakland, is a close second. Its minority population increased from 9 percent in 1945 to over 40 percent in 1990. By contrast, Sonoma County reported only 2 percent minorities in 1945, which increased to only 9 percent in 1990. The composition of the nonwhite populations also varies considerably by county: San Francisco's minority population includes roughly equal numbers of African Americans, Chinese Americans, and Hispanics. But Asian Americans as a whole (including Chinese) comprise over 20 percent of the population and represent the county's largest minority group (Godfrey 1984). Minorities in Alameda County are predominantly African American, and in Santa Clara County, Hispanic.

2. Urbanization is defined by the U.S. Bureau of the Census as "a population concentration of at least 50,000 inhabitants, generally consisting of a central city and the surrounding, closely settled, contiguous territory (suburbs). Also included are persons living in places of 2,500 or more inhabitants outside urbanized areas" (U.S. Bureau of Health Professions 1995: 72).

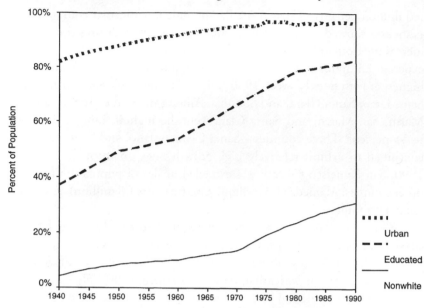

Figure 5.1   Demographic Composition of the Bay Area, 1940–90

NOTE: Educated represents persons of at least 25 years of age with a high school or more education.

SOURCES: U.S. Bureau of Health Professions (1990, 1995), U.S. Bureau of the Census (1940c–90c, 1947e–92e).

Dependent populations. As is the case in the U.S. generally, the Bay Area population is gradually aging. While in 1945, 8.2 percent of the population was 65 or older, the percentage had increased to 11.1 by 1990. Again, there is considerable range across counties, with San Francisco exhibiting a high in 1990 of 16.5 percent and Santa Clara a low of 8.7 percent. Santa Clara is the only county hosting a smaller proportion of elderly persons in 1990 (8.7 percent) than in 1945 (9.0 percent). Because of its burgeoning high-technology industries, Santa Clara has been a magnet for young workers during the past three decades.

At the other end of the spectrum, the percent of population 14 years or younger has changed little over the period of study. On average, slightly over 19 percent of the population were age 14 or younger in 1945 and in 1990. The variation across counties in 1990 ranges from a high of 25 percent in Solano County, home to a rapidly growing number of "bedroom" suburbs, to 13 percent in the city and county of San Francisco.

Income and education levels. The Bay Area is one of the more affluent in the nation. In 1990, the average nominal income per capita in the nine-county area was over $25,000, in comparison with $21,000 for California as a whole and $19,000 for the U.S. The trend toward affluence was marked by particularly large increases in average income of the local population between 1970 and 1980—close to 200 percent in nominal figures and 40 percent in real figures (based on 1967 dollars)—and, to a lesser extent between 1980 and 1990, when the nominal income of Bay Area residents more than doubled and their real income rose over 28 percent.

The percent of the Bay Area population below the poverty line is relatively low.[3] In 1989, an average of 8.5 percent of the population was living in poverty, compared with an average of 12.9 for California and 12.8 for the U.S. as a whole. Again, there is substantial variation across counties. San Francisco is at the high end with over 12 percent living in poverty compared with only 5 percent in Marin. Alameda is second to San Francisco with 10 percent of its population in poverty; the other counties range between 6.6 (Napa) and 7.7 percent (Sonoma).

Education levels in the Bay Area have steadily increased from less than 40 percent having completed high school in 1940 to over 80 percent having completed high school or more by 1990 (see fig. 5.1). As with income, Bay Area residents exhibit slightly higher levels of education than do residents in the state (76 percent) or the nation as a whole (75 percent). There is little variation in this dimension across the nine-county region.

In summary, although the San Francisco Bay Area is a relatively highly urbanized and affluent region that has experienced rapid population increases during many of the decades of the period of study, it exhibits substantial variation along dimensions of importance to our subject. Variance exists in extent of urbanization, in the numbers and types of minority populations, and in the relative size of dependent populations. We exploit this variation—both that occurring over time and across counties—in our analyses.

Financing of Healthcare

Private insurance. We were unable to obtain data on private insurance coverage for residents of the Bay Area over the time period of our study. We

---

3. Federal poverty levels may underrepresent poverty in the Bay Area because of the region's high cost of living.

report instead historical trends in private insurance coverage for the nation as a whole, and note levels of coverage for California for the current time. In 1945 about 22 percent of the U.S. population held private insurance, most covered by Blue Cross/Blue Shield (BC/BS) plans (see fig. 5.2). The total proportion of U.S. residents covered by private insurance steadily increased during the period 1945 to 1975 to a high of 82 percent, after which time it has somewhat declined to levels in the low 70 percent range. Up until 1975, increased coverage was about equally due to the growth in BC/BS coverage and group (employment-based) insurance plans. Self-insurance and HMO plans did not become significant components of private insurance coverage until the early 1970s, when they began to grow, accounting for 6 percent of persons covered in 1975 and nearly 35 percent in 1990 (see HIAA 1996).

Private insurance coverage levels vary significantly by age, race, and, of course, income levels. In 1993, only about 50 percent of African American and Hispanic persons in the U.S. held private health insurance compared with 75 percent of whites. Only 66 percent of persons under 14 years of age had such coverage compared with 81 percent of those between 44 and 64 years of age. And, only 26 percent of persons with incomes less than $14,000 held private insurance compared with over 89 percent of residents with incomes above $35,000 (NCHS 1995; see also, Andersen and Davidson 1996).

Overall, levels of insurance coverage are lower in California than in the U.S. as a whole. In 1994, 85 percent of individuals in the U.S. had some form of health insurance, with 70 percent of them having private rather than governmental insurance coverage. By contrast, only 70 percent of California residents had health insurance coverage, with 60 percent having private insurance (U.S. Bureau of the Census 1995).

Medicare/Medicaid. With the passage of Medicare legislation in 1965—perhaps the high watermark of the Great Society era in the U.S.—the federal government entered into the healthcare sector in a major new role: that of third-party purchaser of healthcare services. Financial responsibility for medical care costs for the elderly (those 65 and older) was accepted by the federal government in the Medicare program and for the poor through the Medicaid program. Virtually overnight, in the interest of increasing equity of access to healthcare services for underserved citizens, massive amounts of new funds flowed into the sector (see fig. 5.2). Funding levels for both programs rapidly increased between 1965 and 1970; the Medicare program exhibited slightly higher funding levels until the 1990s, at which

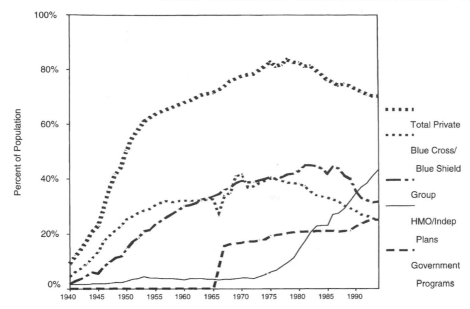

Figure 5.2   Health Insurance Coverage of the U.S. Population, 1940–94

NOTES: Categories are not mutually exclusive or exhaustive.

Government programs include Medicare and Medicaid only. HMO/independent plans include prepaid and employer self-insured plans not underwritten by Blue Cross/Blue Shield or commercial insurance companies. Group consists mostly of employment-based health insurance plans. Total private includes the nonduplicated enrollment in commercial insurance companies (not shown separately), group, Blue Cross/Blue Shield, and HMO/independent plans.

SOURCES: HIAA (1997, 1965), U.S. Bureau of the Census (1975, 1945–96).

time the Medicaid program caught up. Together the two federal programs provided health coverage for nearly 25 percent of the U.S. population in 1994.[4]

Data were collected to show the growth and variation in these federal programs in the Bay Area. Reflecting the variation in the age structure of the resident population, some counties such as San Francisco and Napa had over 14 percent of their population covered by Medicare while other rapidly growing or rural counties, such as Santa Clara and Solano, had only about 7 percent of their population covered. Medicaid (termed MediCal in California) enrollments showed similar variation, reflecting variations in the poverty level: from a high of over 12 percent in San Francisco County to a low of 4 percent in Marin County.

4. The U.S. military provided coverage for an additional 4.3 percent of persons in 1994.

County expenditures. Other public funds supporting healthcare facilities and services are under the control of state and county governments. (Most state healthcare funds are routed through and administered by counties in California.) County-level expenditures on health have shown a steady increase throughout the period of our study, as depicted in figure 5.3. This figure also displays the rapid, dramatic increase in federal expenditures after 1965, as they were experienced in the Bay Area, which by 1990 were more than double county-level expenditures for health services (Medicare and MediCal programs combined).

Concentration of Buyers

Our review of healthcare financing arrangements to this point provides evidence of the increasing concentration in purchasing arrangements. One important trend is the shift from individually funded insurance to

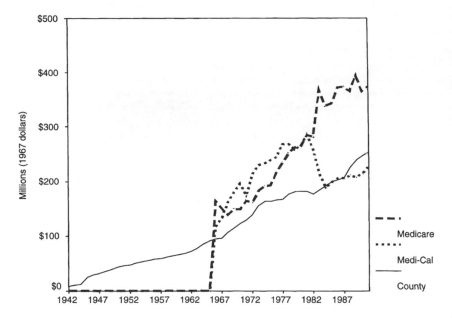

Figure 5.3   Bay Area Public Health Expenditures, 1942–92

NOTES: Medi-Cal is California's Medicaid program.

County consists of direct expenditures made by county level governments for health programs and hospital services (may include intergovernmental funds originating from federal or state levels).

SOURCES: U.S. Bureau of Health Professions (1990, 1995), HCFA (1981–92), U.S. Social Security Administration (1966–72), California Department of Health Services (1968–69, 1970–92), U.S. Bureau of the Census (1942d–92d).

employment-based arrangements, which occurred until the early 1990s. In addition, the increasing importance of public funding for health services just described, both the growth of county and state expenditures and, especially, increases in federal funding levels, are important indicators of increased concentration of purchasing decisions. For many years, this move toward concentration seemed to have little significance. Under the strong guidance of medical providers such as the AMA and AHA, collective purchasers—employers and governmental agents controlling public programs—were content to follow earlier patterns of individual purchasers of healthcare. These actors reimbursed providers for costs incurred and allowed them to determine levels of services and set prices for those services.

Thus, one of the most dramatic and important developments in the healthcare arena in recent years is the emergence of organized and informed purchaser groups willing to negotiate over the price and evaluations of healthcare quality. Such novel activities are now occurring and spreading rapidly as both private companies and public employers have mobilized to become better informed and more aggressive consumers.[5]

Private employers. American business developed an important stake in healthcare costs during the 1950s when health benefits were widely introduced into the collective bargaining process and paying for healthcare services became a routine cost of doing business for many companies. However, it was not until corporate profits began to decline, beginning in 1969 and continuing through the decade of the 1970s, at the same time that healthcare costs continued their inflationary rise, that companies began to become genuinely alarmed about these costs (Bergthold 1990). A number of associations and coalitions of organizations became active at the national level, including the Chamber of Commerce of the United States, the Business Roundtable and its creation, the Washington Business Group on Health. These associations worked to raise the consciousness of their members and to weigh in on national policy discussions but primarily acted to support "the development of local- and state-level business initiatives and coalitions on health" (Bergthold 1990: 76). Such initiatives by business organizations became much more possible and effective with the passage of federal enabling legislation in 1981 allowing states (and subsequently, commercial insurers) to contract selectively with medical providers (see chap. 6).

5. We consider here only the role of such organizations in negotiating prices. Other types of activities (e.g., utilization and quality assurance controls) are discussed in chapter 6.

California became one of the most lively arenas, and the Bay Area, one of the most active venues for business action. Large individual companies at first experimented with adding deductibles and copayments, then began to exchange information about their experiences. In 1989, ten of the largest of these corporations with headquarters in the Bay Area formed the Bay Area Business Group on Health. This coalition quickly recognized the benefits to be attained by collective negotiation and developed a broad agenda of reform. The intent was not to obtain volume discounts, in the sense of forcing the health plans to reduce premiums for one set of buyers and raise them for others, but rather to lay the foundation for joint efforts to lower administrative costs, resolve questions of adverse selection, reduce excess capacity and duplication in provider networks, and otherwise reduce the costs of the healthcare system as a whole (Robinson 1995). In short, the Bay Area Business Group on Health (as of 1995, the Pacific Business Group on Health, or PBGH), has not only functioned as influential actor in the material-resource environment in its role as purchaser of healthcare services but also has assumed important governance functions (see chap. 6).

In its narrower economic role as hard-bargaining purchaser, the coalition has been very effective throughout most of the 1990s. Currently consisting of an alliance of 17 large firms covering over 2.5 million employees and dependents, in 1994–95 PBGH was successful in achieving for its members an average HMO premium reduction of 9 percent attributable to collective negotiations (Robinson 1995: 126). But during the most recent period (1998), premium increases have reoccurred.

Collective negotiation of health plans by private businesses has also been fostered by the state. In 1992, the State of California established a purchasing pool to enable small businesses to attain the advantages of scale in negotiating for medical care for their employees. This purchasing alliance, termed the Health Insurance Plan of California (HIPC), functions as a successful example of the pooling of private purchasers envisioned under President Bill Clinton's failed Health Security Act of 1993–94.

Public employers. At about the same time that private businesses were mobilizing, the California Public Employees' Retirement System (CalPERS), which provides health insurance for nearly one million people, began to use its purchasing power to negotiate contracts with HMOs. They developed a standard benefit package that was mandated for all contracting HMOs—a package that the PBGH later adopted as the basis for its own collective negotiations (Robinson 1995). Between 1992 and 1996, CalPERS has negotiated HMO contracts with premium increases in the 1 percent range, compared with the earlier average of 5 to 10 percent (Casalino 1997). But, again, premiums are on the increase, rising to 9.7 percent for the year 2000.

Composition of health insurance. Considering these public and private developments in combination, we have witnessed a substantial increase in purchasing concentration and, what is more important, the use of the bargaining power that such concentration makes possible. In 1994, "pooled" purchasers of healthcare services constituted over 27 percent of the healthcare market in the Bay Area, compared with 58 percent nonpooled purchasers and 21 percent uninsured.[6] Included in the categories of "pooled" insurance are Medicare and MediCal, CalPERS, the PBGH negotiating alliance, and HIPC. And the recent growth in these programs is quite remarkable. Considering only the nonfederal purchasing groups, the numbers of lives covered in the Bay Area by these purchasers has increased from 1.2 million in 1994 to 1.6 million in 1996. Most of this growth is due to increases in the numbers of employers participating in PBGH. After years of embracing a "price-taking" role in healthcare markets, employers have begun to exercise an effective "price-negotiating" role.

Changes in Characteristics Affecting Supply

Concentration of Providers

Physicians. For more than a century, physicians have been the key providers of medical services in this country (Freidson 1970a; Starr 1982). Their exclusive right to order prescription medications, to perform specified therapeutic procedures such as surgery, and to admit patients to specified healthcare facilities, is supported not only by widely held popular belief systems but also by legal statutes and licensure provisions. Thus they act as exclusive providers of significant medical services as well as gatekeepers to institutions and to services provided by other more specialized and restricted providers. They also serve in a coordinative and directive capacity to a host of other professional and paraprofessional practitioners (Freidson 1970b).

6. These data were obtained from the following sources: CalPERS (1994, 1997), California Department of Health Services (1997a, 1997b), California Managed Risk Medical Insurance Board (1997), HCFA (1995, 1997), HIAA (1996), PBGH (1997), Robinson (1995), and U.S. Bureau of the Census (1945–96).

Throughout the first part of our study period, from 1945 into the 1960s, the ratio of physicians to population was relatively stable. Public concerns were raised about what was perceived to be a shortage of physicians, and foreign medical graduates flowed into the U.S. in increasing numbers. In an attempt to increase the relative numbers of physicians, but also to provide American citizens with greater opportunity to practice medicine, Congress passed the Health Professions Educational Act in 1963. This legislation supported the creation of new medical schools and the expansion of existing schools. Beginning in the early 1960s, the proportion of physicians began an increase that has steadily continued into the 1990s (see fig. 5.4). As a result of the program, the ratio of active, nonfederal physicians per 100,000 population in the U.S. increased from just under 120 in 1960, to 170 in 1980, and to over 206 in 1990. Although originally intended as a manpower augmentation program, over the long run the increasing supply of physicians has had an important influence on organizational arrangements by increasing the level of competition among physicians (see chap. 6).

While the population of the Bay Area has increased nearly threefold between 1945 and 1990, the numbers of physicians in the region has grown nearly three times faster than the rate of population increase. In 1990, the Bay Area had an average of 303 active, nonfederal physicians per 100,000 residents. This ratio is one of the highest in the nation. There is substantial variation across the nine counties in physician-patient ratios. San Francisco has a particularly high ratio of physicians (660). Marin County has the next largest concentration (440). The lowest physician-population ratio (140 per 100,000) is found in Solano County.

Like the nation as a whole, the Bay Area has experienced a steady decline in the proportion of general practitioners to all physicians throughout the period of study (see fig. 6.3). Whereas in the mid-1950s generalists made up about 23 percent of the physician workforce, by 1990, the average proportion in the Bay Area was 9 percent. In spite of federal efforts since the 1970s to increase the number of generalist physicians, only two counties in the Bay Area show an increase in their relative numbers between 1980 and 1990, from 13 to 14 percent in Napa County and from 4.9 to 5.3 percent in San Francisco. There exists, however, a substantial range across the counties in the proportion of general practitioners, from a low of 5.3 in San Francisco to a high of 26 percent in Sonoma, the least urbanized county in the region.

We have already reported in chapter 3 a variety of data indicating that physicians' services have become more concentrated during the last fifty

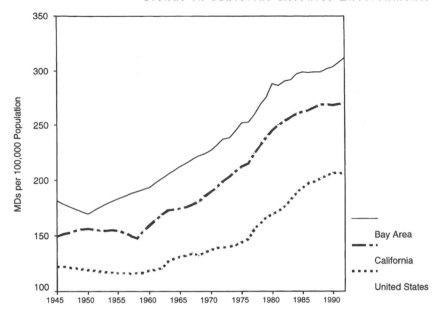

Figure 5.4 Physician-to-Population Ratios in the United States, California, and the Bay Area, 1945–92

NOTE: Physician-to-population ratios based on active, nonfederal MDs.

SOURCES: U.S. Bureau of the Census (1975, 1945–96), PHS (1960, 1962), AMA (1942, 1950, 1959–73, 1974–77, 1981–97), U.S. Bureau of Health Professions (1990, 1995), California Department of Finance (1997).

years. This trend is evident in the increasing numbers and size of medical groups, PPOs, and HMOs, which combine larger numbers of physicians into more highly organized and centralized provider units.

Hospitals. Economists have developed a standard measure, known as the Herfindahl-Hirschman Index (HHI) after its creators, to measure the degree of market concentration in an industry.[7] Market concentration is operationalized in terms of the size of market share—for hospitals, the number of beds—controlled by each provider relative to the total market in the area. The HHI index is calculated in such a manner that

7. The Herfindahl-Hirschman Index (HHI) is operationalized as:

$$\sum_{i}^{N}(S_i/S)^2$$

where S_i defines the size or market share of the i'th organization and S defines the total capacity or market for the N organizations in the region.

an index of 1 indicates a completely monopolistic market and 0 indicates a perfectly competitive market. In the absence of detailed patient service data, it is always difficult to estimate the size of the market served by any given organization. Our approach to this problem was to employ a variable market-radius approach that allowed the area dimensions to vary according to consumer concentration. Patients in urban regions have been found to be more sensitive to facility distances than those in suburban or rural areas. For hospitals located in rural areas, we used a radius of 35 miles since it serves as the federal government's criterion for deciding whether a facility is the sole provider in a region (OTA 1990). For urban and suburban areas, we applied 10 and 15 mile radii, respectively.

Figure 5.5a depicts how the HHI index of concentration has varied over the study period for Bay Area hospitals. As is indicated by the historical path of the index, the hospital market became decidedly more competitive during the period 1945–73. This trend leveled off in the late 1970s and slightly reversed itself after 1981, because of a movement toward greater consolidation of facilities.[8]

Home health agencies. The HHI measure of concentration was also calculated for home health agencies. For these providers, we employed the number of patients served by each agency as a measure of market share. We used the same variable radius approach to define service boundaries as we did with hospitals. Figure 5.5b shows the HHI index for HHAs for the period 1978–92.

While data are lacking on the concentration of HHAs for the period prior to 1978, we observe some general similarities between the behavior of this population and that of hospitals. Both underwent a period of declining concentration (increasing competition) followed by a period of increasing concentration. For hospitals, the period of greatest competition occurred about 1970 while for HHAs, it occurred about 1985. Beyond 1980, however, the HHI for the two populations behaves somewhat differently. Hospital markets show signs of slightly increasing or leveling off in concentration while HHA markets fluctuate greatly, moving toward lower levels of concentration until 1985, then higher levels until 1988, and thereafter to lower levels again.

8. It is important to recognize that the index does not take into account reductions in competitive pressures that might occur as a result of memberships in multihospital systems or other forms of cooperation (or collusion).

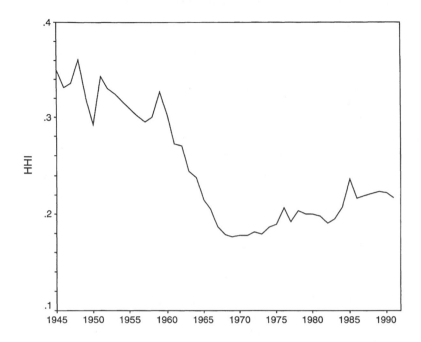

Figure 5.5a　Bay Area Hospital Market Concentration, 1945–92

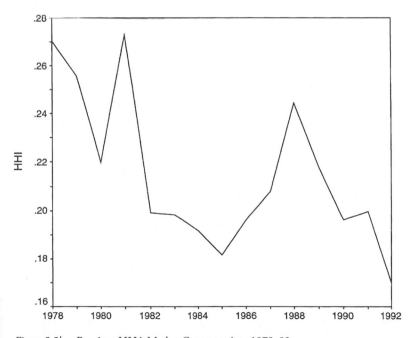

Figure 5.5b　Bay Area HHA Market Concentration, 1978–92

Changes in Technology

The importance of technology, broadly defined, in stimulating increased demand and improved supply of healthcare services can hardly be exaggerated. We consider in chapter 6 the more general buildup of a scientific research base to support medical practice, providing details on funds expended and the timing of these developments. Here, we present data from the U.S. Patent and Trademark Office on the profile over time of new patents issued for drugs and medical purposes between 1945 and 1995 (see fig. 5.6).[9] Patents represent a specific type of indicator of technological expansion; they are less reflective of developments in basic science and more indicative of commercially relevant innovations. Figure 5.6 reveals a relatively substantial rise of patenting from the early 1960s through the mid-1970s, then a leveling off until very rapid increases again occur after the early 1980s.

We believe the strong upward trajectory of the graph reflects two underlying processes: first, an increase in the energy and resources devoted to medical innovation, and second, heightened attention to the commercially relevant aspects of scientific and technical advances. For example, university scientists and their host institutions are much more likely today to seek patents for their discoveries than was the case a decade or two ago. This reflects both a greater focus of universities on commercially relevant technologies and an increased industry funding of university research (see Powell and Owen-Smith 1998).

Much of the decentralization and development of specialized healthcare organizations that we have described in chapter 3 has been facilitated by technological innovations. The increasing use of surgicenters, rather than full-scale hospitals, and the greater reliance on home health and other lower-cost substitutes for inpatient care depends greatly on new therapeutic techniques and equipment.

While we lack systematic data to chart its rise, another highly significant technological development during the past few decades involves the area of information processing. Innovations in this area have been applied to aid clinical diagnosis and the improved tracking of patient data, but their business applications (e.g., the monitoring of costs, insurance benefits, and patient billing) have been of far greater significance for organizational change. The complex networks of health plans, providers, and patients

9. Trends were calculated as 3-year moving averages to smooth fluctuations caused by procedural changes and structural reorganizations in patent administration (see U.S. Patent and Trademark Office 1962–1964, 1977). Refer to footnotes in table 5.6 for specific data sources.

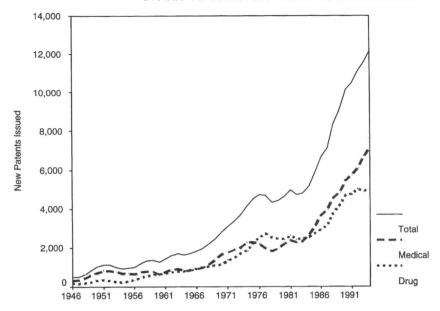

Figure 5.6   Medical and Drug Patents Issued in the United States, 1946–94

NOTES: Includes utility patent classes associated with medical equipment, supplies, and techniques, and drug and bio-affecting compositions.

Trends calculated as 3-year moving averages to smooth irregularities caused by procedural changes and reorganizations in patent administration (sce U.S. Patent and Trademark Office, 1962–64, 1977).

SOURCES: U.S. Patent and Trademark Office (1998a, 1998b).

that have developed during the past few years would be inconceivable in the absence of these computer-aided record-keeping systems.

In summary, while the demand for healthcare services has greatly increased in the Bay Area because of rapid increases in the area's population, supply, in the form of physician density, has increased even more rapidly. The structure of the market has been affected greatly by changes in the degree of concentration of both purchasers and suppliers of healthcare services. Purchasers, in the form of both government agencies and private and public employers, have become much more concentrated in the past few decades and have begun to exercise their purchasing power to improve benefits and reduce costs. Suppliers display a mixed picture. Physician services have become more highly concentrated as individual physicians increasingly enter into various types of groups and networks. On the other hand, medical organizations, such as hospitals and HHAs, have generally become less concentrated and more competitive during the study period.

And technical innovations have encouraged demand and changed delivery systems but have also facilitated the development of physically decentralized but interrelated and highly complex delivery systems.

Rise in Healthcare Expenditures

Demand, supply, industry structure, and technological considerations all come together to affect expenditures for healthcare. As we have already suggested, expenditures for healthcare services have increased. Indeed, in the United States during the second half of the twentieth century, national health expenditures considered as a proportion of gross domestic product (GDP) have continuously risen (see fig. 5.7). From the end of World War II, increases have occurred with noticeable acceleration in rate during the mid-1950s and again, quite steeply, after 1965. Between 1960 and the early 1990s, national healthcare spending as a proportion of GDP nearly tripled.

Also, from as early as the 1950s, annual increases in healthcare prices regularly exceeded the consumer price index (CPI) (see fig. 5.8). The excesses were relatively modest until the mid-1970s and after 1980, periods when medical care costs have greatly outpaced the CPI. This persistent

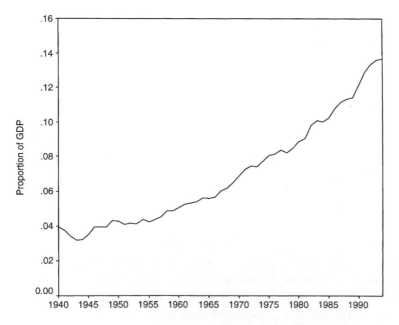

Figure 5.7   National Health Expenditures as a Proportion of GDP, 1940–94

SOURCES: U.S. Bureau of Economic Analysis (1997), U.S. Bureau of the Census (1975, 1945–96).

upward trend has been attributed to a variety of causes, including increases in the technical sophistication of treatments, the demand for services, and the cost of a given unit of service (Payton and Powsner 1980). In addition to rapid increases after 1980, the yearly gains in healthcare costs have fluctuated more widely during this recent period, adding the issue of uncertainty to that of inflation.

Given this "bottom line" of continually rising expenditures and in-flationary costs in healthcare services during the past half century, it is not surprising that much attention has been devoted to issues of cost containment by providers, politicians, the public, as well as analysts. It is useful to note that while the phenomenon of increased expenditures and costs has been continuing and ever present throughout the period of our study, the issue has received variable attention and has elicited diverse responses. Consumption of monies in the form of health expenditures is, of

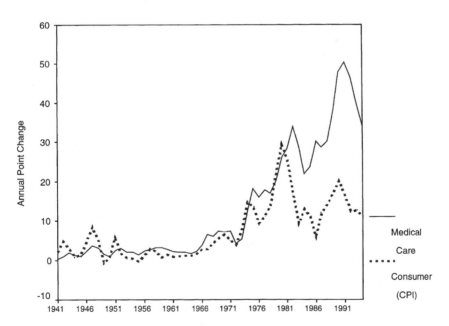

Figure 5.8   Annual Point Change in Medical and Consumer Price Inflation in the United States, 1941–94

NOTES: Annual point change is the annual increase or decrease in the price index from the previous year (with index set at 100 points in 1967).

Medical care price index includes medical care services, equipment, drugs and prescriptions, and other medically related goods and services.

SOURCES: U.S. Bureau of the Census (1975, 1945–96).

course, an important element of the material resource environment. At the same time, however, *responses* to cost escalation—how the issue is framed, how increases are interpreted, and what remedies are sought—are greatly affected by the institutional environment. In chapter 6 we will examine how interpretations of and reactions to rising costs have varied during the three institutional eras.

Resource Environments and Healthcare Organizations

Resource Partitioning

We are primarily interested in the effects of the material-resource environment on the dynamics of our focal organizational populations. Our interest represents an important departure from the conventional focus of health economics on either costs or aggregate utilization of services, in that we want to learn how the various resource variables affect the life chances of different types of provider organizations. To make this connection, we adopt and adapt the ecological concepts of niche and resource partitioning.

A *niche* describes "combinations of resource abundances and constraints in which [population] members can arise and persist" (Hannan and Freeman 1989: 50). Two approaches to assessing niches are: defining structural characteristics of forms that inhabit them and focusing on levels of relevant environmental conditions. The width of a niche can vary so that narrow niches support specialized organizations and wider niches support generalists.

Resource partitioning assesses how members of a population differ in their use of resources. Carroll (1985) and Freeman and Lomi (1994) have adapted this concept from population biologists to address how the material resources available to support populations may be partitioned. Carroll suggested that in mature markets, competition among oligopolistic generalists in the "core" of a niche tends to free resources in the niche "periphery," which are then exploited by smaller, specialist organizations. As a result of this partitioning, specialist organizations are able to exist comfortably alongside generalists.

While previous researchers have used the concept of partitioning to explain differences in the vital rates of subtypes of organizational forms, this approach does not seem well suited to the case of healthcare organizations such as hospitals. The decline (relative to population size) over the last half century in the numbers of generalist hospitals has not been associated with any apparent freeing of resources for specialist hospitals, which, as noted in chapter 3 (fig. 3.3), have experienced even more rapid decline (see also Alexander and Amburgey 1987). Rather, new entrants into the markets previously dominated by hospitals have typically not been new subtypes of hospitals, but different kinds of organizations.

To use the concept of resource partitioning in our own study, we shift the level of analysis from the organizational population to the organizational field. Rather than focusing on competition among the subforms of populations, we examine the extent to which different populations of organizations compete for or make use of differing resources within the common field they occupy.

Institutional Effects on Resource Environments

The concept of institutional environment refers to the belief systems and the regulatory and normative structures that prevail in a given organizational field. We believe that these features are extremely important in shaping the structures and behaviors of human activity, including organizations, and we will devote much attention to them in subsequent chapters.

All organizations operate in both institutional and material-resource environments. While it is possible and, we think, useful to distinguish between these two facets of environments analytically, it is also important to recognize how they interact. We see institutional environments as exerting important influence on material-resource environments, not only because rules and norms constrain the ways in which resources are used, but also because cultural belief systems influence the goals that govern actions, the choice of means for accomplishing them, and the meanings associated with material artifacts. In short, we expect institutional environments to have both direct and indirect effects on organizations, the latter by interacting with resource environments.

To examine this possibility, we employ the notion of "institutional eras" introduced in chapter 1. These eras represent our attempt to characterize the broad trajectory of changing types of social actors (both individual and organizational), belief systems (institutional logics) and governance structures (normative and regulative systems) that have operated in the healthcare sector during the second half of the twentieth century. The three eras identified are:

- *era of professional dominance* (1945–65), when professional providers, especially physicians, were unchallenged in establishing institutional logics and in controlling governance systems;

- *era of federal involvement* (1966–82), which was marked by the massive infusion of governmental funds, the introduction of a new logic emphasizing equity and access, and the increased reliance on public regulatory controls;

- *era of managerial control and market mechanisms* (1983–present), which was characterized by the increasing influence of managerial logics and by greater reliance on market controls.

We will provide both empirical justification and a more nuanced description of these eras in chapter 6. Here we seek to examine the ways and the extent to which the broader institutional context mediates the effects of material-resource variables on organizational processes.

Entries into Organizational Populations

Arguments and Predictions

Earlier in this chapter, we identified a number of characteristics of the material-resource environment that may influence organizational foundings and closures. We now develop more specific predictions about which factors may be important in explaining how and why new organizations of a specific type were founded. (Factors associated with organizational exits are considered in the next section.) We base these predictions on findings from previous studies as well as our understanding of the differences among the populations studied. We analyze foundings in three of our populations: hospitals, home health agencies, and renal dialysis centers.[10] In order to take advantage of the variance exhibited in environmental characteristics across the nine-county Bay Area as well as over time, we conduct this analysis at the county level.

We anticipate that HHAs will tend to enter niches that are differentiated from those of hospitals, while ESRDCs will target types of niches that combine characteristics of the other two provider populations. These predictions derive not only from substantive considerations, which we review below, but also from the contours of competition confronted by

10. We did not have sufficient cases to conduct this analysis for HMOs. As for multihospital systems, we also lack sufficient cases and, in addition, we would not expect this population to be responsive to the same types of factors as the other three populations of provider organizations.

each of the provider forms. Medical care researchers have suggested that hospitalization and home healthcare are increasingly viewed as substitutable goods (Moller, Goldie, and Jonsson 1992). Government policymakers and health plan administrators have begun to take this substitutability into account as they weigh inpatient versus outpatient options for a broad range of services. For both hospital and home health organizations to survive in the same field, then, significant resource partitioning between the two populations may be required.

The services provided by ESRDCs, on the other hand, are highly specialized and, increasingly, can be performed in a variety of locations: within hospitals, specialized centers, or patients' homes. Moreover, the significant level of federal funding for end-stage renal disease (see chap. 2) has created a highly munificent resource environment, allowing hospitals, HHAs, and ESRDCs to coexist in the same bountiful niche. Accordingly, we expect this population to occupy a niche whose resource dimensions overlap significantly with those supporting hospitals and HHAs.

Various dimensions comprise potential bases of resource partitioning and can influence foundings. We expect demographic characteristics such as the educational level and the age structure of the populations residing in each of the nine counties in the Bay Area to differentially affect entry of the various forms. Previous research (e.g., Aday et al. 1993; Millman 1993) has shown that highly educated consumers are more likely to seek preventive services and those that preserve patient autonomy, consistent with the use of home health programs and less hospital care. Thus we expect areas in which populations are more highly educated to support the entry of HHAs but to deter the entry of hospitals.

The relation between education and dialysis programs is less clear. In its early years, prior to ESRD Medicare legislation (Public Law 92–603), transplantation and dialysis selection procedures favored the wealthier and better-educated patients (Evans, Blagg, and Bryan 1981). Following the passage of PL 92–603 in 1972, the playing field was leveled so that treatments included the poor and less-educated. Since our systematic data for ESRDC entries do not begin until 1970—only two years before the extension of Medicare benefits—we do not expect to see any bias toward entry of ESRDCs in counties with higher education levels. Indeed, since lower education levels serve as an indirect indicator for some epidemiological factors that predispose individuals toward kidney disease, we may see an inverse relation between dialysis center entries and education.

Demographic age structure may also influence foundings. We expect that HHAs will be more likely to thrive in niches containing a higher proportion of the elderly, given their emphasis on providing chronic care services. Hospitals, by contrast, are expected to be more likely to enter areas containing a younger populace since these are the years of childbearing and childrearing with the higher probability for contagious diseases and trauma injuries. As for ESRDCs, given the prevalence of chronic kidney disease among seniors (Evans, Blagg, and Bryan 1981), the resource niche for this population is likely to resemble that of HHAs on this dimension.

We anticipate differences in the geographic niches of these organizational forms as well. HHAs are especially suited to serving suburban and rural areas, where access to other forms of medical care becomes more difficult for infirm patients and seniors, while hospitals are more likely to be attracted to urban centers. Because of the specialized character of transplantation and dialysis services provided by ESRDCs as well as the relatively rare nature of the disease, we expect them to also target urbanized regions.

Another major dimension of resource environments is the level of financial resources. One of the most salient types of funding affecting our three organizational populations is the amount of Medicare funding received. We expect HHA and ESRDC entries to be more responsive to Medicare funding levels than hospitals entries. Although all three provider forms rely on Medicare funds to a considerable extent, the dependence of HHAs and ESRDCs is particularly pronounced given the demographic and historical factors previously described (see chap. 2). Hospital entries, on the other hand, have more frequently been supported by other federal programs, such as the Hill-Burton facilities construction program, which affected hospital entries during the period prior to 1970 (see chap. 4).

The predicted effects of the four dimensions of material-resource environments just described are summarized in table 5.1. In addition to this attempt to map the basic contours of the resource environment, two other classes of factors will be evaluated for their impact on provider entries: industry structure and institutional environments.

The concept of industry structure is intended to take into account the effects of other organizations of the same type on the likelihood of new entries. It serves as a reminder that resource environments are shaped not simply by the presence and distribution of resources but also by the presence and distribution of other organizations consuming those resources. We explore three specific measures that allow a nuanced examination of various facets of industry structure: organizational density, organizational concentration, and contagion.

Table 5.1 Demographic, Geographic, and Funding Bases of Resource Partitioning for Hospitals, HHAs, and ESRDCs

		Hospitals	HHAs	ESRDCs
Demographic	Education	Less	More	(Less)
	Age	Younger	Older	Older
Geographic	Urbanization	Urban	Suburban/rural	Urban
Funding	Federal programs	Other programs	Medicare	Medicare

Organizational ecologists consider organizational *density* to be an indicator of both legitimation and competition at the population level (Hannan and Freeman 1989; Hannan and Carroll 1992).[11] When properly scaled by demand-side factors (e.g., size of consumer base), the level of organizational density in a niche—the number of similar organizations operating in the same area—offers a reasonable measure of competitive intensity. We will employ county-level ratios of provider density to inhabitants in a number of our models. Our expectation is that the competitive effects of density will inhibit entries for all populations.

Organizational *concentration* refers to the tendency of providers in a niche to be represented by a few large players as opposed to numerous small ones—that is, an oligopolistic rather than a more competitive market structure. While this structural characteristic is often inversely correlated with density, there are many scenarios in which divergences occur from this relationship. Consider the difference between a market in which five hospitals each have 20 percent of the bed capacity (HHI = 0.20) versus one in which one hospital has 80 percent while the other four hospitals divide up the remaining 20 percent (HHI = 0.65). Because of data limitations in our records of organizational size, we have restricted ourselves to exploratory analyses of market concentration (see figs. 5.5a and 5.5b).[12]

Contagion refers to the dependence of the entry rate on recent previous entries (e.g., those in the preceding year). "Positive" contagion suggests a social bandwagon effect, in which potential market entrants view the sizable number of previous entries into a market as a sign of favorable environmental conditions. "Negative" contagion signifies the presence of a contemporaneous competition effect, in which entries are seen as a sign of

11. But when organizational histories are left-censored, as ours are, and competition is highly localized, it is unclear whether these dynamics may be disentangled. Moreover, the lack of controls for demand-side fluctuations renders simpler density models suspect as indicators of competition.

12. Our organizational size data for HHAs are limited to the time period between 1978 and 1992. No comparable size data were available for ESRDCs.

particularly vigorous rivalry for resources that discourages potential participants from entering. We believe the niche width of an organizational form affects the type of contagion encountered in entry processes. Generalist forms, such as hospitals and, to a lesser extent, HHAs, that inhabit a broader resource niche are more likely to experience positive contagion, since these forms can adjust their service profiles and avoid head-to-head competition with existing providers. Specialist forms, such as ESRDCs, on the other hand, are expected to be more subject to negative contagion because of the narrow boundaries of their resource niche.[13]

Finally, we will examine the extent to which changes over time in the institutional environment, assessed as the period effects of our three institutional eras, affect the relation between material-resource factors and population entries. In a preliminary examination of these data (Ruef, Mendel, and Scott 1998), we observed that the manner in which market structure affected organizational entry varied dramatically depending on institutional conditions. Higher levels of market concentration, measured by the HHI concentration index, tended to deter hospital entry during the eras of professional dominance and federal involvement, while greater concentration served as an inducement to entry under conditions of managerial and market controls in the third era. Similar results were observed for HHAs, with oligopolistic (high concentration) industry structures deterring entries in more regulated markets but failing to serve as barriers to entry in the deregulated conditions observed more recently.

In the following analyses, we consider whether these findings extend to another measure of industry structure: organizational density. In particular, we examine whether the competitive intensity associated with density varies under conditions of market reform (era three), as compared to previous institutional arrangements.

Estimation Methods and Results

The estimation methods employed are described in detail in Appendix C. In general, we count the discrete number of annual entry events in each county and examine the influence of resource factors and institutional eras on these

---

13. In addition to these measures of organizational provider concentration, we control for the density of active physician providers in each county. Physician density is a complex variable, since it has implications for both healthcare supply and competition. On the one hand, organizations such as hospitals and ESRDCs are heavily dependent on physicians as labor; on the other hand, high availability of physician services has been shown to have adverse competitive effects on acute-care and other facilities (see Longo and Chase 1984).

events. Our models are applied using the nine Bay-Area counties as the units of analysis; that is, counts include any entries into an organizational population within each county and covariates are also measured at this level.

The three columns of table 5.2 report the results for entries into each of the three focal organizational populations. Urbanization did not have significant effects on hospital or ESRDC entries, but, as expected, HHAs showed a slightly greater tendency to enter suburban and rural locations. Education exhibited the predicted effects: counties with higher than average education were more likely to support HHAs and less likely to support hospitals (the corresponding impact on ESRDC entries was negative but not statistically significant). Also, as expected, counties with a higher proportion of dependents under the age of 14 were more likely to support hospitals and less likely to support HHAs or ESRDCs. The proportion of senior citizens exhibited a significant effect only for ESRDCs: the presence of seniors was associated with the creation of more dialysis centers.

Table 5.2 Models of Entry into Bay Area Hospital, HHA, and ESRDC Populations

Variable	Organizational Population		
	Hospitals (1946–1992)	**HHAs** (1967–1992)	**ESRDCs** (1970–1991)
Supply and Demand:			
Education	−0.054 (0.019)**	0.047 (0.012)**	−0.020 (0.022)
Minor population ($\leq$ 14)	0.061 (0.029)*	−0.087 (0.033)**	−0.147 (0.065)*
Senior population ($\geq$ 65)	0.049 (0.083)	−0.007 (0.047)	0.171 (0.105)#
Urbanization	0.660 (1.042)	−1.574 (1.157)#	2.441 (2.024)
MediCal expenditures ($ mil)	−0.019 (0.020)	−0.014 (0.009)#	0.021 (0.015)#
Medicare expenditures ($ mil)	0.001 (0.020)	0.023 (0.009)**	0.013 (0.015)
County expenditures ($ mil)	0.047 (0.027)*	0.019 (0.013)#	0.009 (0.025)
Physician density	−0.297 (0.310)	−0.188 (0.158)	−0.362 (0.341)
Industry Structure:			
County-level density[a,b]	−0.422 (0.173)**	−0.584 (0.188)**	−2.146 (0.947)*
Contagion (lagged entries)[a]	0.224 (0.183)	0.115 (0.073)#	−0.696 (0.383)*
Overdispersion (ϕ)	n/a	0.250 (0.140)*	n/a
Number of cases	423	234	198
Number of events	63	235	48
−2 Log likelihood (d.f.)	339.50 (11)	556.58 (12)	216.16 (11)

NOTES: # p < .10; * p < .05; ** p < .01 (one-tailed test)

a. Covariate is lagged by one year.

b. Covariate is computed on per capita basis (per 100,000 inhabitants).

Turning to the funding variables, Medicare expenditures were positively associated with entries of HHAs and, to a lesser extent, ESRDCs (the latter effect is only marginally significant at the 0.11 level). As noted in our earlier discussion, these more specialized organizations may be seen, in part, as the creatures of this federal program. County expenditures for healthcare were positively associated with the entry of hospitals and HHAs. Unexpectedly, MediCal (Medicaid) expenditures had a somewhat dampening effect on HHA entries. This may be because the variable serves as a proxy for (is highly correlated with) unmeasured poverty effects.[14]

Density, the number of other similar organizations in the same county, is our indicator of competitive intensity. As expected, its effect on entries is negative for all three populations: the higher the levels of competitive intensity, the fewer the entries. Contagion, the number of entries of similar organizations in the previous year, showed positive effects on the entry of HHAs, and negative effects on ESRDCs. This is consistent with our arguments concerning the mediating effects of niche width. Contagion is positive for the form (HHAs) occupying a broader niche width and negative for the form occupying a narrow niche.

In summary, the results for organizational entries are supportive of our thesis that the three organizational populations engage in resource partitioning to some extent. Hospitals are drawn more to areas exhibiting lower education levels and greater numbers of young children, and they are more dependent on local (county-level) funding. HHAs, on the other hand, are more likely to develop in suburban areas with higher education levels, fewer children, and higher levels of Medicare funding. The resource niches of ESRDCs share some characteristics with hospitals (e.g., in terms of patient education) and other characteristics with home health agencies (e.g., in terms of dependent populations).

Exits from Organizational Populations

We also collected data on organizations undergoing dissolution and, hence, exiting from their populations.[15] In general, we expect that the same factors operating to invite organizations into an area will operate to retain organizations already existing. But it is important to take into account the inertial characteristics of organizations generally and healthcare providers in

---

14. Direct indicators of poverty could not be included in the entry models because of problems of statistical multicollinearity with other measures.

15. ESRDCs are excluded from the following discussion because the number of exits (13) for this population was insufficient for analysis.

particular. While characteristics of the contemporary resource environment are likely to be especially salient for the prospective decision to create a new facility, their effects are likely to be dampened once resources and manpower have been invested in an organization. In addition, a sizable literature points to the ways in which existing organizations can effectively buffer their technical core from environmental uncertainty, variation, and equivocality (Thompson 1967; Scott 1998). Given these theoretical considerations, we expect organizational exit processes to be far less susceptible to the influence of changes in the material-resource environments than entry processes.

These same kinds of arguments suggest that specific internal organizational attributes, as well as environmental factors, affect exits. For the sake of parsimony, we focus on only three internal attributes: organizational age, size, and integration.[16] Ecologists have long recognized that organizational size and age are important factors associated with the survival of a given organization. Given the widely studied liabilities of "smallness" and "newness" (for a summary of the evidence, see Baum 1996), we expect older and bigger organizations to be less likely to fail than younger and smaller units. In general, we would expect integration (horizontal or vertical) to improve the survival chances of an organization since it connects the organization to a broader support system of financial, informational, and technological resources (see Ruef, Mendel, and Scott 1998). All of these (control) variables are measured at the organization rather than the county level.

Table 5.3 reports the empirical results on those factors that affect the likelihood of hospitals and HHAs surviving as members of their respective populations.[17] Increased age has a deterrent effect for HHAs while larger size reduces the likelihood of exit for hospitals. HHAs or hospitals integrated with other units were much more likely to survive than independent forms.

Only three material-resource variables had a significant effect on exits, confirming our expectation that organizational exits would be less responsive to their contemporary environmental conditions. Education has effects that mirror those reported for entries: hospital exits are more likely to occur in counties with more educated residents while HHAs are less likely to

16. Based on both substantive considerations and issues of data availability, we will also be selective about which organization-level covariates are employed in conjunction with which organizational forms. Given the greater importance of capital factors for hospitals, we focus on size and horizontal integration for this population.

17. Since some of the variables are aggregated to the county level while other variables are at the organizational level of analysis, hierarchical linear modeling techniques represent the preferred approach to analyzing these data. But the small number of county-level units (9) prevents us from employing this technique in any serious fashion (see Appendix C for further details).

Table 5.3   Models of Exit from Bay Area Hospital and HHA Populations

	Organizational Population			
	Hospitals		HHAs	
Variable	Model 1 (1945–91)	Model 2 (1945–91)	Model 1 (1966–91)	Model 2 (1966–91)
Organizational:				
Age ($\times$ 10)	0.052 (0.046)	0.049 (0.050)	−0.640 (0.192)**	−0.558 (0.194)**
Size	−0.594 (0.130)**	−0.618 (0.130)**	—	—
Integration	−0.744 (0.347)*	−0.875 (0.359)**	−0.611 (0.234)**	−0.657 (0.239)**
Supply and Demand:				
Education	—	0.051 (0.019)**	—	−0.049 (0.028)*
Minor population ($\leq$ 14)	—	0.147 (0.059)**	—	0.062 (0.102)
Senior population ($\geq$ 65)	—	−0.011 (0.099)	—	−0.042 (0.104)
Urbanization	—	1.373 (1.705)	—	2.220 (2.064)
MediCal expenditures	—	−0.001 (0.012)	—	−0.006 (0.012)
Medicare expenditures	—	0.013 (0.012)	—	0.014 (0.009)
County expenditures	—	0.004 (0.021)	—	−0.007 (0.013)
Physician density	—	0.255 (0.223)	—	0.031 (0.237)
Industry Structure:				
County-level density[a,b]	—	0.480 (0.246)*	—	0.877 (0.212)**
Number of cases	4089	4089	1756	1756
Number of events	66	66	117	117
−2 Log likelihood (d.f.)	648.56 (4)	622.96 (13)	843.72 (3)	818.36 (12)

NOTES: * $p < .05$; ** $p < .01$ (one-tailed test)

a. Covariate is lagged by one year.

b. Covariate is computed on per capita basis (per 100,000 inhabitants).

leave such areas. Contrary to the findings on entries, counties with a higher proportion of children experience greater rates of hospital exits. County-level density exhibits the expected effects for both populations: the greater the density (competitive intensity), the more likely that both hospitals and HHAs are to exit the field.

While it is the general thesis of this chapter that the material-resource environment influences the numbers and types of healthcare organizations in the Bay Area, we attempt to gain additional insight on how decisions are made to open or close hospitals by considering in more detail one of our case examples: Kaiser Permanente. Case Illustration 5.A describes the decisions made by this HMO system to found, expand, and close its hospital facilities. The case history suggests that many types of considerations in addition to material-resource conditions—personal, political, institutional—enter into these decisions.

Case Illustration 5.A   **Entry and Exit of Kaiser Permanente Hospitals**

Of all healthcare systems, Kaiser Permanente (KP) has the most member hospitals in the Bay Area (see fig. 5.A.1). Because KP is a unique system in many ways, its decisions to open and close hospitals may not be representative of the strategies pursued by other organizations. Especially in its formative years, its incongruence with the institutional environment of professional dominance created many obstacles for KP that were distinct from those facing more conventional providers. Yet these constraints gradually relaxed as the norms of the institutional environment became more supportive of managed care programs. Over time, KP's decisions about facility development became more similar to those of other healthcare organizations. In all eras, these decisions were influenced by a combination of both the material-resource and institutional environments, as well as by the personal interests of the human agents involved.

During World War II, KP cared for Kaiser shipyard workers and their families at hospitals built in Oakland and Richmond. Despite AMA opposition, these two hospitals

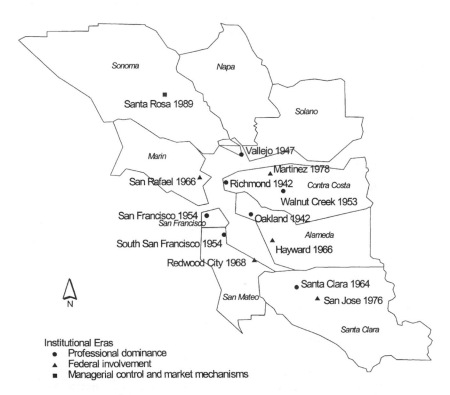

Figure 5.A.1   San Francisco Bay Area Kaiser Foundation Hospitals: Locations and Founding Dates

were supported by the wartime Urgency Committee and expanded rapidly during the war years (Hendricks 1993). Fueled by the pressures of increasing numbers of shipyard workers and the fact that local county medical societies denied KP physicians privileges in community hospitals, KP used a $250,000 loan from the Bank of America to increase its bed capacity (Smillie 1991). Henry Kaiser gave his personal guarantee to bank president A. P. Giannini to back up the loan. This wartime experience convinced Henry Kaiser that in order to survive as a viable healthcare organization, it was imperative that KP own and operate its own facilities.

After the war, as KP opened its health plan to the public, its facility growth was largely driven by its expanding membership. New hospitals (either built by the plan or purchased war-surplus buildings) were opened in San Francisco (1946) and Vallejo (1947). In building its hospitals, KP followed a general rule of having two beds per one thousand health plan members (Smillie 1991). Based on this formula and its growing membership, KP opened new hospitals in San Francisco and South San Francisco in 1954. One of the hospitals constructed during the 1950s, however, reflects more the personal history and personality of Henry Kaiser than the demands of the membership or the rational plans of KP decision-makers.

During the early 1950s, Henry Kaiser's wife Bess became ill and required round-the-clock nursing care, which was provided by a live-in nurse, Alyce (Ale) Chester. Three months after Bess died in 1951, Kaiser married Ale and, motivated in part by Ale's healthcare background, began to take a much more active role in the health plan than he had previously (Heiner 1989; Smillie 1991). This involvement was symbolized by his unilateral decision to build a 100-bed showcase, luxury hospital in Walnut Creek with his own money. At the time, Walnut Creek had only 5000 health plan members, compared to 160,000 in the rest of the Bay Area. Permanente physicians argued that this hospital was unnecessary and simply too big; based on their formula, a ten-bed hospital could serve this area. But Kaiser proceeded undaunted. It took several years for membership in the Walnut Creek area to grow large enough to justify this hospital, and fee-for-service community physicians were allowed to use the facility when it first opened as a way to fill the beds (Smillie 1991).

With membership burgeoning in the 1960s, KP leaders considered seeking access to existing community facilities rather than building new hospitals. One such attempt was made in Santa Clara in 1964, where KP entered into a partnership with community physicians to use a hospital. Conflicts between Permanente and community physicians led to KP purchasing the hospital a few years later (Smoller 1996). After that experience, KP opted for expanding its own system and built hospitals in Hayward (1965) and Redwood City (1968) (Smillie 1991). The Hayward facility was built across the street from an existing community hospital that, although having only 20 percent of its beds occupied, still denied hospital privileges to KP physicians (Yedidia 1987).

In the 1970s, the search for new models of healthcare brought KP to the forefront of health planning and policy. KP continued to serve its members in its own facilities, but AMA opposition no longer served as the motivation for this strategy. Instead, having its own facilities helped KP integrate in- and out-patient services and cope with its more rapid patient turnover and higher acuity levels (because patient stays were shortened, the average patient was sicker) (Williams 1971). New hospitals were opened in San Jose (1976) and Martinez (1978).

In the 1980s, even though it was increasingly clear that the Bay Area was overbedded and new practice patterns were drastically reducing the need for hospital beds, KP erected hospitals in Santa Rosa (1989) and Fremont. The Fremont hospital never opened its doors, however (Smoller 1996; Appleby 1997), and, in the 1990s, KP uncharacteristically considered terminating some of its existing facilities. When its flagship hospital in Oakland required expensive repairs following a major earthquake in 1989, KP explored building a new hospital, but could not justify this approach. Instead, KP contracted with community hospitals in the area to serve its members while the Oakland hospital prepared to close (Wasserman 1996; Appleby 1997).

In its general planning for the 1990s, KP anticipated shuttering a number of its other facilities in the Bay Area. But, like many other hospitals, KP encountered sufficient opposition from community and labor groups to revise its plans. The system now projects closing only four of its hospitals in the next quarter century (Appleby 1997). As in the past, KP's future decisions about its facilities will be influenced by a combination of factors, including the material-resource environment, personal and political processes, and institutional forces.

Effects of Institutional Eras on Resource Environments

Finally, we add period effects to our models, representing the institutional conditions present in each of the three eras. The results for organizational entries are reported in table 5.4.

The first model (cols. 1 and 3) reports the effects of entering the periods (eras) as "dummy" variables. The eras do not show significant direct effects on hospital entries but do significantly impact the entries of new HHA organizations. HHAs were more likely to be founded during the period of market forces than during the period of federal involvement. Note that for hospitals, introducing the period effects does little to alter the effects of the other material-resource variables as reported in table 5.2. Results for HHAs are similarly unaffected when the period variables are added except that some of the funding variables are no longer significant predictors of HHA entries. Once the general temporal variation in entries between period 2 and 3 is controlled for, the impact of expenditure variations within the periods—or across the counties—is minimized. This suggests the possibility that funding changes associated with prospective payment may have significantly and positively affected HHA entry decisions.

More generally, note that for hospitals, there is no significant improvement in overall model fit between the unperiodized model (table

Table 5.4   Models of Entry into Bay Area Hospitals and HHAs, with Period Effects

	Organizational Population			
	Hospitals		HHAs	
Variable	Model 1 (1946–92)	Model 2 (1946–92)	Model 1 (1967–92)	Model 2 (1967–92)
Period 1 (1946–65)	−0.535 (1.053)	−3.440 (1.972)*	—	—
Period 2 (1966–82)[a]	0.349 (0.932)	−3.299 (1.784)*	−1.028 (0.315)***	0.521 (0.576)
Supply and Demand:				
Education	−0.066 (0.023)**	−0.051 (0.024)*	0.034 (0.013)**	0.049 (0.013)**
Minor population (≤ 14)	0.079 (0.039)*	0.112 (0.046)**	−0.069 (0.032)*	−0.095 (0.035)**
Senior population (≥ 65)	0.065 (0.085)	0.090 (0.091)	0.018 (0.050)	0.002 (0.051)
Urbanization	1.082 (1.285)	1.681 (1.427)	−0.349 (1.238)	−1.568 (1.258)
MediCal expenditures	−0.047 (0.032)#	−0.051 (0.035)#	−0.007 (0.011)	−0.006 (0.011)
Medicare expenditures	0.008 (0.027)	0.017 (0.031)	0.006 (0.011)	0.014 (0.011)
County expenditures	0.068 (0.030)*	0.061 (0.033)*	0.010 (0.013)	0.004 (0.013)
Physician density	−0.405 (0.327)	−0.238 (0.319)	−0.096 (0.155)	−0.072 (0.160)
Industry Structure:				
County-level density[b,c]	−0.366 (0.190)*	—	−0.793 (0.206)**	—
1946–65	—	−0.250 (1.336)	—	—
1966–82	—	−0.077 (1.296)	—	−1.880 (0.426)**
1983–92	—	−2.974 (1.272)**	—	−0.595 (0.216)**
Contagion (lagged entries)[b]	0.167 (0.188)	0.116 (0.192)	0.113 (0.070)#	0.110 (0.076)#
Overdispersion (ϕ)	n/a	n/a	0.206 (0.135)#	0.187 (0.129)#
Number of cases	423	423	234	234
Number of events	63	63	235	235
Log likelihood (d.f.)	336.92 (13)	329.68 (15)	545.36 (13)	535.94 (14)

NOTES: # $p < .10$; * $p < .05$; ** $p < .01$ (one-tailed test)

a. Period 3 corresponds to base-line exit rate.

b. Covariate is lagged by one year.

c. Covariate is computed on per capita basis (per 100,000 inhabitants).

5.2) and model 1, which includes periods in table 5.4 (likelihood ratio $\chi^2 = 2.58$, 2 degrees of freedom, not significant). For HHAs, by contrast, the improvement in fit between the unperiodized model and model 1 in table 5.4 is significant (likelihood ratio $\chi^2 = 11.22$, 1 degree of freedom, $p < 0.001$).

In addition to examining these direct effects of institutional eras on organizational entries, we also investigated the possibility of indirect effects via interactions. In exploratory analyses, we examined the interaction effects of eras and various measures of resource environments. The strongest and most stable effects observed were those involving the effects of eras and our measure of competition, county-level density (see cols. 2 and

4 of table 5.4). Model 2 (col. 2) shows how the three eras interacted with density to influence the level of hospital entries. The results show that during era three—the period of heightened market forces—higher hospital density was much more likely to act as a deterrent to the entry of hospitals than during eras one and two. By contrast, for HHAs county-level density exhibited similar effects for both the latter two eras (see col. 4): higher competitive intensity discouraged the entries of HHAs during both the period of federal involvement and the period of increased market forces.

These historical differences between barriers to entry for hospitals and HHAs reveal how social institutions influence the nature of economic competition. Prior to recent market reforms, competitive intensity posed no significant deterrent to hospital entries; as long as cognitive, normative, and regulative frameworks supported the central role of traditional hospitals, these organizations were relatively insulated from pressures stemming from market competition. As these frameworks changed during the era of managerial logics and market orientation, hospitals lost their special position. Home health agencies, on the other hand, enjoyed no such protection. As organizations that threatened the dominance of traditional acute-care providers, HHAs faced high barriers to entry from competition during both the eras of federal involvement and market competition.

Table 5.5 reports results of the same type of periodized models to examine the direct and indirect effects of eras on exits of organizations from each of the two populations. The eras exhibit no direct effects on the exits of either hospitals or HHAs (see model 1, cols. 1 and 3). For hospitals, the effects of size, integration, and minor populations are unchanged, but the effects of education are rendered statistically insignificant. For HHAs, the effects of age, vertical integration, and education are unchanged, but county expenditures become significant: higher expenditures forestall HHA exits.

As with the previous analysis involving entries, we examine the interactive effects of eras and county-level density since this variable was strongly associated with exits. Results show that competitive intensity increases the likelihood of exits for both hospitals and HHAs (model 2, cols. 2 and 4 of table 5.5). But while these effects are significant across both the era of federal involvement and market competition for HHAs, they reached significance for hospitals only during the period of federal involvement.

Thus, there is some evidence in both tables 5.4 and 5.5 that the effect of material-resource variables is mediated by wider institutional conditions. Competitive intensity among hospitals was more strongly associated with

Table 5.5   Models of Exit from Bay Area Hospitals and HHAs, with Period Effects

	Hospitals		HHAs	
Variable	Model 1 (1945–91)	Model 2 (1945–91)	Model 1 (1966–91)	Model 2 (1966–91)
Period 1 (1946–65)	−1.879 (4.265)	−1.395 (4.545)	—	—
Period 2 (1966–82)[a]	−1.354 (4.488)	−1.749 (4.519)	−1.240 (6.453)	−1.707 (6.771)
Organizational:				
Age (× 10)	0.046 (0.050)	0.047 (0.050)	−0.575 (0.191)**	−0.583 (0.192)**
Size	−0.615 (0.131)**	−0.610 (0.133)**	—	—
Integration	−0.921 (0.362)**	−0.926 (0.361)**	−0.676 (0.239)**	−0.686 (0.239)**
Supply and Demand:				
Education	0.022 (0.025)	0.023 (0.025)	−0.077 (0.030)**	−0.078 (0.030)**
Minor population (≤ 14)	0.155 (0.064)**	0.139 (0.068)*	0.011 (0.109)	0.035 (0.116)
Senior population (≥ 65)	−0.053 (0.100)	−0.083 (0.108)	−0.109 (0.106)	−0.099 (0.106)
Urbanization	1.955 (1.744)	1.690 (1.795)	1.445 (2.069)	1.791 (2.126)
MediCal expenditures	0.022 (0.020)	0.025 (0.021)	0.013 (0.014)	0.015 (0.014)
Medicare expenditures	−0.010 (0.016)	−0.011 (0.017)	0.002 (0.011)	−0.000 (0.011)
County expenditures	−0.004 (0.021)	−0.006 (0.022)	−0.025 (0.015)*	−0.025 (0.015)*
Physician density	0.382 (0.243)	0.380 (0.249)	0.173 (0.254)	0.209 (0.261)
Industry Structure:				
County-level density[b,c]	0.549 (0.254)**	—	0.545 (0.244)*	—
1946–65	—	0.392 (0.333)	—	—
1966–82	—	0.700 (0.319)*	—	0.843 (0.496)*
1983–92	—	0.528 (0.605)	—	0.511 (0.250)*
Number of cases	4089	4089	1756	1756
Number of events	66	66	117	117
Log likelihood (d.f.)	618.18 (15)	617.52 (17)	810.86 (14)	810.42 (16)

NOTES: * $p < .05$; ** $p < .01$ (one-tailed test)

a. Period 3 corresponds to base-line exit rate.

b. Covariate is lagged by one year.

c. Covariate is computed on per capita basis (per 100,000 inhabitants).

(discouraging) hospital entries during the period of market competition and with (encouraging) hospital exits during the period of federal involvement. For HHAs, the effect of competitive intensity on both exits and entries peaked during the era of federal involvement.

CONCLUSION

All organizations must acquire and process resources of various types. For service organizations, such as those providing healthcare, among the most important resources are clients to be served. It is for this reason that we have attended closely to the sociodemographic characteristics of the populations in the Bay Area. All organizations compete with other similar and related organizations in providing these services; the number and variety of these other organizations creates the competitive structure within which all operate. Our analyses of these demand and supply features, as well as the structure of the markets within which the services are dispensed, has been informed by the previous work of health economists and industrial organization economists.

We have argued that our different populations of healthcare organizations make somewhat different demands on their environments—that they tend to partition the resource environment, serving somewhat distinctive types of clients and drawing on somewhat different types of resources. Our empirical analysis, focusing on the differences among hospitals, home health agencies, and kidney disease centers, provides support for many of our predictions. We have also shown that the structure of the competitive environment, as measured by density of similar forms, concentration (the numbers of large players), contagion (entries during the previous year) into which organizations attempt to enter or to survive affects their birth rates and life chances.

Finally, we have explored how these processes are affected by changes over time in the wider institutional environment. Our results here are more suggestive than compelling. While we did not observe many significant direct effects of the three eras on organization foundings or failures, institutional conditions were observed to interact with market structure in such a way that organizational density had variable effects on the life chances of hospitals and HHAs depending on which institutional regime was in place.

Six

THE CHANGING INSTITUTIONAL ENVIRONMENT

IN PREVIOUS CHAPTERS, WE used theories associated with organizational ecology, strategy, health, and industrial organization economics to frame our study. Now we add and attempt to integrate institutional theory with these perspectives. As must be clear by now, however, we view institutional theory as not just another competing perspective to be added to the mix, but as a framework within which these other approaches can be housed. Institutions define the context within which social structures can be created and sustained and social behavior can be shaped. By specifying the rules, the governance structures, and the meanings that constitute and are carried by social actors, institutions provide the "ground" supporting and defining the "figures" that carry on social life.

Organizations exist and operate not only in material-resource environments, but also in a world of beliefs, rules, and ideas that are referred to as *institutional environments*. While it is possible to separate these two environmental facets analytically, material-resource environments are greatly affected by the institutional context, as we have emphasized. What constitutes a "resource" and whether and how it can be used and combined are matters determined, at least in part, by institutional beliefs and rule systems. But the effects of institutional environments on organizational structure and behavior are not only indirect, through their effects on material-resource elements. Institutional environments also influence organizations more directly through the kinds of archetypes they develop for actors, the logics they legitimate, and the governance systems and rules of social action they support.

Social actors, individuals as well as organizations, both create and modify their institutional environments, as we have noted throughout our discussion. However, once such institutional environments are in place, even if often endogenously created, they operate as an external force, constraining and empowering social actors. We attend to both moments: forces exerted on and by institutions.

In this chapter, we first briefly discuss the development of institutional theory as it has varied across disciplines and over time. We draw from the broad and rich literature depicting the ways in which societal systems generally, and organizations and healthcare institutions more specifically have changed during this fifty-year period.[1] But, to these "thick descriptions" (Ryle 1971; Geertz 1973)—i.e., accounts of the multitude of factors and forces that come together in predictable and unexpected ways to produce a changing pattern of institutional arrangements—we add more systematic, variable-based analysis. To attempt to untangle the knot of complex interrelated factors, we identify a few selected indicators to serve as "tracer" variables, helping us to gauge the timing and magnitude of the different kinds of forces at work in the wider healthcare arena. Thus, as a complement to the qualitative "thick description," we propose to add the quantitative equivalent: a "dense depiction." In particular, the discussion is organized to identify and elaborate the three eras of healthcare presented in earlier chapters.

CONCEPTUALIZING AND STUDYING INSTITUTIONAL ENVIRONMENTS

Three Institutional Elements

Institutional theory displays a lively and lengthy intellectual history, having been an active school of thought since the 1870s that has affected not only sociological scholarship but also political science and economics (for a brief history, see Hodgson 1991; Scott 1995: chaps. 1 and 2; Thelen and Steinmo 1992: chap. 1). Scott (1995: 33) offers a broad, inclusive definition of the concept of social institutions: "*Institutions* consist of cognitive, normative, and regulative structures and activities that provide stability and meaning to social behavior." As such, institutions operate as important components of the environments of all organizations. Attention to these aspects reminds us that organizations are not only production and technical systems, affected by the flows of material resources; they are also social systems, greatly influenced by cultural rules and normative and legal frameworks.

---

1. For treatments of the more general societal changes, see Parsons (1966), Bell (1973), and Charot (1977); for changes in organizations, see Stinchcombe (1965), Coleman (1974), Chandler (1977), and Perrow (1991); and for changes in medical institutions, see Starr (1982) and Stevens (1989).

Scott's definition identifies three facets or "elements" from which institutions are constructed: cultural-cognitive, normative, and regulative structures. All institutions incorporate one or more of these ingredients, in varying combinations, but institutional forms differ in the priority accorded one or another element, and institutional scholars vary in the attention granted to elements.

Economists and legal scholars emphasize the importance of the *regulative* environment: the structure of rules, backed by sanctions and enforcement agencies, that regulate commerce and govern exchange relations (e.g., North 1990). The "new" institutional economists stress the importance of governance mechanisms (for example rule and authority systems), operating at both the organizational field and organizational levels, that arise to reduce "transaction costs" (Williamson 1975, 1985).[2] And ecologists, such as Singh and colleagues (Singh, Tucker, and House 1986) and Baum and Oliver (1991), have examined the effects of public regulatory structures on the survival rates of social service organizations.

Political scientists and most sociologists have, until recently, stressed the importance of *normative* systems, including more informal and diffuse rule systems that operate to structure expectations and establish and enforce a system of mutual obligations (e.g., Parsons 1960; Selznick 1949; Stern 1979). As we emphasize, such structures are particularly important in governing behavior in highly professionalized sectors.

The "new" institutional sociology, which borrows heavily from the "new" cultural studies in anthropology and the work of cognitive psychologists, directs attention to the importance of *cultural-cognitive* systems, including beliefs, orienting frames, and scripts for guiding choices and behavior (Geertz 1973a; Berger and Luckmann 1967). At the micro level, many of these ideas were introduced into organizational studies by March and Simon (1958), who emphasized the ways in which shared beliefs ("decision premises") constrain choice and the importance of "performance programs" and routines for regulating participant behavior. At the macro level, Meyer and Rowan (1977) were the first to point out the ways in which organizational structures are shaped by widely held belief systems ("rational myths") that specify the form that schools or hospitals or factories should exhibit in order to be regarded as legitimate players in their respective institutional settings. Organizations are obliged to conform to the socially defined organizing recipes or templates if they wish to receive resources and normative support from others in their environment. Thus, institutional

2. We consider and test selected arguments developed by institutional economists in chapter 8.

arrangements are composed not simply of regulative rules—specifying who is allowed to behave in a given way—but also of constitutive rules—specifying what types of actors (and acts) are allowed to exist or take place at all (Searle 1969, 1995: chap. 2).

DiMaggio and Powell (1983) observed that organizations experience pressure to conform to their institutional environments because of the operation of "coercive" pressures from political institutions, "normative" pressures from occupational and professional constituencies, and "mimetic" pressures from other organizations with whom they compare themselves. Scott (1995) has pursued this insight by suggesting that each of these mechanisms is associated with a different type of institutional order: the coercive with *regulative* structures; the normative with the *normative* system; and the mimetic with the *cultural-cognitive* order. Moreover, these orders coexist, interact, and often exhibit diversity such as to cause tension and change.

In addition to recognizing the new emphasis accorded to cultural-cognitive beliefs and knowledge systems, three other developments merit recognition. Most earlier work stressed the uniformity and stability of institutional pressures (e.g., DiMaggio and Powell 1983) while later work has recognized the extent to which many institutional environments are inconsistent, fragmented, and ambiguous (see Friedland and Alford 1991; Scott and Meyer 1991; Edelman 1992), and capable of changing over time (Fligstein 1990). In addition, early work emphasized the tendency of organizations to conform automatically to the requirements of institutional constraints while more recent work has recognized that organizations often attempt to influence, evade, or resist institutional dictates (Oliver 1991), particularly when the environment is not highly unified (Goodrick and Salancik 1996). Third, most early studies of institutional fields have examined the origins and developmental processes involved in building up a stable institutional order. Only recently have investigators turned their attention to the factors that operate to undermine and lead to destructuration processes (e.g., Davis, Diekmann, and Tinsley 1994; Thornton 1995).

Our own work benefits from and attempts to reflect these trends. We do not overlook the importance of the regulative and normative features stressed by early institutionalists, but we also include within our framework the newer cultural-cognitive facets. In taking this approach, we agree with Greenwood and Hinings (1996), Hirsch and Lounsbury (1997), and Stinchcombe (1997) that researchers need to reconcile the "old" and "new" institutionalisms. In particular, new institutionalists have tended to overlook or underemphasize both the play of power and moral conviction in the building and dismantling of institutional arrangements.

Earlier institutionalists were more attuned to the ways in which power was employed not only to design structures that advantaged some groups over others but also to construct rules and norms that justified and legitimated these advantages (Selznick 1949; Stinchcombe 1968). Even though power in the service of interests is not the only force supporting or overturning an institutional arrangement—there are also efficiency concerns, status and prestige processes, and the force of habit and convention—it should not be overlooked. Similarly, earlier institutionalists also accorded more weight to moral authority and to the centrality of values (Selznick 1957; Parsons 1990). As Stinchcombe (1997: 15) emphasizes: "The guts of institutions is that somebody somewhere really cares to hold an organization to the standards and is often paid to do that." We should not forget that institutions often embody moral standards upheld by some constituency and that these efforts may even be pursued apart from any parochial interests.

Far from assuming the existence of organizational conformity to these changing forces, we examine empirically the effects of institutional change on our focal populations of organizations and, through the lens of our case studies, consider the ways in which selected organizations conform to, reinforce, and take advantage of but also seek to influence, evade, defy, and manipulate their environment. And, because we view the second half of the twentieth century as a period of profound change in the healthcare sector, we devote considerable attention to detailing both the breakdown of previous arrangements and the attempt to craft new ones.

Three Institutional Components

As previewed in chapter 1, we identify three components that are employed to support a more detailed investigation of the changing nature of institutional environments in the healthcare sector. They are institutional logics, institutional actors, and governance structures.[3] We view these components as intrinsically interdependent, although analytically distinct.

Institutional Logics

Institutional logics refer to the belief systems and associated practices that predominate in an organizational field. As Friedland and Alford (1991: 248)

---

3. Our views of how these categories map onto the three institutional elements may be of interest. Actors are particularly reflective of the cultural-cognitive elements insofar as they embody the constitutive definitions that specify capabilities within the field. Institutional logics are made up of both cognitive and normative elements: belief systems about what is and ought to be. And governance structures consist primarily of normative and regulative elements.

note, institutional logics provide the "organizing principles" that supply practice guidelines for field participants. Logics specify what goals or values are to be pursued within a field or domain and indicate what means for pursuing them are appropriate. Thus, logics tap into both the cultural-cognitive and normative dimensions of institutional environments. The logics are only salient to the extent that they affect action within the field—sometimes being carried by established participants, sometimes by outsiders who influence behavior within the field. While there often are dominant logics that reflect the consensus of powerful institutional actors, secondary or repressed logics representing other, subordinated interests may over time become more influential or even superordinate. In our discussion, we emphasize secondary logics that act as precursors to institutional change, although it is also important to recognize that not all challengers are successful.

Early institutional theorists tended to restrict their examination of institutional logics to the study of schools or other types of public service organizations operating outside of competitive sectors. Such organizations were argued to be primarily responsive to "institutional" rules rather than to imperatives of producing quality outcomes or operating efficiently (see Meyer and Rowan 1977; DiMaggio and Powell 1983). But more recent analysts have come to recognize that *all* organizations operate in institutional environments and collectively develop beliefs and norms to guide their activities, including their technical work. After all, there are various ways to organize productive activity of whatever kind and differing ways to compete effectively. A subset of these will come to prevail and be regarded by participants as the "appropriate" or "natural" way to carry out the functions in question (see Fligstein 1990; Orru, Biggart, and Hamilton 1991; Powell 1991; Scott 1995; Whitley 1992). Previous studies that have focused primary attention on cognitive-cultural factors in the creation of organizational fields include DiMaggio's (1991) study of the effect of organizational archetypes and cultural norms on the formation of the field of art museums and Suchman's (1995a) study of the role of lawyers in developing and diffusing a common pattern of organizational templates for semiconductor firms in Silicon Valley.

How does one chart changes in shared understandings, in cultural beliefs? How can one capture the cognitive reframing of a set of activities? There is no simple or single answer, and so we employ a variety of indicators, all of which serve to assess changes in underlying belief systems. Shifts in the content of professional journals, in the circulation of popular magazines, in the ways in which financing is arranged, in who is regarded as a legitimate healer—these are some of the markers employed to capture changing institutional logics.

Institutional Actors

Institutional actors, individual and collective, both create (produce) and embody and enact (reproduce) the logics of the field. Viewed as agents, they are capable of exercising power to affect and alter existing systems and rules. Viewed as carriers, individuals and organizations embody and enact the institutionally defined structures, capacities, and rights with which they are endowed. Their identities and capacities are created through constitutive processes. Their interests are shaped by their location in the field; and, in turn, they endeavor to have these interests reflected in the governance structures. Data obtained through our organizational case studies provide some insight into the circumstances under which organizations are able to behave proactively and exert influence, as well as enact and embody institutions.

We have already devoted considerable time and attention to defining and describing the numbers and types of institutional actors that make up the healthcare scene (see, in particular, chaps. 2 and 3) and we will describe below some of the new corporate and "integrated" systems that are developing (see chap. 8). Changes in the composition of the principal "players"—both individual and organizational—occupying a given domain provide one important type of evidence regarding alterations in what interests are represented and what and how work is done. As discussed in chapter 3, these changes also may be interpreted as shifts in the relative legitimacy of the organizational populations. Prevalence is a useful indicator of cognitive legitimacy (Hannan and Carroll 1992).

Evidence has already been provided concerning the extent and timing of these changes in the Bay Area. As previously discussed, such changes represent "internal" field-level processes but also constitute an alteration in the wider "external" context: the distribution of organizational types is an important feature of the environment for each organizational population and each organization in the arena. These more endogenous effects were considered in chapters 4 and 5, while here we focus on influences originating at or outside of the field level.

Governance Structures

As Abbott (1988: 59) has observed, "jurisdiction has not only a culture, but also a social structure." Institutions are made up not only of various types of social actors and belief systems but also of normative and regulative structures that exercise oversight and enforce compliance. Governance structures refer to all those arrangements by which field-level power and authority are exercised involving, variously, formal and informal systems, public and private auspices, regulative and normative mechanisms.

Many frameworks for analyzing societal level governance structures have been proposed. We are particularly attracted to a set of recent analyses that insist that, while societal-level structures exhibit important, common overarching features, substantial variation often exists in governance structures and mechanism across societal sectors (Schmitter 1990; Campbell, Hollingsworth, and Lindberg 1991). To recognize this possibility allows us to comment on the general features of governance structures in American healthcare and better compare this field to other sectors.

We start with a typology devised by Streeck and Schmitter (1985), who propose four models of governance regimes. They are, simply described, as follows:

Community model: Families or clans governed by customary practices enter into exchanges and compacts with other units based on respect and trust. Internal leadership is based on ascriptive status and the principle motives governing action are identification with the group and solidaristic goods.

Market model: Firms or parties engage in competition with one another for material resources or votes. Exchanges are governed by contracts and participating units attempt to maximize their private good, seeking power and/or wealth.

State model: Governmental agencies exercise legitimate control over specified areas under a rule of law and backed by the power of coercive sanctions. Collective goods are protected and conflicts or differences are formally adjudicated.

Association model: Functionally defined interest associations having a monopoly status within a sector exercise normative-legal control over a specific jurisdiction. Associations engage in concertation of interests within the sector and develop pacts with groups in other sectors based on mutual recognition of status and entitlements. (Streeck and Schmitter 1985: 3–12)

In effect, Streeck and Schmitter have added the association model to three other conventionally recognized forms of governance. They argue that the association model is increasingly acknowledged as a mode of control and coordination that is neither "market" nor "hierarchy" but supports the development of what they term "private interest governments" in selected sectors.

    This typology—in particular, the latter three models—appears to have particular utility in characterizing changes in governance regimes within the healthcare sector over the past fifty years.[4]

Interconnections of Components

Complex interdependencies exist among the components of institutional environments. Institutional actors carry but also create logics, and actors are, variously, the subjects of power wielders within and claimants and petitioners attempting to benefit from and alter governance structures. Governance structures instantiate the dominant logics but may change more slowly than ideas and interests.

    While there will be important exceptions, in general we expect changes in logics to occur first, allowing for the construction of new types of social actors—new roles and new types of organizations—and the development of new governance structures. Logics lead the way, because they are largely based on ideas. Ideas are often generated within a field by the "creative odd ones" who formulate new concepts, models, and designs. On the other hand, new logics can be imported into the field from other arenas, as proponents cross boundaries. Campbell (1997: 17) has described how the introduction of new actors alters patterns of interaction that, in turn, cause participants to gain new perspectives on their situation. In this manner, "changes in interaction may precipitate changes in interpretation," that is, in logics. When the new ideas and interpretations diffuse and become widely accepted—and often they do not—they can become the basis for social movements and reform programs. The most successful of these become institutionalized, replacing former truths and, over time, become taken for granted as "how things are" and "the ways these things are done."

    New types of actors cannot come into existence in the absence of a supportive ideological base (Stinchcombe 1965; Aldrich and Fiol 1994). Social visionaries, intellectuals, and entrepreneurs create new possibilities: new designs for structures and new ways of acting. They propose new templates or archetypes for roles, groups, and organizations (Greenwood and Hinings 1993). But these ideas must find a receptive audience: their "time must come." More importantly, the new ideas and ways of acting must be instantiated in routines, roles, and social organizations if they are to persist over time. As we have seen in the case of Kaiser Permanente,

---

    4. The community model was in force in the U.S. healthcare sector during the middle of the nineteenth century.

new forms can exist in protected, special circumstances for a time without enjoying broader support (see chap. 2). But if they are to survive and diffuse, they must find wider acceptance, and governance structures must be modified to accommodate them.

Changes in governance structures tend to lag the introduction of new ideas and actors, since they usually require the buildup of pressure and political will. As logics are more fluid than the codified rule systems that they produce, there can be a lag between an evolving logic and the more static governance regime. When major legislation occurs or a new policy is created by, for instance, a professional association, the resulting change may appear to be abrupt. It usually seems so, however, because the period of preparation and buildup of pressure is less visible to outside observers. Thus, logics and social actors interact to create governance structures; and these structures, in turn, constrain and empower actors and actions (Giddens 1984; Sewell 1992).

We turn now to the task of operationalizing and applying these ideas regarding institutional environments to the study of the healthcare field. Inasmuch as the escalation of healthcare costs has been among the most salient issues during each of the three eras, we examine how it was framed and interpreted by each of the logics and associated with the development of different kinds of actors and governance structures.

CHARTING CHANGE IN HEALTHCARE INSTITUTIONAL COMPONENTS

Institutional Eras in American Healthcare

To this point, our assessment of institutional factors has been based on the serviceable but relatively blunt notion of institutional "era": the idea that institutional systems and beliefs tend to coalesce into relatively coherent complexes that vary in composition and meaning over time. As discussed previously (see chaps. 1, 2, 4, and 5), the eras we have identified for the healthcare field in the United States are professional dominance (commencing prior to the onset of our study and continuing up to 1965), federal involvement (1966–82), and managerial control and market mechanisms (1983–present).

The delineation of the three periods takes into account a number of factors but is based primarily on changes in *governance structures:* the dates denoting significant legislation affecting the healthcare field. The end of the first and the beginning of the second era was inaugurated by the passage of the Medicare and Medicaid programs in 1965, an event that signaled a major transformation of governance in that the federal government for the first time became a major player in the healthcare delivery arena. Similarly, the beginning of the third era was ushered in with the passage of two bills, the Omnibus Budget Reconciliation Act (OBRA, 1981) and the Tax Equity and Fiscal Responsibility Act (TEFRA, 1982), which introduced new types of incentives and rules governing healthcare financing. (These legislative actions are described in more detail later in this chapter.)

As we will see, the eras map rather neatly onto three of the general types of governance structures identified by Streeck and Schmitter (1985). The first era is characterized by the *association model,* professional associations providing the central governance mechanisms for the field. We concentrate attention on physicians' organizations as the strongest exemplars of orga-nized medicine, but many other occupational and industry groups created bodies to represent and enforce their interests actively in this sector. The power and privileges of these associations was backed by public authority, whose agents endorsed and enforced licensure and other forms of monopoly power. Professional groups have remained strong throughout all eras, but physicians were exceptionally unchallenged during the first era.

The second era reflects more clearly the *state model.* Since the dawn of the modern national state, governmental structures have provided a framework of authority within which more specialized, "private" actors operate and pursue their ends. The ability of public agencies to "rely on legitimate coercion" (Streeck and Schmitter 1985: 20) places them in a special category of governance structure. While ever present, public authorities at the federal level became much more influential and more directly involved in governance activities within healthcare during the second era.

The third era corresponds to the *market model,* as corporations and business associations become much more active, and marketlike incentives and controls are emphasized. New organizational forms of various types—medical groups, HMOs, integrated healthcare systems—emerge or expand, in part because they offer providers a better way to compete in a sector increasingly driven by market forces. Professional associations and their governance systems become less influential, and state agencies realign policies to emphasize deregulation and competition.

We use these eras as the organizing framework for discussing the interplay of logics, actors, and governance structures but also acknowledge and detail the extent to which multiple forces richly interact across eras.

Evidence of Discontinuous Change

This periodization of three major eras fundamentally assumes that the U.S. healthcare sector has been punctuated by discontinuous and, at the field level, "revolutionary" change (see chap. 3). But all three institutional logics have been present since at least the beginning of our study period and detectable in legislative events predating the two major regulatory initiatives we use to demarcate the eras.[5] To what extent do these legislative events accurately reflect episodic, stepwise shifts in governance structures and underlying institutional logics, as opposed to a gradual, incremental tempo of change?

We evaluated these assumptions in two ways. First, we compared whether a long-term transformation in healthcare organizations, such as increasing privatization, is better explained as a linear, continuous trend or by discontinuous time markers. Appendix B describes these analyses for hospitals, HHAs, and ESRDCs in the Bay area. Second, building on the description of these periods in the second half of this chapter, we constructed longitudinal measures of the primary institutional logics in the U.S. healthcare field (see chap. 9). We then examined these trends to determine if the extent and timing of discontinuous change correspond to our periodization.

With both approaches, we find substantial corroboration of the three eras as delineated. Also evident, however, is the importance of charting the varying impact of these shifts across sectors and dimensions of a field and of considering multiple indicators and sources of change.

Utility of Multiple Indicators

We attempt to describe the principal incidents and factors at work in shaping each era, as well as the emergent ideas and actions that came to undermine existing beliefs and practices and foster change. In some cases, elements central to one era continue into the next, comprising part of a new institutional pattern. Our objective is to identify a limited set of quantitative indicators or markers allowing us a better opportunity to trace the ebb and flow of these forces. These indicators serve both to demarcate the eras as well as to reveal the somewhat arbitrary placement of the temporal boundaries.

5. For example, the Medicare and Medicaid Acts of 1965 were preceded by other federal efforts at the provision of health insurance, such as the child and maternal health programs and the military CHAMPUS system. Similarly, the HMO Act represented a noteworthy advancement of managerial and market logics nearly a decade previous to the prospective payment system legislation of the early 1980s.

Identifying a number of different indicators enables us to distinguish among the many factors at work, to determine which changed earlier or later, and which exerted crucial influence. While we cannot completely disentangle the dense thicket of factors and forces at work in transforming healthcare systems, we seek to isolate some of the most significant variables and determine their timing and effects. In a later chapter (chap. 9), a subset of principal indicators is identified and employed to capture significant changes in the underlying institutional logics and to assess their effects on populations of healthcare organizations.

Our discussion is organized by era. We first consider some of the principal indicators used to identify each era and then examine evidence of factors operating at that time that appear to undermine existing institutional arrangements and serve as precursors to the next era.

The Era of Professional Dominance (1945–65)

Principal Indicators

Governance structures. Physicians have long been regarded as having created the strongest and most effectively organized profession in U.S. history (Freidson 1970a; Starr 1982; Abbott 1988). In particular, the American Medical Association (AMA) has served as the archetype of the dominant professional association, serving as watchdog, as advocacy and lobbying body overseeing legislative activity affecting physicians' interests, as legitimating agent controlling access to hospital privileges, patient referrals, and malpractice insurance, and as governance body, enforcing norms against advertising, fee-splitting, and the "corporate" practice of medicine. While the early history of medical care in the U.S. was marked by a wide diversity of contending types of practitioners, by the beginning of our study period in the 1940s, the field had come under the secure control of allopathic physicians, whose county-based societies governed the conditions of local practice and whose state and national organizations exercised an effective veto over unwanted legislative action (Garceau 1941; *Yale Law Journal* 1954; Campion 1984). The strength and political unity of organized medicine prior to the beginning of our study in 1945 and continuing on through the 1950s provides the major criterion by which we anchor the era of "professional dominance" in healthcare.

The proportion of physicians belonging to the AMA provides a serviceable indicator of the growing strength of physicians. Membership in the

AMA gradually increased throughout most of this era, embracing almost 70 percent of active physicians at the peak of its power in the 1950s (fig. 6.1). Membership in the California Medical Association closely parallels that of the AMA. Bay area physicians reveal similar general trends, although there is considerable variability across the nine-county region with higher levels of membership occurring in rural counties, such as Solano and Napa, and lower levels, in urban counties like San Francisco.

Note that the meaning of this indicator, like many others we will employ, is not restricted to one institutional element or component. Physicians represent a cognitively constituted role endowed with distinctive characteristics and capacities. Incumbents of this role, both individually and collectively, also exercise impressive normative powers. Through their influence on the state, they are able to leverage additional regulative powers. The growing numbers of physicians signify increases in the prevalence of

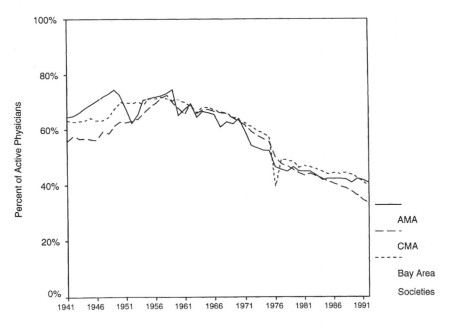

Figure 6.1   Membership in General Physician Associations, 1940–92

NOTES: Bay Area Societies include the eight local county medical societies (Alameda–Contra Costa, Marin, Napa, San Francisco, San Mateo, Santa Clara, Solano, Sonoma).

Membership in the national (AMA) and state bodies is independent, but membership in the state association (CMA) and county medical societies is linked.

SOURCES: American Medical Association (1997), California Medical Association (1941–96), U.S. Bureau of Health Professions (1990, 1995).

this type of institutional actor, and, through their professional association, these actors have constructed a significant governance structure.

The most striking feature characterizing this era was the unity and power of physicians, expressed principally through the medium of the AMA. The AMA worked actively and effectively at all levels to influence and attempt to control size of the workforce, training programs, titles, modes of working, and relevant organizational arrangements in both educational and medical care delivery systems. Control over numbers and qualifications of workers was attained through the licensure process, operated by the AMA in conjunction with state-level public agencies. Control over organizational structures and procedures of both training and practice settings, in particular, hospitals, was effected by means of accreditation processes (see Freidson 1970a; Starr 1982; see also, chap. 7). In short, the professional association of physicians served as a singularly significant governance structure, overseeing the conduct of activities within the healthcare sector.

We focus attention on the professional association of physicians since we believe it to have been, by a considerable measure, the most powerful collective body representing professional interests in the healthcare arena (see Freidson 1970b). But other professional groups, including nurses and hospital administrators, also developed professional associations to reflect and advance their interests.[6]

Because of its political influence during this period, the AMA was able to resist many potentially competing sources of control. Throughout the era, financing arrangements for covering the costs of medical care were organized in such a manner as to minimally interfere with the physician-patient relationship. The great majority of insurance coverage took the form of either Blue Cross/Blue Shield, seated in nonprofit associations, or commercial insurance (see fig. 6.2 and fig. 5.2). Both of these types of insurance carriers issued indemnity coverage, in which patients were reimbursed for the costs of selected aspects of care, an arrangement that maximized physician autonomy and minimized the influence of the "third party" payors. During the era of professional dominance, financial intermediaries exercised, at best, minimal governance of healthcare delivery.

Public agencies were largely quiescent during this period. Medical associations were able to derail numerous attempts by socially liberal political activists to enact national health insurance. For example, they

---

6. We describe the accrediting role of the American Hospital Association in greater detail in chapter 7.

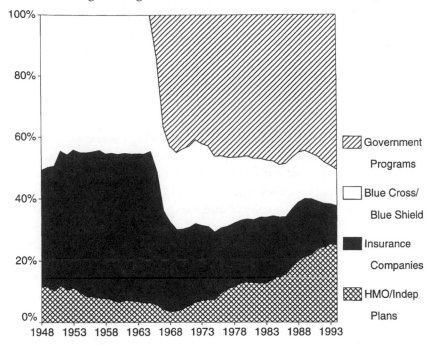

Figure 6.2   Health Insurance Benefit Expenditures in the United States by Type of Insurer, 1948–94

NOTE: Government programs include Medicare and Medicaid only. Insurance companies include commercial insurance carriers. HMO/independent plans include prepaid and employer self-insured plans not underwritten by Blue Cross/Blue Shield or commercial insurance companies.

SOURCES: HIAA (1959–96), OMB (1997), U.S. Bureau of the Census (1975), *Health Care Financing Review* (1987, 1995), Carroll and Arnett (1981, 1979).

dissuaded President Franklin Roosevelt, a champion of many revolutionary social reforms, from putting forward such legislation.[7] And President Harry Truman's plans for a national health program unveiled in 1946 were eventually scuttled by cries against "socialized medicine" led by the AMA (Starr 1982: 280–86; Weeks and Berman 1985).

Except for specialized populations (e.g., military veterans, Native Americans, inmates of federal prisons), the federal government was not directly involved in paying for or providing medical care during this era. Throughout the period, federal-level agencies were relegated to providing

7. Roosevelt, speaking of health insurance in 1943, remarked to a key Senate chairperson, "We can't go up against the State Medical Societies; we just can't do it" (Starr 1982: 279).

infrastructural support and to overseeing the marginalized efforts of public health officers (Starr 1982: bk. 1, chap. 5). State-level agencies worked in close collaboration with professional groups to enforce licensure laws. It was primarily at the local community level, of municipal and county government, in which the public sector was directly involved in financing and managing service delivery systems.

Logics. We have argued that a distinctive primary logic was associated with each era; in the first, it was *quality of care,* as determined by physicians. We have only qualitative and indirect evidence of the importance of this value during the first era. We believe that the medical profession presented itself as centrally committed to quality of care, using this value as justification for their resistance to the "corporate" practice of medicine and as the basis for their insistence that patients' choice of physician should be unrestricted. The importance placed on quality of care was a major factor fueling the vast expansion of medical research and related technologies during the 1950s and 1960s, as every patient was believed to be entitled to the latest and best therapeutic devices and procedures (see Bennett 1977; Bloom and Randolph 1990; Strickland 1972).

This value has been especially evident in the strong predilection of U.S. physicians to specialize in their medical practice. Many physicians viewed specialization and its link to advanced training as an important means of exploiting scientific and technical advances in order to deliver the highest quality of care. Of course, specialization also served other values. It aided the interests of physicians seeking increased status and earning power as well as the interests of medical schools and teaching hospitals committed to expanding the scientific base of medicine as well as their own domains (see Stevens 1971). Figure 6.3 shows that the relative number of full-time specialists grew very rapidly throughout the era of professional dominance, surpassing general practitioners in 1960, and reached a level of over 60 percent of physicians in private practice by 1965. This primary logic of healthcare quality was ascendant during the first era, but remains strong up to the present time.

Healthcare costs began to increase from 1945 onward (see fig. 5.7); and began to exceed the consumer price index regularly after 1950 (see fig. 5.8). During the 1950s, these developments were fairly readily subsumed under the logic of medical quality, with the perspective that cost increases did not signify problems but rather "the success of [the medical establishment] in bringing quality health care to the American people" (Payton and Powsner 1980: 239). As cost escalation persisted and led to calls for action, the

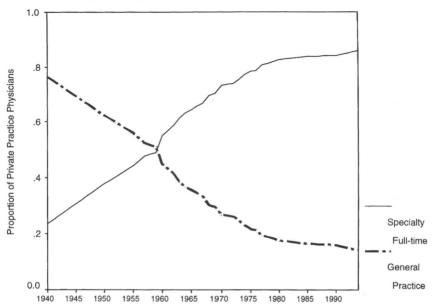

Figure 6.3   General and Specialist Practitioners in the United States, 1940–94

NOTE: Private practice defined as office-based, active nonfederal MDs.

SOURCES: PHS (1962), U.S. Bureau of the Census (1945–96).

assumption, consistent with the logics of the era, was that "voluntary sector self-discipline was preferable to government intervention" (Payton and Powsner 1980: 259). The changing logics, actors, and governance arrangements constructed to deal with the problem of increasing costs are well illustrated in the evolution of health planning regimes (see Case Illustration 6.A).

Secondary logics (i.e., those of lesser scope, salience, and centrality) often exist alongside dominant logics. Such logics act sometimes to support, sometimes to undermine primary logics. An example of the former coexisting with the value of quality of care during the first era was that of the *voluntary ethos,* a complex of beliefs linking hospitals and other healthcare organizations to charitable work and to community service.

As healthcare systems expanded in the United States through the first half of the twentieth century, organized provision of medical care became structured primarily into two arenas: nonprofit, "voluntary" health systems serving the majority of Americans, and local (municipal or county) public systems for the poor and indigent (Boychuk 1994). Both systems were tightly linked to local community institutions and funding sources.

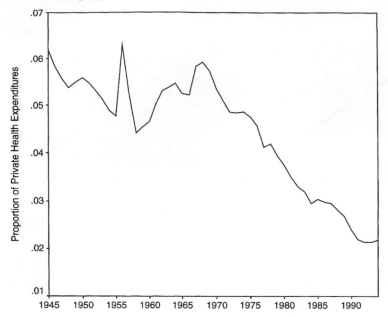

Figure 6.4   Private Philanthropy for Health and Hospitals in the United States, 1945–94

NOTE: Philanthropic funding shown as a proportion of total national private (i.e., nongovernmental) health expenditures.

SOURCES: American Association of Fundraising Councils (1997), U.S. Bureau of the Census (1975).

Private, nonprofit hospitals were deeply embedded in their communities, receiving financial assistance from local philanthropic groups and support from community elites who served on their governing boards and oversaw auxiliary services mobilizing volunteers (Belknap and Steinle 1963; Burns 1990; Faxon 1949; Perrow 1963; Pfeffer 1973; Rosen 1963). A useful indicator of this ethos is the level of private philanthropic giving in the sector. Figure 6.4 shows that private philanthropy was at its height during the two decades following World War II, declining in importance after 1965 relative to other sources of private funding.[8] Private nonprofit organizations were more likely to be "donative," depending on donor contributions, than "commercial," depending on the collection of fees, during the era of professional dominance (Hansmann 1987: 30).

8. The unusual "spike" in philanthropic contributions in 1956 is due to an unexplained, one-time $270 million increase in the amount contributed to hospitals and health in that year. Although the total amount of philanthropy for health and hospitals continues to increase, it has done so at a rate far less than the rise in total private health expenditures (see fig. 6.4).

More generally, the prevalence of nonprofit organizations in this sector (including the early major medical insurance plans of Blue Cross and Blue Shield, which operated as nonprofit insurance carriers) has long signified the dominance of a service ethic as opposed to a commercial orientation (Marmor, Schlesinger, and Smithey 1987). As for the public facilities in this arena, the large majority of these hospitals and related care units were municipal and county facilities, being watched over by local civic bodies and politicians. The continuing salience of the voluntary ethos throughout the era of professional dominance is reflected in the attributes of the organizational actors prevalent during this period.

Actors. The principal types of actors during the era of professional dominance were (1) physicians, the great majority of whom were engaged in individual private practice or small partnership forms; (2) professional associations of physicians, nurses, hospital administrators, and numerous other occupations; (3) hospitals, including nonprofit voluntary forms and local public facilities, as well as a few for-profit providers; and (4) private nonprofit and commercial insurance carriers.[9] This was, as some have termed it, the era of "push-cart" medicine. Physicians practiced alone or in very small shared offices. As figure 3.14 reports, there were only 10 medical groups containing more than 6 physicians operating in the Bay area in 1945, the number increasing only slowly until the 1960s. The principal organizational form for delivering more complex health services was the hospital, and most were either independent, voluntary, nonprofit, or local governmental units (see fig. 3.5). Hospitals continued to flourish throughout the first era. As figure 3.15 documents, in the Bay area, hospitals achieved their highest density levels in 1965; other types of more specialized provider forms were not significant players until after this date. And, as already described, third-party insurance carriers were, throughout this period, constructed to be passive players.

Precursors of Change

Institutional arrangements, by their nature, are unlikely to change abruptly. Even when change appears sudden, it is usually possible to find evidence of earlier forces at work. These forces can be of two types: they may be factors undermining the current arrangements, or they may represent precursors to new logics and forms.

---

9. As discussed in chapter 2, collective units such as organizations and associations also function as governance structures.

Onset of Fragmentation. The first era is characterized by the strength and unity of organized medicine, and so it is noteworthy that, as figure 6.1 documents, the AMA—at national, state, and county levels—begins to suffer membership losses from the 1950s forward. How are we to account for this change? We believe a variety of factors operated to bring about a reduction in the power and unity of organized medicine. These include (1) an increase in the relative numbers of physicians (see fig. 5.5), resulting in increased levels of competition among them; (2) increases in the proportion of physicians employed in organizational settings; (3) increases in the relative numbers of women and foreign-trained physicians;[10] and (4) increases in the numbers of specialist physicians (see fig. 6.3). It is notable that 1960, a few years prior to the end of the first era, witnessed both a marked increased in the ratio of physicians to population and the point at which specialist practitioners first outnumbered generalists.

The growth in the numbers and types of specialists within medicine has a twofold significance. On the one hand, it serves as an important indicator of the value placed by American medicine on improving quality of medical care. On the other hand, while the growth of specialties was endorsed by and occurred under the auspices of the AMA, the development of each new specialization was accompanied by the emergence of a new specialty association that competed with and undermined the power and centrality of the AMA and, thereby, the unity of the profession. The proliferation of specialty associations, combined with the decline in membership and power of the general medical association, thus also serves as an important indicator of the increasing *fragmentation* of organized medicine (see Stevens 1971: 211–12).

Between 1917, when the first specialty board (for ophthalmology) was incorporated, up to 1991, when the latest board (for medical genetics) was approved, 24 primary boards had been established. Each represents the successful effort by a collection of specialists to secure recognition for, and to standardize training in, a specialized area of practice. While the number of primary boards has only gradually increased since the beginning of our study period in 1945, the number of general and, especially, subspecialty certificates has increased rapidly since 1970 (see fig. 6.5), and continues throughout eras two and three. Each of these subspecialties has its own

---

10. Foreign-trained physicians were often discouraged from joining the AMA. Women may or may not have also met barriers but have joined in much smaller numbers than men. During the early 1980s, for example, when 48 percent of the men in the profession were members, only 27 percent of the women were members of the AMA (Starr 1982: 427).

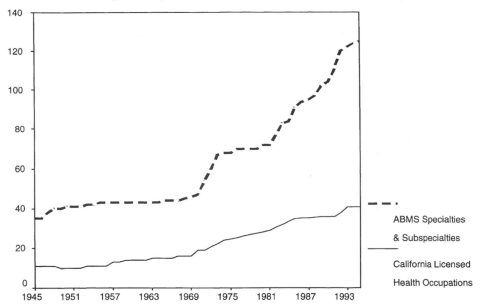

Figure 6.5 American Medical Board Specialties and California Licensed Health Occupations, 1945–95

NOTE: ABMS specialties and subspecialties include the number of medical specialty boards and their respective general and subspecialty certificates.

SOURCE: American Board of Medical Specialties (1996), California Department of Consumer Affairs (1971–95), McCready & Harris (1995), Newman (1991).

association of loyal physician members (ABMS 1996).[11] Increases in specialization and in specialist associations have paralleled decreases in AMA membership.

This fragmentation within the structure of the medical profession has been mirrored in the licensure of health occupations in general, which in the U.S. occurs predominantly at the state level of government. In California, physicians and surgeons were able to institute a lasting state-sponsored regulatory regime only after a good deal of struggle from the 1870s to the turn of the century. In the period that followed, only a handful of mainstream (e.g., dentists, pharmacists) and alternative practitioners (e.g., chiropractors, osteopaths) obtained new licensing boards (McCready

11. As a federation of associations, the American Board of Medical Specialties (ABMS), provides advisory and coordinative functions but has not attempted to supplant the AMA as the voice of organized medicine. Founded as the Advisory Board for Medical Specialties in 1933, the ABMS was reorganized into its current form in 1970. It has remained in a mainly advisory capacity, however, with respect to its constitutive boards (ABMS 1996).

and Harris 1995). From 1945 to 1969, during the height of the medical profession's dominance, the total number of licensed occupations grew by only five, from 11 to 16 (see fig. 6.5), and most of these involved newly sanctioned paraprofessional groups (e.g., vocational nurses, physical therapists, and mental health workers). The roles of these "allied" health occupations generally fit within the traditional hierarchy of care that places doctors at the pinnacle.

The 1970s, however, witnessed an explosion in the number and range of healthcare providers acquiring official licensure, a phenomenon that has continued to the present (California Department of Consumer Affairs 1971–95). As with medical specialties, which as described also began to expand at the same time, many fledgling vocations developed around advances in medical technologies (for example, hearing aid dispensers, electroneuromyographers, and respiratory care technicians). Although broadening the range of specialized roles in medical care, these providers still roughly fall within the established occupational order. But several of the recent occupations (e.g., physician assistants and nurse practitioners) define their work and expertise in ways that encroach on and erode the exclusive discretion of physicians in the delivery of care. Moreover, this latter period has included the introduction, and reintroduction, of alternative health practitioners (e.g., acupuncturists and midwives, respectively) whose jurisdictional claims over professional knowledge directly challenge the authority and purview of traditionally organized medicine. Currently in California, over 40 officially approved health occupations share in the provision of, and increasingly in the direction over, medical treatment and services.

Mirroring these trends in fragmentation, there is much evidence to suggest that, from the 1970s onward, the power of organized medicine to control developments within the healthcare sector has been significantly reduced (see Starr 1982; Campion 1984; Krause 1997). Many of the most important developments in health policy were (unsuccessfully) opposed by the AMA. At the very least, the health professions—of which the AMA remains the leading example—have been obliged to share their governance functions with new and different participants, first with public agencies and, in the third era of managerial control, with private corporations.

Increasing federal role. The fragmentation of physician power is but one factor allowing change in the institutional arrangement in place during the first era. Another factor conducive to change was the development of a secondary institutional logic during the era of professional dominance that helped to pave the way for the emergence of the era that followed. This logic held that there was a public interest in both the quality and availability of medical care. Given the medical profession's resistance to any form of national health insurance or program, this logic had its chief expression during the first two decades after World War II in federal support for health research, facilities construction, and medical education and training.

Beginning during the nineteenth century, the U.S. government had provided health care and facilities for military personnel and veterans, and a modest program in medical research at the Marine Hospital Service gradually evolved in 1938 into the National Institutes of Health. As late as 1945, the Rockefeller Foundation and a handful of other private philanthropies provided most of the financial support for medical research but, following the war, federal support rose rapidly; the budget for the National Institutes of Health increased from $180,000 in 1945 to over $400 million in 1960 (Starr 1982: 342–46). Funding for national laboratories was only one aspect of federal support for biomedical research. In addition, federal support grew rapidly during this period for research conducted by scientists outside government, principally those working in universities and medical schools. These research programs, which were based on investigator-initiated proposals reviewed for scientific merit by a committee of peers, "not only advanced knowledge, but significantly enhanced teaching programs to the eventual benefit of medical practice" (Fredrickson 1977: 161). As figure 6.6 indicates, national expenditures on medical research began their climb in the decade following World War II, and the public—mostly federal—component increased very rapidly during the decade 1955–65, although more gradually thereafter (Strickland 1972).

The other major facet of federal support for medicine during this period involved programs directed toward increasing the availability of healthcare—specifically, medical facilities and physicians' services—to the American public. Support for the construction of medical facilities, typically hospitals and especially in rural areas, was provided under the Hospital Survey and Construction Act, passed in 1946 (see also chap. 7). The legislation, better known as the Hill-Burton program, was careful to limit political, particularly federal, discretion regarding decisions on which projects were to be funded. A formula was devised for allocating money among the states based on their population, number of existing beds, and per capita income; states, in turn, estimated regional needs and responded to grant requests prepared by individual applicants. Between 1947 and 1971, $3.7 billion was disbursed under the program (Saward 1977; Starr 1982). Total expenditures on health facilities from all public and private sources during

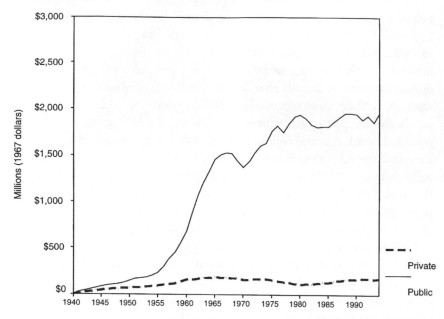

Figure 6.6   Expenditures for Medical Research in the United States, 1940–94
NOTE: Figure does not include R&D expenditures of private pharmaceutical firms.
SOURCE: U.S. Bureau of the Census (1975, 1945–96).

the period of study are reported in figure 6.7. These data reveal two waves in public funding, with the first rapid increase in federal funding occurring after 1947 and a second, larger wave starting in the late 1960s. Private funding for facilities paralleled public until about 1960, when it surpassed governmental funding and continued to increase until 1975.

The second major program, passed late in the era, provided federal support for increasing the supply of physicians. As described in chapter 5, the Health Professions Educational Act (HPEA) of 1963 led to a rapid expansion in the number of physicians by supporting the construction of new, and the enlargement of existing, educational facilities (Thompson 1981; fig. 5.4). Although intended both as a means of expanding opportunity for professional employment and improving access to medical care for underserved populations, this program had the unanticipated effect of increasing competition among physicians in subsequent eras.

During the era of professional dominance, the logics supporting public involvement in medicine restricted governmental support to the funding of infrastructures—such as support for research or service and training

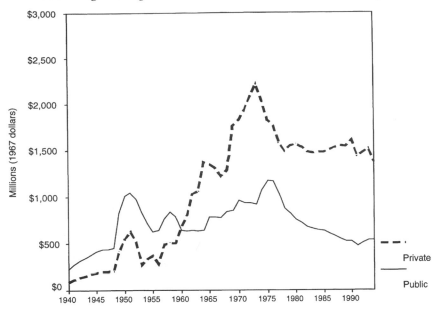

Figure 6.7   Expenditures for Medical Facilities Construction in the United States, 1940–94
SOURCE: U.S. Bureau of the Census (1975, 1945–96).

facilities. Professional interests strongly resisted more direct involvement in payment for medical care. Moreover, as noted, the programs were designed to allow public payment for research and facilities but to restrict severely governmental involvement in decisions as to how these funds were to be distributed among claimants. These programs involved centralization of funding in the absence of centralized programmatic controls, a frequently observed pattern of governmental activity in "weak" national states (Meyer 1983; Scott and Meyer 1983, 1991).

Nevertheless, aided by hindsight, we can observe that the Hill-Burton program and the HPEA represented two important early initiatives by which the federal government became involved in health planning activities, a major focus of federal attention during the second era. This is apparent from an inspection of figures 6.8a and 6.8b, which display two "policy maps"—one for the nation, one for California—in which we attempt to encapsulate the major legislative and policy events during the study period. The tables distinguish among four regulatory arenas: (1) *professional licensing and monitoring* of occupations and services; (2) *health planning,* including support for facility construction; (3) *rate setting,* including pub-

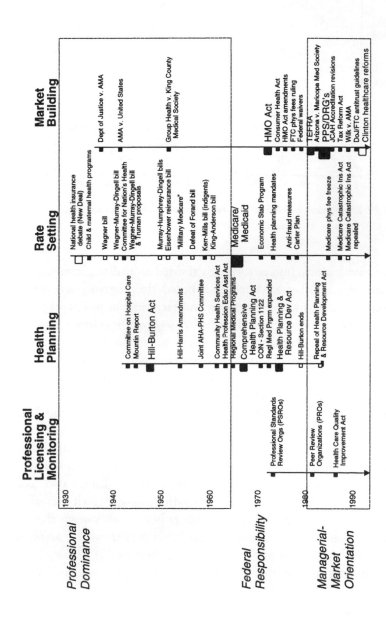

Figure 6.8a U.S. Regulatory Policy in Healthcare Services, 1930–93

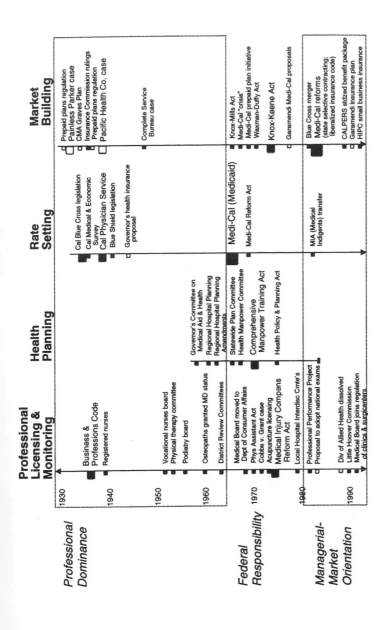

Figure 6.8b California Regulatory Policy in Healthcare Services, 1930–93

NOTE: Empty boxes indicate significant non-events, policy failures, or regulatory reversals. Box size reflects relative importance of event.

SOURCES: Bergthold (1984), Brown (1986), Brown and Cousineau (1984), California Task Force (1971), Christianson et al. (1991), Estes et al. (1992), Grant (1988), HIAA (1995), Hospitals and Related Health Facilities and Services Planning Committee (1968), Keigher (1983), May (1967), McCready and Harris (1995), Payton and Powsner (1980), Robert Wood Johnson Foundation (1994), Starr (1982), Thompson (1981), Tom (1984), Weeks and Berman (1985).

lic reimbursement of medical costs; (4) and *market building*—efforts to encourage competition and provide incentives for cost containment.

The vertical dimension provides a timeline, extending from 1930 to 1990, and distinguishes the three major eras we have identified. Each event is labeled, with its significance suggested by the relative size of the box adjoining the event. An "empty" or blank box indicates a policy failure (e.g., legislative proposals that did not pass) or the ending of an administrative program. The "white spaces" in the maps, revealing the absence of any events in a category, are as revealing as the active arenas, those containing many events. A glance at figure 6.8a, for example, reveals the lack of significant regulatory activity at the federal level (as well as the failure of attempts to engage in such action) during the first era. Institutional eras are defined as much by the absence of events and actors as by their presence. The Hill-Burton Act stands out in sharp relief as the first important regulatory initiative by the federal government in the healthcare arena.

Figure 6.8b reveals that there was more regulatory activity at the state than at the national level in the first era. States during this period were most active in the area of professional licensing. Important legislation related to health financing arrangements was implemented, however, mostly for the purpose of excepting the Blue Cross and Blue Shield insurance plans— community-based organizations governed by professionally dominated, nonprofit private systems at the state level—from the financial requirements and antimonopoly restrictions imposed on commercial insurers (Payton and Powsner 1980; Grant 1988).

Summary

The first era was characterized by a cozy and consistent pattern of professional dominance. Professional associations, particularly those involving physicians, comprised the primary governance regime. The central logics, stressing quality of medical care, provided guidance to the structuring of activities as well as an important legitimating frame to support professional hegemony. They even provided a rationale for medical costs, which began to rise as early as 1945, linking it with improvements in quality of care. The other principal actors—insurance carriers, public agencies— were constituted so as to provide maximum support for and minimum interference with professional autonomy. Public actors primarily confirmed and augmented professional prerogatives, serving as licensing agents at the state level and as sources of funding for research and facilities at the federal level—essential, but peripheral to the delivery of care.

Through close historical inspection, however, signs of change during this period are also visible. Increasing specialization among physicians began to erode their organizational and political unity, and heightened federal activity in providing resources began to create a strengthening presumption of a public interest in healthcare. A liberal political administration coming to power in the 1960s would exploit these openings.

The Era of Federal Involvement (1966–82)

Principal Indicators

Governance structures. The onset of the second era is marked by the passage of the Medicare/Medicaid bill, the crowning achievement of President Lyndon Johnson's Great Society agenda. With this legislation, the U.S. government became a major player in the healthcare arena for the first time. The passage of this legislation in 1965 ushered in a major period of expanded governmental involvement in healthcare services, first in the role of purchaser and subsequently, when the escalation of healthcare costs precipitated a crisis in public finance, as regulator. We consider both roles.

Funding is obviously an important general resource required by all organizations and, thus, is properly considered to be an aspect of the material-resource environment (detailed in chap. 5). But the nature of funding sources and their associated programmatic definitions and restrictions provide important information regarding changes in institutional logics and governance structures. Programs carrying public funding have a different meaning from those that rely on private funds, and even when public financing is involved, great differences can occur in the extent to which the programmatic decisions are centralized or decentralized (Scott and Meyer 1991). Such considerations can greatly affect the structure of organizational fields. For example, DiMaggio (1983) has shown that the increased centralization in federal funding for the arts acted to increase the overall structuration of that organizational field.

Federal funding for healthcare services was for many years limited to supporting basic health research and, with Hill-Burton and HPEA legislation, expenditures for health and educational facilities. With the limited exception of funds for specially targeted client groups, state and local sources provided the bulk of public funding for healthcare services in the United States. Change occurred abruptly, in 1965, with the passage of the Medicare and Medicaid acts. With this landmark Great Society legislation, the federal government became the largest single purchaser of healthcare services. And, for the first time in the United States, public expenditures for health and medical services began to approach the level of private expenditures (see fig. 6.9). This watershed legislation, designed to provide greater equity of access to healthcare services for the elderly and indigent, signaled in a dramatic manner the onset of the era of federal involvement. Beginning in 1965 the Medicare program expended funds in the San Francisco area at roughly twice the level of local (county) expenditures, with Medicaid expenditures not far behind (see fig. 5.3). And governmental programs suddenly became a significant source of health coverage in this country (fig. 6.2).

With the large, rapid infusion of new funds into the sector, the Medicare and Medicaid programs exacerbated what, for some years, had already been perceived to be a problem: the elevation of medical care costs. This condition continued at about the same level well into the 1970s, but in this era increasingly came to be framed as a *public* issue, requiring attention from the federal government.

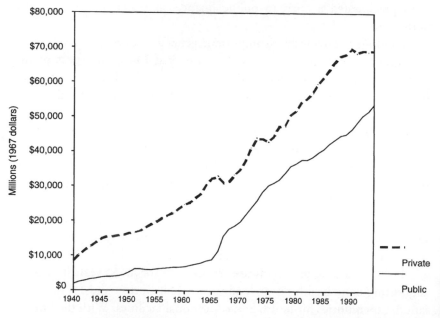

Figure 6.9   Expenditures for Health and Medical Services in the United States, 1940–94
SOURCE: U.S. Bureau of the Census (1975, 1945–96).

It is largely for this reason that the rapid rise in federal funding was accompanied by a substantial increase in the number and types of regulatory bodies operating at the federal level. The number of agencies increased particularly rapidly between 1950 and 1955 (the period following the introduction of the Hill-Burton program) and again during 1965–75, following the passage of Medicare/Medicaid (see fig. 6.10). During this period, federal agencies were created not only to administer the funds allocated under Medicare/Medicaid but to monitor health quality and, in particular, to attempt to rationalize the numbers, locations, and types of medical facilities. Existing local and regional agencies engaged in health planning were coopted and their efforts redirected to attempt to curb costs (see Case Illustration 6.A; Payton and Powsner 1980). Figure 6.8a displays the burst of regulatory activity at the national level that erupted during this second era, involving new legislative initiatives in all four categories: licensing, health planning, rate setting, and market building.

Health agencies at the state level, in California, grew more gradually between 1950 and 1970, after which time their rate of growth increased (see fig. 6.10). The spurt in health policy activity at the federal level in the mid-1960s did not cause waves in California until a few years later. Figure 6.8b shows the major, related activities that were spawned at the state level, in California. This lag between federal and state action is even more clearly seen when we examine the total numbers of pages devoted to "health" and "medical" topics in federal and California statute indexes (see fig. 6.11). Federal statutes in these categories markedly increased beginning in 1965 whereas, in California, state legislation did not begin to expand rapidly until after 1975. Similarly, it was not until after 1970 that Bay area health planning bodies began to increase in numbers (see fig. 6.10). Although state agencies had been more numerous than federal prior to 1955, the federal programs rapidly overtook them. Federal and state programs grew in a parallel manner between 1955 and 1965 in part because programs like Medicaid were operated as partnership programs. State agencies did not begin their rapid expansion until after 1970, in the Nixon era, at which time a number of federal programs were devolved to state and local levels. During the second era, federal, state, and local governmental agencies substantially increased their size and capacity to exercise oversight functions. Physicians and other health professionals had acquired a new partner in governance.

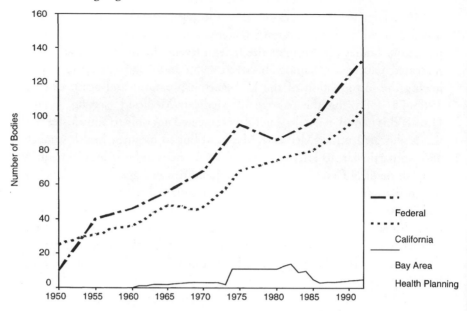

Figure 6.10   Health-Related Regulatory Bodies in the United States, California, and the Bay Area, 1950–92

NOTE: Federal government includes department, bureau, office-level units, and independent boards and commissions. California government includes all agencies, except office-level units. Bay Area Health Planning is restricted to bodies at the local level and includes voluntary and comprehensive planning committees, health services agencies (HSAs), professional standards review organizations (PSROs), and community and employer health coalitions.

SOURCES: U.S. Office of the Federal Register (1950–95), Newman (1991), California Department of General Services (1970–95), California Secretary of State (1940–75), California Office of the Governor (1975–91, 1992–96), California Hospitals and Related Health Facilities and Services Planning Committee (1968), BACHPC (1971–76), U.S. Congress (1974), AHA (1986, 1992), U.S. Chamber of Commerce (1984, 1985), PHS (1981).

It is neither feasible nor necessary for us to attempt to review developments in all of the four regulatory streams charted in figures 6.8a and 6.8b. Rather, we selected one area, health planning, for detailed discussion (see Case Illustration 6.A). The evolution of the governance structures in the area of health planning illustrates a general pattern of change, but also provides evidence of some of the more nuanced developments in the institutional environment of healthcare organizations. While health planning is most clearly associated with the era of federal involvement, it preceded and outlived this period and has reflected the logics, both dominant and secondary, of each era.

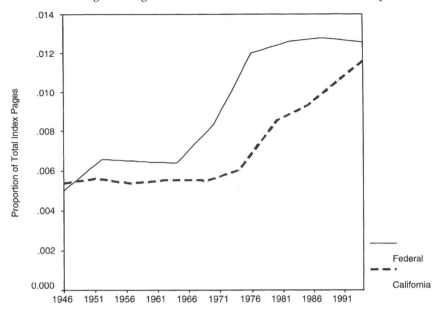

Figure 6.11 Health-Related Index Pages in United States and California Statutory Codes, 1946–94

NOTE: Page counts are limited to "Health," "Medic," and "Public Health" headings and are standardized by the total number of pages in each index per year.

SOURCES: U.S. Superintendent of Documents (1946–94), Larmac (1945–94).

Case Illustration 6.A Health Planning: Refractions of Changing Logics

Over the fifty-year course of our study, health planning structures exhibited change along numerous dimensions: the composition of actors, the salience of planning for different organizations, the centrality of planning as a set of institutional logics, and the cognitive content of the term's meaning. We discuss these changes as they developed in five health planning regimes operating between 1930 and 1980 (see table 6.A.1 for a summary). At times, the establishment of a new set of structures replaced preceding arrangements, but at other times, the previous structures continued to exist alongside the newer forms. In addition, local, state, and federal actors were involved in health planning, sometimes working in concert, sometimes at cross-purposes. Such processes lead to varying degrees of regulatory fragmentation and complexity within the overall governance structures of the field and, at times, to outright conflict.

Private, Philanthropic Regime (1930–46)

In the period predating our study, health planning was dominated by private philanthropic organizations, such as the Kellogg, Commonwealth, and Rockefeller

Table 6.A.1 Health Planning Governance Regimes, 1932–82

Regime	Year	Associated Report	Associated Legislation	Sources	Structures Established	Geographic Scope	Salience	Cognitive Content
Private philanthropic	1932	Committee on the Costs of Medical Care	n.a.	Philanthropic foundations	n.a.	n.a.	Delivery system-wide	Systemwide integrated planning
	1944	Committee on Hospital Care	n.a.	AHA, philanthropic foundations	n.a.	n.a.	Hospitals	Bed capacity distribution
Hospital bed rationalization	1947	n.a.	Hospital Survey and Construction Act (Hill-Burton)	Federal government	State-level hospital advisory council	State	Hospitals	Bed capacity distribution
Voluntary coordination	1961	Joint Committee of AHA and U.S. Public Health Service	1964 Hill-Harris Amendment to Hill-Burton	AHA, federal government	Local areawide, voluntary planning agencies (HFP)	Local Bay Area	Hospitals	Integration to increase efficiency
	1965	n.a.	Hospital and Related Health Facilities and Service Planning Committee (SB 543)	California state government	Local areawide, voluntary planning agencies (HFP)	Local Bay Area	Hospitals and related facilities	Integration to increase efficiency
Comprehensive community-based	1966	n.a.	Comprehensive Health Planning and Public Health Service Amendments (PL 89-749)	Federal government	Local comprehensive health planning committees (CHP)	Local Bay Area	Delivery system-wide	Equity and access, participation
Cost containment	1974	n.a.	Health Planning and Resources Development Act (PL 93-641)	Federal government	Local health system areas (HSA)	Local subarea (North Bay, West Bay, East Bay, Santa Clara)	Hospitals	Cost-containment, certificate-of-need (CON)

NOTE: n.a. = not applicable.

SOURCES: May (1967), Weeks and Berman (1985), BACHPC (1971–76), California Hospitals and Related Health Facilities Services Planning Committee (1968).

Foundations, as well as professional provider groups such as the American Medical Association (AMA) and the American Hospital Association (AHA). This private, philanthropic regime emphasized "intimate, organic relationships" and encouraged the formation of regional hospital systems (May 1967). Although lacking in coercive power, these actors did exercise significant normative influence on the professional and community groups. The role of planning was to provide information and support to strengthen these local, informal cooperative systems, while not infringing on the independence of communities or the autonomy of professional actors.

Hospital Bed Rationalization Regime (1947–60)

The federal government's passage of the Hill-Burton Act in 1946 initiated a new era of health planning that identified a more central role for both states and the federal government. The act required that each state develop a comprehensive plan for hospital facility construction with the goal of insuring a rational, geographic distribution of hospital beds. With this legislation, for the first time the federal government entered the healthcare delivery arena in a significant way, dispersing more than $3.7 billion between 1947 and 1971. The Hill-Burton regime witnessed the creation of a set of formal mechanisms to allocate public resources for hospital construction. It also created a direct partnership between federal and state authorities, forging a linkage that, over time, would increase in significance. Most observers of the program believe that, while the program did serve to reduce differences among the states, its primary effect was to shunt funds toward middle-class communities (since communities were required to raise two-thirds of the funds involved) and to increase the average size of existing hospitals (Thompson 1981; Starr 1982).

Voluntary Coordination Regime (1961–65)

During the late 1950s, a joint committee of the AHA and the U.S. Public Health Service initiated a more integrated approach to planning. The committee's 1961 report recommended the expansion and formalization of voluntary community planning efforts. By 1966, the number of these voluntary areawide planning committees had grown from 9 to over 80 (May 1967).

In California, legislation passed in the early 1960s created three regional hospital advisory committees and a statewide structure of voluntary heath facility planning committees. By 1968, this network had expanded to include 52 of California's 58 counties. The Health Facility Planning Council (HFPC), with boundaries contiguous with the nine-county Bay Area, was established in 1965 but was limited in that it focused exclusively on hospitals and its recommendations were not backed by sanctions of any sort. Also, its recommendations sometimes conflicted with the statewide Hospital Advisory Council, which held the legal authority to distribute the state's Hill-Burton funds.

In addition to adding a new layer of committees, this period was also marked by the introduction of certificate-of-need (CON) regulation in many states. These procedures were developed by a coalition of Blue Cross, hospital, and public health interests as a way of educating "the public to the increasing quality and expense of good hospital care and thereby lead to public acceptance of rising costs" (Payton and Powsner 1980: 204).

Comprehensive Health Planning Regime (1966–73)

In 1966, the federal government passed the Comprehensive Health Planning and Public Health Service amendments. This legislation created a virtual mandate for comprehensive health planning and extended its scope beyond facilities to include planning for services and manpower. Payton and Powsner (1980: 211) point out that "regionalized health planning was only one of a number of contemporary commitments to greater discipline in the use of public resources," other areas receiving attention being schools, housing, and transportation systems. This legislation coincided with the passage of Medicare and Medicaid and, hence, was imbued with the ethic of providing accessible basic health services to the entire community. For the first time, insuring access and equity to the underserved became a major objective of health planning efforts.

The amendments generated a new set of institutional actors and governance structures that were not consistent in geographic scope or mission with the previous set of facilities-planning organizations created by the state. For instance, the Bay Area Comprehensive Health Planning Council (BACHPC), created in 1968 by federal action, coexisted alongside the state's Bay Area HFPC until 1970, when the two entities were merged.

Health planning also began to incorporate consumer and alternative health logics during this regime (Lee 1976; Blum 1976; Fink 1976). In the Bay Area, for example, the targets set in 1971 for the first areawide regional health plan included environmental health as a major concern, as well as social issues related to health services, facilities, and manpower. And, in 1972, goals for the BACHPC included a public better and more directly involved in decisions affecting its health (BACHPC 1971, 1972).

Cost-Containment Regime (1973–82)

The fifth, and final, health planning regime, formally recognized in 1974 with the passage of the federal Health Planning and Resource Development Act, emphasized cost-containment. The legislation established a nationwide system of Health Service Areas (HSAs), which were given the authority to administer CON procedures. These procedures, originally developed by health professionals to justify increasing costs, were redirected by governmental agencies to control rising costs. CON represented an attempt to increase the authority of the planners in controlling unwarranted expansion (Melhado 1988). Health facilities planning expansion or the addition of major equipment were required to justify these expenditures by providing evidence of unmet needs in the communities served.

In the Bay Area, the BACHPC was subdivided into four HSAs, and considerable confusion and conflict ensued between the new agencies, the earlier council, and county officials. By 1976, state legislation was passed to create a formal state-level governance structure for the HSA system, and the CON program was expanded to cover any capital investment over $150,000. Yet evidence soon began to accumulate that CON procedures did not succeed in controlling the escalation of costs (e.g., Salkever and Bice 1976; Sloan and Steinwald 1980). In 1982, the Reagan administration disbanded the national Health Systems Agencies.

By the end of the 1970s, public planning regimes were considered ineffective—particularly since they were now evaluated solely as a tool for containing costs. In the 1930s, the government had been a bystander, as officials took the position "that voluntary sector self-discipline was preferable to government intervention" (Payton and Powsner 1980: 259). The result was that professional self-interests held sway. During the era of federal involvement, the regimes created involved the addition of bureaucratic layers at first intended to encourage, then, later, to require the rationalization of local delivery systems. Although not formally involved in health planning, healthcare corporations and coalitions of health purchasers have continued the cost-containing regime (see chap. 8).

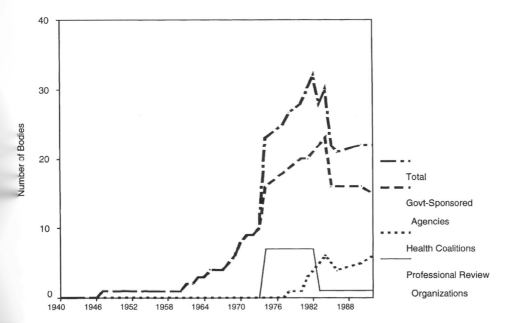

igure 6.A.1 Bay Area Health Planning Bodies by Type, 1940–92

OTES: Figure includes both local and state-level agencies with Bay Area jurisdiction.

overnment-sponsored agencies are comprised of voluntary and comprehensive planning ommittees, health services agencies (HSAs), and state planning boards and commissions. Health oalitions include community and employer health coalitions, councils, and purchasing groups. rofessional review organizations consist of professional standards and peer review organizations 'SROs and PROs).

URCES: Newman (1991), California Department of General Services (1970–95), California Secretary of ate (1940–75), California Office of the Governor (1975–91, 1992–96), California Hospitals and Related ealth Facilities and Services Planning Committee (1968), BACHPC (1971–76), U.S. Congress (1974), ɪristy (1993), AHA (1986, 1992), U.S. Chamber of Commerce (1984, 1985), PHS (1981).

Summary: The Many Meanings of Planning

Figure 6.A.1 charts the rise and fall of various types of health planning bodies having jurisdiction in the Bay Area from 1945 to 1995. We note the rapid increase of governmental agencies from 1965 to 1985, then a marked decline. We also observe the rise of the new coalitions of health purchasers in the 1980s, which began to assume important planning and regulatory functions. Note that the structures associated with one governance regime do not quickly disappear but often linger on, creating a layering of health planning bodies.

We also chart the rise and fall of a set of keywords related to health planning in *Modern Healthcare,* a major journal targeted to medical care administrators (our search was limited to article title and subject indices). Figure 6.A.2 records the percentage of articles published during the period 1966–95 containing the keyword "health planning." While these data were not available for the first two decades of our study period, they tell a story quite consistent with our brief survey: health planning as a significant governance tool began to develop during the late 1960s and reached its apex during the decade of the 1970s, after which time it became less prominent.

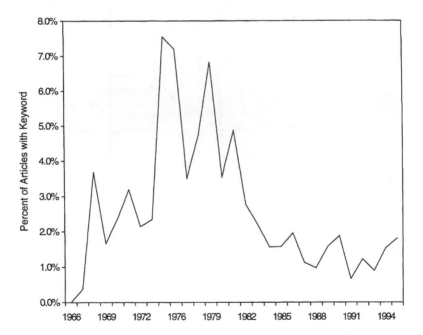

Figure 6.A.2   Health Planning Articles, *Modern Healthcare,* 1966–95

NOTES: Keywords are phrases included in an article's title, abstract, or database subject headings.

Article counts for each keyword are standardized by the total number of articles per year. Data for 1974 omitted because of change in journal format.

SOURCES: MEDLINE periodicals database (National Library of Medicine, 1998).

Since the meanings and mechanisms associated with the term "planning" have changed over time, we examined the relationship between "planning" and several other keywords. Table 6.A.2 reports the frequency with which ten terms appear in the titles and subject index in combination with the term "planning" during three periods: 1966–74, the dominant period of community health planning activities; 1975–80, the transition period in which attention turned primarily to planning as a tool for cost-containment, and 1980–85, the early years of market competition. The first three keywords reveal a conception of planning as oriented to the needs of the wider community with a focus on hospitals as the primary players. The second three reflect the shift from a voluntary community focus to a regulative, agency-centered agenda; and the last four show the increasingly negative connotations associated with planning and the involvement of business coalitions and corporate care systems in the planning process. We note that the first cluster of terms is concentrated in the first period 1966–74, the second, in the period 1975–80 and the third, in the period 1980 to 1985, a pattern consistent with our historical review.

Table 6.A.2 Modifications in Meanings of Health Planning, *Modern Healthcare*, 1966–85

Associated Terms	1966–74	1975–79	1980–85
Community needs	9	1	1
General health care system	10	0	0
Hospitals as major participants	10	1	5
Certificate-of-need	0	12	6
HSA state agencies	3	11	7
Health care legislation	5	8	3
Health planning (negative)	0	1	8
Healthcare systems (corporate)	0	0	5
Market, competition	0	2	2
Business coalitions	0	0	7

SOURCE: MEDLINE periodicals database (National Library of Medicine, 1998).

Logics. The principal logic underlying these new programs was the Great Society vision of enhanced *equity of access* to healthcare services—increasingly viewed as a right of all citizens (Callahan 1977). Healthcare was only one of many arenas within which liberal reformers attempted to secure greater equality of opportunity and outcomes. Other notable federal initiatives addressed problems of income inequality and racial injustice. Thus, while the new logics resonated with ideas held by some participants in the healthcare field, they were largely imported into the field as part of a broader public philosophy (Marmor, Mashaw, and Harvey 1990). In healthcare, reforms were targeted to involve two categories of citizens—the elderly and the indigent—that were recognized as having high unmet needs.

The Great Society programs served the new logic of increasing access for underserved groups but did not directly challenge the previously existing professional logic stressing quality of care as defined by professional standards. Physicians' and hospitals' interests were represented in the legislation. Freedom of provider choice was protected; "fiscal intermediaries," typically Blue Cross and Blue Shield, buffered providers from dealing directly with governmental agencies paying the bills; and hospitals and physicians were to be reimbursed for "usual and customary" costs, reflecting community standards of care (Starr 1982: 375).

Throughout this period, however, and especially after 1970, observers focused their attention on increasing costs. Many actors, especially economists, began to challenge the notion that health was to be valued above all other considerations. High quality and broad access to medical care were, of course, desirable, but at what cost (Fuchs 1974)? As described below, a search for new governance mechanisms to rein in healthcare expenditures became a leading priority for reformers. Gradually, the logic of cost containment worked to undermine the professionals' pursuit of quality and the government's interest in access. Both quality and access began to be framed as relative rather than absolute values—desirable but costly, worthy but not at any price.

Actors. The era of federal involvement was accompanied, as we have seen, by the rapid proliferation of a host of new federal and state agencies engaged in some aspect of healthcare funding, oversight, or planning (see figs. 6.11 and 6.A.1). Armies of bureaucrats were assembled to staff these new agencies. In addition to the managers, statisticians, and accountants, the new staff members included professional social scientists, especially in the latter decades, economists.

Associated with the federal initiatives were a number of innovative medical delivery forms, not included among the organizational populations we surveyed, which embodied and attempted to implement the logic of increasing access to underserved populations. These included maternal and infant care programs, neighborhood health centers, and community mental health centers (Stevens 1971). We did not collect specific data on these providers, but a useful indicator of the new level of activity stimulated by these and related initiatives is provided by the increase observed in the proportion of nonmilitary physicians employed in federal programs. This workforce increased from just over 20,000 physicians in 1965 to over

30,000 physicians by 1969 only to decrease again to earlier levels after 1975. These physicians were primarily involved in staffing the new federal domestic programs engaged in direct health delivery (see AMA 1959–73, 1974–79, 1981–98).

With respect to the organizational actors in our five populations, it is early in the federal era that hospitals achieved their highest density in the Bay area only to begin their long, slow decline after 1968 (see fig. 3.3). It was also during this era that the other, specialized populations—home health agencies, renal disease centers, and health maintenance organizations—first appeared or began their significant increase in numbers. In this same era, multihospital systems—a rarity in 1945—began to grow rapidly (see chap. 8). The influx of public funds in very large amounts appears to have had substantial effects on the number and variety of organizational actors. A secure and growing source of funds and the development of a regulatory framework of rules and guidelines constitute conditions conducive to the creation of organizations, as institutional theorists have long observed (Meyer and Rowan 1977; Scott and Meyer 1983).

In addition to examining the effect of these changes in the institutional environment on populations of organizations, it is instructive to consider the variety of reactions by individual organizations of diverse types. Our case studies provide some insight into these processes (see Case Illustration 6.B). The four organizations selected for more intensive study responded in quite different ways to the changing institutional governance regimes. We attribute much of the variance in organizational response to the degree of congruence between each organization and the structure of the healthcare field. That is, organizations more congruent with the field—in normative beliefs, practices, and structures—were affected by changes in governance in ways intended by the new policies or programs. By contrast, organizations that were incongruent—deviating from prescribed practices and structures—responded in unexpected or unintended ways (Caronna, Pollack, and Scott 1997).

Case Illustration 6.B **Responses to Governmental Initiatives in the Era of Federal Involvement**

We consider the responses of our four organizational cases to two federal programs and policies: Medicare/Medicaid and the cost-containment efforts of the early 1980s. The varied reactions of the cases illustrate the complex ways in which these institutional changes affected organizations, and the ways their effects were mediated by each organization's congruence with the field.

Responses to Medicare/Medicaid

Our four cases exhibited a diversity of reactions to Medicare/Medicaid legislation passed in 1965. Congruent with the norms of the field and legislators' beliefs about what a healthcare organization should look like, SJH experienced little difficulty incorporating these programs into its financing and services. By 1970, the new federal programs funded 47 percent of the patient population, and the hospital operated at full capacity for several years (Visions 1984). In contrast, Stanford physicians complained that designers of the program failed to consider the needs of specialized providers like tertiary care hospitals because reimbursement did not fully cover the costs of care provided by academic medical centers (Walsh 1970; Knox 1979). SUH increased prices charged to private patients to subsidize Medicare/Medicaid patients, who made up 34 percent of its patient population in 1966, and undertook major revisions in pricing policies to make costs more consistent with the federal reimbursement formulas (Palo Alto–Stanford Hospital 1967).

Medicare/Medicaid had a less direct impact on KP finances and services than on other health care organizations. Only 5 percent of KP's patient population in 1965 was over 65 and, by the nature of its membership plan, no members were uninsured or indigent and thus eligible for Medicaid (KP 1965). However, KP viewed the legislation as threatening because it made no provision for organizations with prepaid insurance plans (Yedidia 1987). KP feared that, if forced to conform to fee-for-service reimbursement for even a small proportion of its members, its allegiance to the principle of prepayment would be violated and its very identity challenged. Eventually, KP and other prepaid groups secured modified reimbursement policies that allowed them to participate (Smillie 1991).

Like Kaiser Permanente, the Palo Alto Medical Clinic had a prepaid plan for elderly patients already in place four years before Medicare passed in 1965. Unlike KP, however, PAMC simply phased out its own plan and reverted to fee-for-service reimbursement for its Medicare patients (Fortney 1980). The new programs were less threatening to PAMC than to KP because the clinic offered both prepaid and fee-for-service plans. Medicare reimbursement was not entirely inconsistent with its several modes of health care financing, and PAMC responded by incorporating Medicare funding into those parts of its program that were more congruent.

These diverse responses reveal that Medicare/Medicaid was not perceived as a beneficial new program—a "cash cow"—by all field participants, even though it infused large amounts of guaranteed federal funding into the healthcare sector. For some field participants, the funding was deemed insufficient to cover the costs of providing care; for others, it required extensive adjustments in their mode of operation as a condition of participation.

Responses to Cost-Containment Programs

The cost-containment efforts of the early 1970s (see Case Illustration 6.A) were accompanied by significant changes for some of our healthcare organizations. Because cost containment introduced new field-level norms and expectations, previously congruent organizations confronted new demands and some incongruent organizations, such as KP, suddenly found themselves to be in conformity with field requirements—not because they had changed, but because the field had changed around them.

In the early 1970s, San Jose Hospital entered a time of "retrenchment and consolidation" and operated at a loss for the first time in 25 years (Visions 1984). In attempting to cope with cost-containment efforts, SJH helped found an experimental HMO funded in part by a grant from the HMO federal program, closed its nursing school, and sold a branch facility to the county. Hospital Director John C. Aird noted in 1976 that hospitals were "moving quite rapidly away from a total autonomous 'free-enterprise' . . . type of activity toward becoming a regulated, quasi-public industry (Visions 1984: 42). In the same year, the hospital hired a second full-time director responsible for the day-to-day operations of the hospital so that Aird could devote his time to strategic planning, development activities, and dealing with the increased complexity of regulation (Visions 1984).

Cost-containment programs adversely affected Stanford University Hospital's clinical and research efforts. By the early 1960s, research had become a dominant force in shaping academic medical centers. But as federal research funding began to diminish during the early 1970s, just as cost-containment efforts began to increase, Stanford and other academic medical centers experienced financial difficulties. Responding to these problems, SUH founded the Office of Medical Center Finance, which consolidated the financial management efforts of the hospital, outpatient clinics, and medical school (Andreopoulos 1993). In 1971, leaders also proposed that the clinical faculty be organized into a corporate group practice. This plan, however, was not implemented until much later, in 1994.

Unlike SJH and SUH, Kaiser Permanente actually benefited from cost containment. Based on its structure and policies, KP was judged to have met the requirements developed by HSAs and so was in conformity to this regulatory program. In addition, KP and other HMOs were exempt from CON programs (Smillie 1991). As KP's congruence with the new directions of federal policy became apparent, it was increasingly regarded, not as a deviant organization, but a pioneering model of the HMO—the organizational form expected to usher in a new and improved era of healthcare delivery by improving services and containing costs.

Like the hospitals, Palo Alto Medical Clinic responded to cost-containment programs with changes in its financing and structure. In 1970, PAMC joined with several other area clinics to form the United Medical Clinics (Casalino 1997). This enlarged medical group practice developed a prepaid health plan for Pacific Telephone employees in 1970 and formed a new HMO with Blue Cross in 1975 (Casalino 1997). Unlike the changes in the hospitals, these developments were driven less by a need to cope with an increasingly constrained financial environment and more by a desire to take advantage of opportunities to expand those portions of the organization which, at an earlier time, had been judged deviant but were now regarded as legitimate.

Conclusion

These federal programs and policies reveal the different ways organizations respond to their environments and the wide range of effects governance structures can have on actors. The "field" does not provide a uniform environment for all its component organizations and these organizations do not respond in the same manner to the challenges and opportunities provided. The differences we have observed stem both from the different locations in the field, that is, different types of organizations, as well as from differences in their congruence to the prevailing norms of the field.

Precursors of Change

New secondary logics. While the political accommodation to medical interests resulted in access being combined with quality concerns in the 1960s, the hegemony of professional medicine was beginning to wane during the succeeding decade. Two important secondary logics appeared in the 1970s, which, in our view, helped to weaken the control of professional providers and pave the way for the new market-oriented logics associated with the third era. One of these, *consumer health,* was closely connected to a broader social movement espousing rights for subordinated groups—minorities, women, the disabled, as well as clients who were viewed as powerless vis-à-vis professionals. The second involved the increasing acceptance of *alternative health perspectives and providers.*

   Consumer health. The consumer health ideology challenged the notion that "the doctor knows best" and the view that the responsibility for a person's health rests primarily with the physician rather than with the patient. Adherents pointed to the "diminishing returns on health from the system of acute, curative, high-cost, hospital-based medicine" and emphasized the "increasing evidence that personal behavior, food, and the nature of the environment around us are the prime determinants of health and disease" (Knowles 1977: 58–59). Many activists attempted to reframe the traditional view, shifting attention from illness to health and from medical care to a healthful lifestyle. In addition, more educated and sophisticated patients were increasingly critical of the long waits and impersonal atmosphere of traditional healthcare settings and called for more convenient hours and "user-friendly" service delivery systems (Herzlinger 1997).

   A useful indicator of the acceptance and timing of this consumer health movement is provided by the growing number of popular magazines devoted to health-related issues. *The Reader's Guide to Periodical Literature* offers a cumulative index to periodicals of general interest published in the United States since 1900. Prior to 1965, only one or two magazines dealing with health issues reached a sufficiently wide public to be listed in the guide. But this situation altered rapidly thereafter, the largest increases occurring during the mid-1970s. By 1990, 13 health-related publications

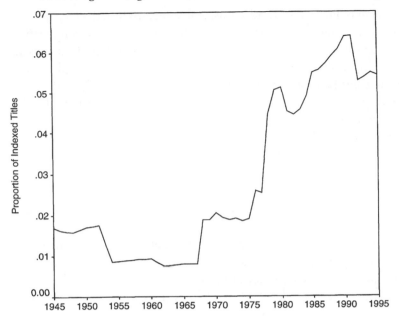

Figure 6.12 Health-Related Titles in the *Guide to Periodical Literature,* 1945–95

NOTE: Periodical counts are standardized by the total number of titles indexed each year.

SOURCE: *Reader's Guide to Periodical Literature* (1945–95).

were listed (see fig. 6.12).[12] In percentage terms, the representation of healthcare publications increased from under 2 percent in 1945 to over 6 percent of all general interest publications in 1990.[13]

In addition, the consumer health movement was able to ground these ideas in judicial decisions and legislative and regulatory changes. A number of court cases during the 1970s established the patients' right to informed consent, access to their medical records, and participation in therapeutic decisions. According to Starr (1982: 389), "few other developments so well illustrate the decline of professional sovereignty in the 1970s as the increased tendency of the courts to view the doctor-patient relationship as a partnership in decision making rather than a doctor's monopoly." In 1970, California moved its state medical licensing board from the

12. Early health publications included *Todays Health* and *Hygeia.* Publications from the 1980s period include: *Aging, Children Today, Current Health, Family Health, Health, Organic Gardening, Prevention, Today's Health,* and *World Health.* We counted publications only if oriented toward or exhibiting a significant health-related component.

13. The total number of periodicals also increased throughout the period of study, but after 1975 an increasing proportion of them were devoted to consumer health.

Department of Professional and Vocational Standards into the Department of Consumer Affairs, and in the mid-1970s, reorganized the composition of the medical board to shift leadership from medical professionals to functional specialists, such as administrators and lawyers, with physicians acting as consultants to the board (Grant 1988; McCready and Harris 1995). On the federal level, the U.S. Congress passed the Consumer Health Information and Promotion Act in 1976.

Alternative health. A related secondary logic emerging around the same time involved alternative conceptions of health and healers. This development encompassed a bundle of belief systems and new types of actors that challenged the medical profession directly at the fount of its legitimacy; namely, its scientific claims to an exclusive base of knowledge pertaining to health and healing. The more conservative factions of the movement rediscovered and placed new emphasis on preventive medicine, a long-standing but neglected area of medical practice. Others turned to folk wisdom and to experienced, but nonprofessional healers such as midwives and lay-healers (see Ruzek 1978). And still others increasingly embraced methods of healing outside the purview of orthodox Western medicine and science, such as traditional Chinese and Indian Ayurvedic systems or more controversial therapeutic modes, including aromatherapy and psychic healing (NIH 1994; Monte 1993).

Organized medicine was able to suppress or eliminate competing practitioners throughout most of this century. "Rival healing professions and perspectives gradually disappeared, were relegated to 'fringe' status, or were swallowed up by the biomedical paradigm" (NIH 1994: xxxviii). Christian Scientist practitioners, for example, have withered in influence and numbers, and osteopaths have survived by moving closer to orthodox medicine. In contrast, chiropractors managed to maintain a cohesive professional identity and distinct service niche on the periphery of mainstream medical care (see Baer 1987; Wardwell 1992; Moore 1993).

Beginning in the late 1960s and intensifying to the present, there has occurred a resurgence of interest in and use of a variety of alternative therapies and practitioners. Recent systematic data, although scarce, attests to the prevalence of these practices. A national survey conducted in 1991 found that approximately 1 in 4 Americans had used "unconventional" therapy to treat one of ten common medical conditions; and, in a similar survey in 1998, 40 percent of respondents indicated that they had used some form of alternative healthcare during the past year (Eisenberg et al. 1993; Astin 1998). In terms of authorized practitioners, California, for example, extended its first license for acupuncture in 1975. By 1978, almost 900 acupuncturists had been licensed, and the numbers have steadily grown by 200 to 300 each year, reaching more than 4000 in 1994. Chiropractic licensing was established in California in 1922. The number of licenses in the state for this specialty had declined noticeably since the 1950s but also began a rapid increase during the late 1970s (see fig. 6.13).

Although certainly a national trend, the available evidence suggests that the acceptance of alternative healers developed earlier and has spread more broadly in the western United States generally (Eisenberg et al. 1993), and California and the San Francisco Bay area more particularly, than in almost any other region of this country. Data on the number of employed chiropractors in the civilian labor force illustrate this pattern.[14] For the United States as a whole, there were 8.5 employed chiropractors per 100,000 population in 1950. That figure increased to 9.0 in 1980 and jumped to 19.3 in 1990. Comparable figures for California for the same years were 21.2, 16.4, and 31.7; and for the Bay area, 15.7, 13.9, and 39.2 (PHS 1954, 1963; Ruggles and Sobek 1997).

Thus, two competing secondary logics began to emerge during the 1970s. While the central new logic associated with the era of federal involvement was attention to equity of access, this value was applied in such a manner as to complement rather than undercut the existing logic of professional dominance. Yet emerging secondary logics were less compatible with and served to undermine the hegemony of the professional norms and beliefs. The emphasis on alternative providers weakened physicians' claims to a monopoly of medical knowledge, and a renewed attention to prevention helped to increase public acceptance of the new forms promoting health maintenance. The logics emphasizing consumer rights and choice also helped pave the way for public acceptance of more market-oriented approaches to healthcare delivery, transforming patients to consumers to customers.

Rise of health and business administration. Precursors of change were reflected in the professional composition of healthcare administrators, as well as clinical practitioners. Since the turn of the century, there has occurred a gradual but inexorable shift in the nature of healthcare organizations

---

14. Census data on employed chiropractors in the civilian labor force and those for licensees at the state level in California are roughly consistent. But census enumerations of employed civilians in many allied health occupations (including chiropractors) are often considerably lower than estimates of practitioners from the corresponding professional associations, which may include persons in the Armed Forces, as well as some who are retired, inactive, or devoting a major portion of their time to other occupations (see PHS 1954: 35–36).

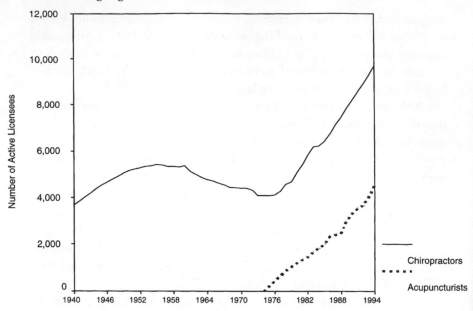

Figure 6.13   California Licensed Chiropractors and Acupuncturists, 1940–94

NOTE: Licensing by the State of California for acupuncturists began in 1975 and for chiropractors in 1922.

SOURCES: California Board of Chiropractic Examiners (1925–84), California Department of Consumer Affairs (1971–95, 1998).

from the "communal" patterns of an earlier, philanthropic, and paternalistic mode of organizing to a more "associative" and rationalized model (Starr 1982: 148; see also Burns 1990). Accompanying this transition has been the transformation of administrative authority from untrained, lay leadership toward increasing reliance on professionally trained managers. It was not until 1934 that the first program in hospital administration attached to a university was established, at the University of Chicago (Weeks and Berman 1985: 226). Several other university-affiliated programs were founded during the mid-1940s. These early training programs for healthcare administrators were located almost exclusively in schools of public health, emphasizing the distinctive nature of healthcare organizations. And, as is so often the case in the rationalization of a field of practice in the U.S. context, a foundation—the W. K. Kellogg Foundation—played a major role in promoting the development of these graduate education programs (Weeks and Berman 1985: 224).[15]

15. Abraham Flexner, whose report helped significantly to advance reform efforts of medical education during the second decade of the twentieth century, was a representative of the Carnegie

In the mid-1960s, the nature and locus of training programs for healthcare administrators started to undergo an important change. Programs began to appear for healthcare managers that offered advanced degrees in business administration (MBAs) rather than in health administration (MPHs or MHAs). In some cases, business schools developed special programs in health services administration. In others, business schools entered into "joint ventures" with schools of public health, offering qualified graduates an MBA.

Figure 6.14 provides evidence regarding the timing and progress of both these trends from 1949 to 1995. The numbers of professional degree programs in health services administration grew slowly until about 1965, after which time they steadily increased up to the present. But also, beginning at about the same time, we observe the increasing proportion of such programs that offer the MBA as an alternative to the MPH. It appears that training for the administration of healthcare organizations is, increasingly, being subsumed under the more generic category of business administration. Note, too, that our figures understate the strength of this trend, since they do not reflect the large number of healthcare organizations that are staffed by graduates of conventional programs of business administration.

Summary

After a period of providing infrastructural support, during the era of professional dominance, the federal government elected to become a major player in the healthcare arena. The passage of the Medicare/Medicaid program in 1965 marked the commencement of the era of federal involvement unleashing a flood of federal funds for medical services. Existing professional governance structures were joined by a complex array of federal and state funding and regulatory agencies, which became increasingly active during this period.

A professional emphasis on quality of care was joined with a public concern for equity of access. The two logics could coexist peaceably early in the second era because the federal role was defined as increasing the size of the pie, not fundamentally transforming the system or modifying physicians' prerogatives. Public programs were designed to accommodate professional interests. Nevertheless, the introduction of massive amounts of federal funding stimulated the emergence of several types of specialized

---

Foundation (Starr 1982: 119). DiMaggio (1991) has chronicled the role played by the Carnegie Foundation in professionalizing the field of museum directors.

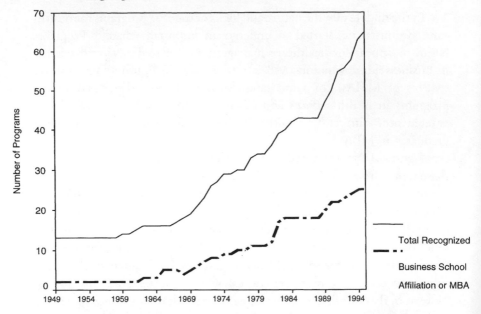

Figure 6.14   Recognized Health Administration Training Programs in the United States, 1949–95

NOTES: From 1949 to 1967, recognized programs include members of the Association of University Programs in Hospital Administration (AUPHA), and after 1968 accredited programs of the Accrediting Commission on Education for Health Services Administration (ACEHSA), which began operation that same year.

Business school affiliation or MBA include programs located in a graduate school of business, maintaining a joint program or formal connection with a graduate school of business, or offering an MBA degree at the time of or after recognition by the AUPHA or ACEHSA. Seventeen programs had a business school affiliation or offered an MBA degree prior to accreditation.

Figure does not include four programs with missing data.

SOURCES: ACEHSA (1995), PHS (1968).

provider forms, as entrepreneurial administrators seized the opportunity to carve out selected portions of the service portfolios of existing diffuse, hospital providers.

Well entrenched interests and ideologies, such as physicians' claims to be the sole arbiters of medical care quality, do not disintegrate in the absence of internal fractures and external challenges. We have provided some evidence of both. Beginning in the late 1960s, the medical profession showed increasing signs of fragmentation along several dimensions. And, somewhat later, social movements developed that acted to empower both patients and physicians' competitors, opening up more room for legitimate choice in the medical arena. The long-standing hegemony of physicians was challenged by the emergence of the consumer movement, which stressed the rights and responsibilities of patients to see after their own health, and by the rise of alternative medical beliefs and practitioners. During this same period, healthcare administrators became increasingly professionalized and less subordinated to the medical mystique. Finally, as health expenditures, especially public outlays, for services escalated rapidly during the 1970s, cost containment began to overshadow the concern for equity and even to challenge the value of quality.

The new arrangements associated with the second era proved to be relatively short-lived, largely because neither professional nor public regulatory controls were successful in stemming the rising costs of medical care, which had come to be defined as the central issue affecting healthcare. In combination, these developments helped to pave the way for a widened role for market forces in the healthcare sector.

The Era of Managerial Control and Market Mechanisms (1983–present)

Principal Indicators

We begin this section by discussing the logics associated with the third era and then describe changes in the governance structures. This order seems preferable here because changes in logics began to seep into healthcare approximately ten years prior to their codification in governance arrangements.

Logics. While the formal onset of the era of managerial control is marked by federal legislation passed in 1982–83, it is important to understand the foundational ideas—the new institutional logics—on which these revised governance mechanisms rested. Early in the 1970s, intellectuals in the health policy arena began to construct the conceptual frameworks that became the basis for new and different approaches to care delivery. In addition, different values were coming to the fore: the former priorities, to insure healthcare quality or to build comprehensive community health systems and insure access for all, were being replaced by the overriding concern to control ever escalating costs (Brown 1986). The early 1970s witnessed the appearance of new kinds of actors and new ideas into the health policy arena (see fig. 6.8a, column on "market building"). Economists began to question the authority and wisdom of public health and public administration experts; planning and regulatory approaches were being challenged as reformers urged reliance on competitive mechanisms. Market solutions were touted over governmental regulatory controls; *efficiency* was enshrined as a central value.

It is important to recognize that these policy changes, like the earlier logic emphasizing equity, did not originate within or single out the health-care sector but were part of a broader political movement—this time to rein in big government and strengthen reliance on market-type controls. But it is also essential to point out that, unlike previous attempts to introduce general economic reforms in the United States, the healthcare field was not treated as an exception, as a realm to be insulated from market reforms. Indeed, cost concerns made it a prime target.

Shifting incentives. The new philosophy was spearheaded by Charles Schultze (1969, 1977), a financial economist and director of the Bureau of the Budget under President Richard Nixon, who pointed to the general failure of governmental interventions in numerous sectors and called for the replacement of "regulatory and administrative agencies with private markets operating under suitably devised incentives" (Melhado 1988: 41). This broad challenge was taken up in the medical care arena by physician-reformer Dr. Paul Ellwood (1971, 1972), who proposed the development of "health maintenance organizations" (HMOs) as an alternative mode of healthcare provision. While the basic organizational template had long existed in the form of prepaid group practices, such as Kaiser Permanente, Ellwood relabeled the model and emphasized the importance of shifting incentives from rewarding practitioners for providing more care to encour-aging them to provide less by practicing preventive (health-maintaining) medicine. Ellwood was successful in obtaining the backing of the Nixon ad-ministration, and federal legislation endorsing and subsidizing the creation of HMOs was passed in 1973.

Melhado (1988) points out that two streams make up the competitive health policy movement. The first, and earlier strand, emphasized "cost sharing"—the attempt to restrain consumption by increasing the cost of care to consumers through the use of co-payments and deductibles in health insurance policies. The second, "competitive health plans," exem-plified by HMO-type approaches, involved attempts to alter the structure of incentives governing the behavior of providers. Melhado (1988: 65) notes:

> Advocates of plans differed from advocates of cost sharing in supposing that incentives had to be applied directly to the providers (by reorganization of their institutions), not indirectly (by changing the economic incentives of consumers). Cost sharing seeks to reform the demand side of the market; competitive plans, the supply side.

Although market-driven approaches were being devised and promoted early in the 1970s, they did not become an important force in healthcare until a decade later.[16] Ideas and their institutional embodiment in new laws, organizational actors, and governance systems most often do not emerge overnight but take time to develop. As Casalino (1997) points out, several essential ingredients to support the new delivery organizations were already in place at that time, including the existence of many large third-party payors, both public and private; the presence of successful closed-panel health plans, which had been ruled by the courts to be legal; and the growing surplus of physicians and hospitals. Still, HMO-type medical plans did not develop rapidly, largely because of the heavy service provision requirements imposed on HMOs by legislators during the first decade of their existence (Brown 1983b).

The competitive reform movement continued to grow and gain adherents through the 1970s. When Ronald Reagan was elected president in 1980, supply-side economists and market enthusiasts came to dominate the upper echelons of policy making. At the beginning of the decade, the foreword to *A New Approach to the Economics of Health Care* announced:

> Health policy analysts are beginning to think of the health care sector more as an economic system. The focus on the health policy debate is on changing the incentives in medical care delivery and financing to encourage a more efficient allocation of resources, reflecting cost-conscious consumer and provider choices. (Baroody 1981: xvi)

Alain Enthoven also published his influential treatise *Health Plan: The Only Practical Solution to the Soaring Cost of Health Care* in 1980, extolling the virtues of managed care. Economists had begun to make substantial inroads, changing the discourse concerning healthcare. "As more nearly competitive arrangements developed in the 1980s, competitive theory made them comprehensible and palatable and provided the language and concepts for understanding them" (Melhado 1988: 26).

Managerial logics. At the heart of these substantial shifts in institutional logics has come the development that currently poses the greatest and most pervasive challenge to the traditional organization of the healthcare sector: the logic of managerial authority and corporate control. The scope and depth of this new logic is suggested by the observation, repeatedly made,

---

16. In Appendix B, we describe our attempt to determine whether the two regulatory events singled out to demarcate the eras exhibited significant effects on privatization of hospitals, HHAs, and ESRDCs. In order to assess whether the HMO Act of 1973 was of similar importance, we entered this event into the analyses, finding no significant effects (see model 3 in table B.2 and model 2 in table B.3).

that even those organizations retaining their conventional, nonprofit status have been compelled to adopt the new organizing principles—to engage in strategic planning, unbundle service packages, identify cost centers, and create for-profit affiliates to operate alongside the nonprofit entities—if they are to survive in the new world (Alexander and D'Aunno 1990; Fennell and Alexander 1993). As Shortell and colleagues (Shortell, Morrison, and Robbins 1985: 219–20) observe:

> The transition is captured in both language and symbols. Observers speak of an "industry" rather than a "system" and there has been movement from a "cottage industry" to corporate consolidation, from health care as a social good to health care as an economic good, from a production orientation to a marketing orientation, from advertising as anathema to billboards dotting highways emphasizing the advantages of one provider over another. To this one might add a fundamental managerial transition from an emphasis on operational management to an emphasis on strategic management.

Many discursive discussions inform us that important changes have occurred in logics related to healthcare, but our interest is in attempting to document more precisely the timing, magnitude, and locus of these changes. Change does not proceed evenly; some participants are more likely to be in the vanguard of some movements while others are inattentive or reluctant to embrace the new directions. In this instance, we expected to find that healthcare managers would be in the forefront of adopters and physicians should be slower to recognize and respond to these changes.

To secure tracers of these developing logics, we examined two leading healthcare publications, one directed toward administrators and one toward physicians. *Modern Healthcare* is one of the oldest and most influential journals directed toward medical managers. Originating in 1912 under the title *Modern Hospital,* it is noteworthy that the new title was adopted in 1974. The *Journal of the American Medical Association* (*JAMA*) was selected as an influential publication directed toward physicians. As with our analysis of health planning (see Case Illustration 6.A), we used a medical periodicals data base to search for instances of articles mentioning particular keywords closely linked with the new logic.[17] The keywords selected were *"provider," " managed care,"* and *"industry."* The generic term "provider" was introduced by economists to refer to any source of services, disregarding (treating as interchangeable) various types of practitioners and settings. The term "managed care" has developed to refer to the new emphasis on actively

---

17. We employed the MEDLINE computerized database (National Library of Medicine 1998). The search utilized abstracts as well as article titles and subject indices.

controlling access to and utilization of services to insure cost-effective practice. And the term "industry" has come to be applied to the healthcare sector as a way of discounting its distinctive features and emphasizing its commonalities with other industrial and commercial arenas. The counts for each keyword, grouped into five multiple-year periods from 1966 to 1995 were standardized by dividing by the total number of articles for the journal in each period.

Figures 6.15a and 6.15b graph the results of this search procedure for each of the two targeted journals. We observe that, as expected, there is increased use of the three terms in both sources over the period surveyed. The period 1980–84 appears to be the inflection point at which most change commences although it is noteworthy that changes in the journal oriented to physicians occur somewhat later, the most visible effects being evident during the period 1985–89. Moreover, it is important to recognize that the new market logics appear to be much more salient to managers than to physicians. The proportion of articles reflecting the new logics is roughly three times greater in *Modern Healthcare* than in *JAMA*. It appears that mainstream medical discourse was relatively less centered on these managerial logics than their administrative counterparts.

We examined one other set of documents, the curricular offerings of medical schools, to further explore the penetration and acceptance of logics

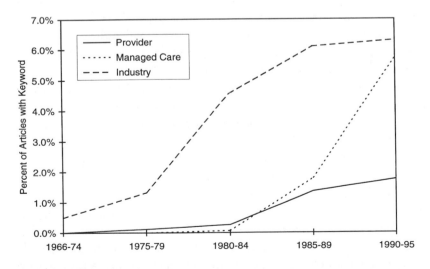

Figure 6.15a Managerial-Market Oriented Articles, *Modern Healthcare*, 1966–95

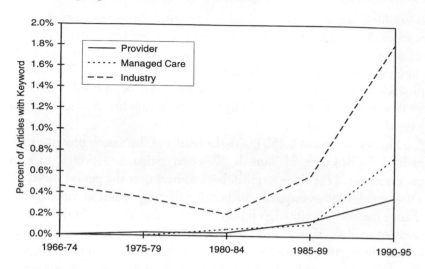

Figure 6.15b   Managerial-Market Oriented Articles, *Journal of the American Medical Association,* 1966–95

NOTES: Keywords are phrases included in an article's title, abstract, or database subject headings.

Article counts for each keyword are grouped into five multiple year periods and are standardized by the total number of articles in each journal per period.

SOURCE: MEDLINE periodicals data base (National Library of Medicine, 1998).

in different, and potentially more resistant, parts of the field. Curricula are the product of accumulated professional consensus and compromise concerning the knowledge, skills, and beliefs deemed essential to a field: a central repository of cultural knowledge and moral authority in society (Meyer 1977). Professional educational programs do not readily attend to or incorporate changes in their surrounding social circumstances even when these developments can profoundly affect the lives and working conditions of their trainees. We anticipated that professional schools engaged in the training of physicians would be slow to reflect changes in the world of professional practice.

To investigate this possibility, we collected data during the period 1942–95 from the two medical schools located in the Bay area—the Stanford University Medical School and the Medical School of the University of California, San Francisco (UCSF)—on course offerings primarily concerned with the "business," "economics," or "organization" of medical care. In either school, a course of this type had yet to be included by 1995 in the required "core" courses for medical students. With respect to elective courses, Stanford offered its first such course in 1942; by 1967 there were four, and by 1990 eight courses among the hundreds of electives offered. Most of these courses were offered under the Department of Preventive Medicine, renamed the Department of Family, Community, and Preventive Medicine, and, more recently, the Department of Health Research and Policy. UCSF has been even slower to respond: its first two elective courses in these subjects appeared in 1969, and this remained the number offered through 1995. These data hint at some difference between a private (Stanford) and public (UCSF) school, but, more important, suggest that medical schools, far from being in the vanguard, have barely begun to acknowledge the most recent logics as part of their curricular offerings.

Governance structures. We mark the formal onset of the era of market competition by the passage of federal and state legislation during the period 1981–83. Competition among providers was encouraged by two important bills—the Omnibus Budget Reconciliation Act (OBRA) passed in 1981 and the Tax Equity and Fiscal Responsibility Act (TEFRA) passed in 1982. OBRA introduced changes in the Medicaid program that allowed states to move Medicaid patients into managed care programs. California was among the first states to take advantage of this enabling legislation and, in 1982, passed bills allowing "negotiated contracting by the state and private insurers with hospitals and physicians" (Bergthold 1990: 69).[18] California's quick response was possible largely because of the work of the Roberti Coalition, a consortium of more than a dozen business coalitions and the California Chamber of Commerce, that was alarmed by the rise in healthcare premiums paid by employers and had mobilized to lobby legislators. TEFRA allowed managed care organizations to enter into "true risk contracts" for Medicare beneficiaries—contracts allowing provider plans to accept the full risks, and potential rewards, of contracting (Morrison and Luft 1990). TEFRA also directed the Department of Health and Human Services to develop a prospective payment system for Medicare patients.

Congress enacted the Prospective Payment System (PPS) in 1983 as part of the Social Security Amendments of that year. PPS tied Medicare payment for hospital services to diagnostic categories that indicated which types of patients were to be admitted for care and provided hospitals with a set amount of funds per patient (weighted by diagnostic category) to cover treatment rather than reimbursing them for costs entailed. Hospitals

18. Companion legislation allowed health insurers, both private and public, to contract with "closed panels" of physicians and hospitals, in addition to HMOs. These provisions contributed significantly to the emergence and rapid growth of preferred provider organizations (PPOs) (see Casalino 1997; and related discussion in chap. 2).

providing more services than those covered by prepayment formulas would bear the loss; those providing fewer services, could retain the savings. As Feldstein (1986:7) observes: "The incentives facing hospitals changed. It was now in the economic interest of hospitals to provide less rather than more services." The PPS was similar in principle to the capitation arrangements developed in earlier prepaid plans in the private sector, except that the reimbursement level took into account the type and severity of illness (diagnosis).

The period 1975 to the early 1980s also witnessed the dismantling of the earlier health planning efforts and a (temporary) reduction in the size of their associated bureaucratic structures, as described above (see Case Illustration 6.A and fig. 6.10). Indeed, the changes in governance structures were marked as much by the dismembering of previous control systems as by the creation of new regimes. Particularly important in this regard were changes in antitrust laws.

Changes in antitrust laws. The application of antitrust law—the American government's characteristic approach to regulating economic activity— to the healthcare field has been viewed as both an indicator of the general shift toward market logics in the sector (Light 1991), as well as a crucial mechanism for bringing about this transformation (Havighurst 1986). Prior to the 1970s, antitrust challenges within the healthcare field were "almost unheard of" (Furrow et al. 1995: 186).[19] The few convictions that did occur represented "little more than moral victories" for alternative providers, as most of organized medicine's professional authority and structures restricting competition, especially at state and local levels, remained intact (Starr 1982: 305–6; see also Furrow et al. 1995, chap. 10).

Not until two landmark cases in the mid-1970s, which explicitly discarded the assumption that the "learned professions" were exempt from antitrust laws and legally recognized a substantial impact of general medical care delivery on interstate commerce,[20] would antitrust become widely applied to healthcare. The medical profession's protected monopoly position and long-standing legal defenses against competition rapidly began to unravel. During the late 1970s, the Federal Trade Commission (FTC)

---

19. Notable early antitrust actions against overt physician attempts to destroy nontraditional forms of practice did occur, such as the Department of Justice's prosecution of the AMA and local medical societies in the early 1940s and a similar rebuffing by the courts of physician persecution of the Group Health Co-operative of Puget Sound in 1951 (see *AMA v. U.S.* 130 F.2d 233 [D.C. App. 1942]) and *Group Health Co-operative of Puget Sound v. King County Medical Society*).

20. *Goldfarb v. Virginia State Bar* 421 U.S. 773 (1975) and *Hospital Building Co. v. Trustees of Rex Hospital* 425 U.S. 738 (1976), respectively.

gathered evidence and ruled against medical and specialty societies for restricting advertisement and restraining price competition. In addition, the dominance of providers on Blue Cross and Blue Shield boards of directors encountered antitrust challenges,[21] as did conventional state laws against prepaid health plans and the corporate practice of medicine (Light 1991; Furrow et al. 1995).

The 1980s witnessed an intensified campaign to apply antitrust laws in the healthcare sector. A 1982 court ruling broadened the scope of antitrust implementation beyond traditional medical providers by finding price-fixing potential in the structure of a "health foundation," a precursor form to PPOs,[22] helping to raise antitrust as a fundamental concern for future innovations in the organization of healthcare delivery. By the mid-1980s, antitrust pressures had led to changes in the Joint Commission's accreditation of healthcare organizations, allowing for the first time the granting of clinical privileges and staff membership to nonphysician practitioners (Havighurst 1986; Light 1991). And the FTC's successful challenge of two horizontal mergers of acute care hospitals established even closer scrutiny of mergers in healthcare institutions.[23] In sum, the monopoly position of physicians, long justified by the value placed upon quality of care, could not survive a transformed institutional environment emphasizing the importance of cost containment and efficiency (see Schmidt 1998).

Purchasing coalitions. The appearance of health coalitions and, more recently, organized purchasing groups has heralded another important change in healthcare toward market and private modes of governance. Early third-party purchasers of healthcare services included "the Blues" (Blue Cross and Blue Shield), which developed during the 1930s to provide insurance coverage to middle-class patients to help defray the costs of hospital and physicians' services. Commercial carriers entered the field soon thereafter. Both approaches, however, as discussed earlier, provided indemnity benefits that reimbursed the subscriber for a portion of medical expenses incurred, and so did not involve any direct relation between the fiscal intermediary and the physician (see Starr 1982: 290–310). Governance functions by these groups over professional providers were held to a minimum. Similarly, when employers increasingly began to provide medical coverage during World War II as a part of their benefit package, these plans (with important

21. See *Barry v. Blue Cross of California* 805 F2d 866 (9th Circuit 1986).
22. *Arizona v. Maricopa County Medical Society* 457 U.S. 332 (1982).
23. *American Medical International, Inc.* 104 FTC 1 (1984) and *Hospital Corporation of America* 106 FTC 361 (1985).

exceptions such as Kaiser Permanente) continued to provide indemnity benefits to employees.

Somewhat later, private employers pioneered the introduction of service benefit plans, so-called prepaid plans that provided payment for services directly to the physician or hospital (chap. 5). Then, during the 1970s, as healthcare costs routinely exceeded the rate of inflation, employers formed local health coalitions, often in conjunction with community, labor, consumer, government, and even provider representatives. At first, they utilized their political influence to attempt to persuade states to establish and enforce ceilings on healthcare costs, as described above in the actions of the Roberti Coalition. Subsequently employers began to negotiate rates directly with providers (Bergthold 1990), and some sought to achieve greater control of the risk-bearing function through self-insurance (Barger, Hillman, and Garland 1985; Carroll and Arnett 1979).

The Pacific Business Group on Health (PBGH), in the Bay area, influenced by the Kaiser Permanente model, became an "early and enthusiastic advocate of managed care" (Robinson 1995: 119). This coalition was effective during the mid-1990s in reducing healthcare premiums for their employer members (chap. 5). In addition to acting as a hard-bargaining purchaser of healthcare services, the PBGH also assumed governance functions usually reserved for provider organizations, professional associations, or state agencies. Adopting a "partner" rather than a "vendor" model, PBGH initially began to conduct employee satisfaction surveys and to promote the coverage of preventive services among providers with whom they had contracts. More recently, PBGH has developed methods for gauging the quality of services in California, using risk-adjusted outcomes for selected clinical areas and has created a research fund to support the development and diffusion of tools for measuring clinical quality. As Robinson reports, the PBGH "has assumed a leadership role with respect to adjusting the standard benefit package, deciding which forms of utilization and quality data HMOs must report, and evaluating the range of possible methods for risk-adjusting payments from particular companies and to particular HMOs" (1995: 128). Such functions carry this purchaser coalition far beyond the simple role of healthcare purchasing agent and into the realm of governance (see fig. 6.A.1).

Thus, by the mid-1980s, after a ramp-up of over a decade, previous planning systems had been sufficiently dismantled, antitrust provisions significantly strengthened, incentive systems realigned, and competitive processes engendered to constitute a different governance system and to foster the construction of new types of social actors.

Actors. We have already noted the entry of several new types of actors, both individual and collective. The third era has witnessed a veritable invasion of economists into the health sector and into policy-making positions in both private and public organizations having an influence on medical care decisions.[24] We have also discussed the new roles being played by employer organizations and coalitions representing the interests of purchasers.

In terms of our five populations of healthcare organizations, the era of managerial control is associated with the continued decline of hospitals and growth of specialized providers (see chap. 3). In particular, HMOs have increased greatly in numbers of providers and, dramatically, in number of enrollees since the mid-1970s (see fig. 3.8). Another significant change in our populations is reflected in the growth of multihospital and integrated healthcare systems and the development of extensive linkages among the members of each of the other populations. We examine these developments in chapter 8.

Yet another clear trend evident among our populations during the third era is the continued decline of public service providers and the increasing proportion of for-profit forms, especially among the specialized providers. HMOs, HHAs, and ESRDCs in the Bay area all exhibit an increasing proportion of for-profit forms since 1980 (see chap. 3).

Regulation of deregulation. What has happened to the public agencies that increased so rapidly during the era of federal involvement? It might have been expected that, with deregulation and the unleashing of market forces, the federal and state regulatory structures would begin to "wither away." Such appears to be the case in the limited instance of health planning bodies and professional review organizations where, as we have noted, governmental agencies sharply declined during the early 1980s (see fig. 6.A.1).

This is not, however, the pattern revealed by state and federal health regulatory bodies more generally. Rather, federal health agencies experienced a brief period of decline between 1975 and 1980, but after 1985 have increased at a rate comparable to that observed during the earlier era of federal involvement. California state health agencies do not experience

---

24. Concomitantly, academic interest in healthcare among economists has also greatly expanded. Fuchs (1996) notes that 132 dissertations were completed within the subdiscipline of health economics in the United States between 1990 and 1994, compared with only 12 between 1960 and 1964.

any decline, but after 1975, their rate of increase is somewhat dampened (see fig. 6.10). These data suggest that between 1975 and 1980, with the introduction of new logics, we observe a period of transition as some agencies and earlier programs are discontinued and agencies disbanded or slowed in growth. But, after 1985, when the new cost-containment regimes are in place, the regulatory bureaucracy again begins to grow. New agencies are created to negotiate and monitor the Medicaid contracts and enforce the PPS reimbursement systems. Thus, it appears that the era of "managed competition" is well named. It is managed not only by the new corporate entities (about which we will have more to say below and in chap. 8) but also by a collection of federal and state oversight bodies that continues to expand up to the present time.

In addition, we call attention to two new types of actors, one individual, the other collective, that we believe reflect important shifts in the underlying archetypes from more professional to more managerial and corporate forms. The first involves the emergence of new types of roles for physicians. The second, a new organizational form for providing health services.

Physician roles. For most of this century physicians have been self-employed, operating in individual offices or in small multiple physician practice settings. This situation has changed dramatically, particularly during the past two decades. Surveys of representative samples of physicians conducted by the AMA show that between 1983 and 1994 the proportion of self-employed physicians in solo practices fell from 40 to 29 percent and those self-employed in group practices from 35 to 28 percent at the same time that physicians practicing as employees increased from 24 to 42 percent (Kletke, Emmons, and Gillis 1996).[25] Employed physicians were more likely to be female, younger, and to lack board certification. For example, 25 percent of physicians under forty years of age were in solo practice in 1987, compared with 40 percent of all practicing physicians (excluding federal employees). By 1991, physicians under age forty in solo practice had dropped to 19 percent (Takagi 1996). Thus, the observed changes in employment status have been accelerating for each new cohort of practicing physicians.

Specialization among physicians has developed primarily around axes defined by their technical and clinical practice, but differentiation has also proceeded along other dimensions. One of the more important for present

25. Note that these figures differ slightly from those reported for overall rates of physicians in group practice in chapter 2, since members of medical groups are comprised of both self-employed and employed physicians (at least by the definitions used in Kletke, Emmons, and Gillis 1996).

purposes is the division between "practice," whether in the form of clinical or research activity, and "administration."

For years, most physicians have been reluctant to assume any type of administrative position. When such functions were required (as in, for example, those residing in the chief of the medical staff of a voluntary hospital), physicians would "rotate through" these positions, returning to the bedside as quickly as possible. As the scale, scope, and complexity of healthcare systems have advanced, however, physicians increasingly face the prospect of either becoming full-time administrators themselves or seeing nonphysicians occupy these managerial positions. The extent to which this type of managerial authority acts to challenge or undermine the physician's clinical decision making—posing the possibility of "proletarianization"—has long been a subject of debate (see Haug 1973; Freidson 1984; McKinlay 1982; Hafferty and Light 1995; Krause 1997). But the recent emergence of managed care systems is experienced by many practicing physicians as constraining, if not directly threatening, their clinical autonomy. As these organizations and their associated managerial positions have gained in authority and begun to encroach on matters formerly reserved to individual physicians, physicians themselves have become increasingly attracted to management.

Information over time concerning the number of physicians occupying administrative positions is fugitive at best.[26] Yet, a telling sign of the increasing attractiveness of these positions to physicians is the creation in 1975 of the American Academy of Medical Directors (AAMD), the first professional society "explicitly and exclusively for physicians with interest in health care management" (Montgomery 1990: 184). Notably, the AAMD was organized by a group of physicians involved in the American Group Practice Association, whose constituents are large group practice associations.[27] The academy not only provides managerial training for its members but has

26. Although available statistics show the number of physicians in administration to have steadily increased, it is difficult to assess by what degree, since the relevant classification schemes and associated data are not consistent over time (see PHS 1962 and AMA 1959–73, 1974–79, 1981–97). In surveys on physician characteristics conducted by the AMA since 1957, MDs can be categorized into a "Major Professional Activity" of "Administrative Medicine." Prior to 1966, physicians could also elect a subspecialty of the same title, which was subsequently eliminated. Later, revisions to the classification structure for "Major Professional Activities" resulted in a tripling of the reported number of MDs in "Administrative Medicine" (AMA 1968), and more recent analyses have shed doubt on the efficacy of these classifications, particularly for emergent and less codified roles such as physician executives (Fennell and Leicht 1998).

27. An older and larger association, the American College of Healthcare Executives, affiliated with the American Hospital Association, includes some physicians but is made up primarily of nonphysician members.

engaged in a sustained effort to form an administrative elite centered around a certified specialty within the medical profession. Having been unsuccessful in its attempt to attain the status of a primary board under the auspices of the American Board of Medical Specialties, the AAMD has created its own certification procedures review body, the American Board of Medical Management. In 1990, the AAMD changed its name to the American College of Physician Executives (ACPE). Membership in this association grew gradually during the first decade, but after 1985—during the era of managerial logics and corporate control—has increased rapidly to over 10,000 physicians at the present time.

To what extent administrative physicians will be successful in bringing medical values to bear in managed care organizations or, conversely, will come to reflect primarily managerial logics remains to be seen. Nevertheless, increases in the proportion of employed physicians together with the growth in the numbers of physicians moving into administrative positions attests to the changes occurring in healthcare systems. Many physicians feel they must endeavor to move toward some type of accommodation with the forces of corporatization.

Large healthcare corporations. Shifting from the individual to the organizational level, a different kind of indicator of the encroachment of business practices and forms into the healthcare sector is provided by the emergence in recent years of large healthcare corporations, stock in which is publicly traded. Attention is restricted to those corporations that are engaged primarily in providing or managing the provision of healthcare services, such as Columbia/HCA and Tenet. In order to develop a relatively stringent measure of the growing success of these forms, we identified those healthcare corporations that have acquired sufficient size to be listed among the largest thousand companies in the United States according to market valuation.[28]

Despite yearly fluctuations in the numbers of such companies and their market valuation, the data reported in figure 6.16 indicate that the general trend is decidedly up. The numbers of healthcare companies making the top 1000 have increased from none in 1975 to over 20 in 1994, and their market valuation has increased rapidly, especially since 1990. We view the rapid

28. The list is comparable to that published in the *Business Week* 1000 annual rankings. However, since *Business Week* did not publish its listing prior to 1986, we regenerated the annual rankings, using the original data source, Standard and Poor's COMPUSTAT industrial and commercial data base, back to 1975 (Standard and Poor 1996). Our count includes healthcare providers, hospital and medical service plans (including HMOs), and management consulting and service firms, if primarily devoted to healthcare. Excluded are pharmaceutical, medical equipment, and indemnity insurance companies.

growth of such for-profit firms as significant in several respects. It represents the introduction of a new and different type of organizational provider into the healthcare sector, one long dominant in other industrial and commercial arenas. Their growth reflects not only the increasing acceptability of these forms to patients and the healthcare sector generally but also the increasing legitimacy of these forms in the eyes of investors and the wider business community. Note that the most rapid rate of growth in these forms occurs during the late 1980s and early 1990s, well into the era of managerial and corporate control.

Precursors of Change

The era of managerial control is rapidly approaching the end of its second decade of existence. While it is too early to discern how long existing arrangements will be in place, let alone the shape of the next institutional

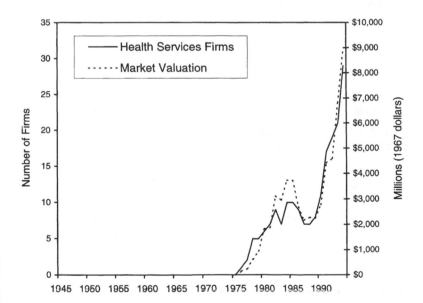

Figure 6.16 Health Services Companies and Market Value among the 1000 Largest American Firms, 1945–94

NOTES: Largest 1000 firms ranked by market valuation.

Market value measured in terms of stock market capitalization (outstanding shares multiplied by average share price).

SOURCES: COMPUSTAT industrial and commercial data base (Standard & Poor, 1996), U.S. Bureau of the Census (1975, 1945–96).

era, a few recent developments may provide some clues to what may lie in the future, as well as point to unlikely directions of change. For example, the major initiative to reorganize the healthcare system put forward in 1993–94 by the Clinton administration, which would have guaranteed a minimum package of health insurance to all Americans and created state-sponsored alliances of insurance organizations to bargain with competing networks of providers, failed its crucial political test. Opposing groups, including the AMA and the insurance industry, were able to persuade legislators that the proposed program was too costly and would result in the creation of an unmanageable governmental bureaucracy to oversee the system (Skocpol 1996). The Clinton health plan was branded as a big government approach ill-suited to a market-oriented milieu: second-era solutions inappropriate to third-era times. It appears politically unlikely that the American system will move in the direction of increased governmental intervention in the direct management of the healthcare system at any time in the near future.

Defenders of the current system point out that many of the proposed reforms and cost-saving measures are in the process of being put in place by private-sector initiatives as employers bargain more aggressively for reductions in healthcare costs and corporate managers design more efficient systems (Enthoven and Singer 1996). But the problem of the large numbers of Americans lacking health insurance or routine access to medical care services remains and, indeed, has become worse. The proportion of persons receiving coverage through employer-based health insurance has continued to decline, from over 61 percent in 1989 to under 57 percent in 1995,[29] while the ranks of uninsured persons has steadily grown, from below 13 percent to more than 15 percent during the same time (HIAA 1998).

But the issue receiving most public attention in recent years has to do with perceived incursions of business interests into medical decisions. The headlines frequently read: "Profits over patients!" The concerns are that, in the interests of cost cutting and profit maximization, providers are sacrificing quality of care and even endangering patients' lives (Anders 1996). Others warn that market-based incentives tend to neglect neces-sary, important, and often underserviced—yet "unprofitable"—portions of the healthcare system, such as trauma and burn units, graduate medical education, and indigent care (Friedman 1996; Thorpe 1997; Mechanic 1994).

---

29. See also figure 5.2 for a similar decline in "group" (mostly comprised of employment-based) health insurance coverage starting from the mid-1980s.

Discharging patients too early from hospitals, demanding cash for additional pain medication, refraining from informing patients about more efficacious, but also more expensive, treatment possibilities, refusal to treat uninsured patients—increasingly common charges such as these have culminated in a contemporary "managed care backlash" (Brodie, Brady, and Altman 1998). There is clearly some point at which market mechanisms are insufficient to govern healthcare delivery decisions and other, regulatory mechanisms are required. The current debate increasingly recognizes the limitations of market reforms. Despite the failure of comprehensive healthcare reform in the early 1990s, piecemeal regulatory initiatives (e.g., the federal Kassebaum-Kennedy bill facilitating the portability of benefits and state restrictions on closed panels and selective contracting) are finding favor with politicians and the public (Moran 1997; Marsteller et al. 1997). Both legislators and health agencies have been emboldened to strengthen rules and procedures to protect patients' rights and interests.

Yet another startling indicator of the changes afoot is the decision by the AMA's house of delegates in 1999 to create union-type affiliates, enabling physicians to organize to better represent their interests in collective bargaining with employers and managed care organizations. Because existing antitrust rules prevent the organization of self-employed physicians, initially only salaried physicians and medical residents will be targeted. But the AMA intends to lobby Congress to pass an antitrust exemption allowing physicians in private practice to organize and bargain collectively. Physicians insisted that "a major reason for favoring unionization was to pressure HMOs and hospitals to improve patient care" (Greenhouse 1999).

Summary

New managerial logics and corporate forms began to penetrate the healthcare field beginning in the 1970s. These initiatives led to and were further encouraged by court decisions and legislation deregulating the industry and establishing incentives for selective contracting and for cost savings. New types of actors, including health economists, purchasing coalitions, and healthcare corporations have become prominent in the arena, and physicians are more frequently employed by and serve as administrators of healthcare organizations. Recent signs suggest, however, that there are limits to reform based primarily on business-oriented criteria and that the American public is unwilling to allow a concern for efficiency and increased profits to erode the quality of medical care they have come to expect.

CONCLUSION

Many types of variables and numerous indicators have been employed in an attempt to capture some of the complexity of changes occurring in the U.S. healthcare sector during the past half century. In chapter 9, we distill some of these indicators, examine their interrelation, and employ them to help account for changes in healthcare delivery systems. Here we conclude by summarizing our conception of the principal changes that have taken place in the institutional environment of the healthcare field during the period of our study. Table 6.1 outlines the principal actors, logics, and governance structures for the three eras. Entries in italics are considered to be the most significant elements.

The central actors—those defining the discourse and determining the logics of the field—change over time from 1945 to 1995. During the first era, these actors are the medical professionals, aided by local elites and governmental units and supported by private insurance companies. They exercise uncontested, legitimized authority over the core activities of the field, defining the central value to be quality of care as specified by professional criteria. Their authority is supported by state licensure. Care settings are primarily independent, nonprofit, "voluntary" organizations or local public facilities. Governance structures are those enforced by professional norms, which encourage voluntary coordination of services.

During the second era, professional providers remain central actors,

Table 6.1   Actors, Logics, and Governance Structures in the Healthcare Sector across Three Insitutional Eras

Eras	Institutional Actors	Institutional Logics	Governance Structures
1945–65	*Independent physicians* Community hospitals Local/state governments Private insurance	*Professional authority* *Quality of care* Nonprofit, voluntary ethos	*Professional associations* State licensure of health occupations Voluntary health planning
1966–82	*Federal government* State governments Medical profession Multihospital systems	*Equity of Access* Consumer health movement Alternative conceptions of health	*Regulatory controls* Mandatory health planning Mandatory peer review Rate setting
1983–Present	*Healthcare corporations* Purchasing groups Specialized healthcare organizations	*Managerial-market orientation* Cost-containment Efficiency	*Market building* Selective contracting Prospective payment

but they are joined by agents of the federal government, supported by state agencies. The federal government enters the arena under the banner of achieving equity of access to healthcare services for all citizens, particularly the most needy. And, federal agencies begin to take a more proactive role, in cooperation with physicians, in insuring healthcare quality by mandating peer review procedures. State agencies become empowered largely through their partnership with the federal government in the funding and management of the Medicaid program, although, as medical care costs continue to rise, states become increasingly active in attempting to regulate healthcare rates and services. Consumers begin to demand a larger role in making decisions about their health and a wider range of choice of providers and therapies.

The third era is characterized by the appearance and increasing influence of several new types of actors: healthcare corporations, both for-profit and nonprofit, groups of public and private employers who come together to strengthen their bargaining position in negotiating healthcare contracts for their employees, and a variety of new, specialized types of healthcare organizations, the majority of whom operate as for-profit forms. The logics have shifted from an emphasis on quality and equity to cost containment and efficiency. Managed care is the new mantra. Federal, state, and local governments are active in novel ways, attempting to encourage competition through deregulation and to modify incentives offered to providers, emphasizing cost containment. While they engage in less direct regulation, they continue to be active in managing competition.

Seven

INSTITUTIONAL ENVIRONMENTS AND ORGANIZATIONAL LEGITIMACY

THIS CHAPTER FOCUSES ON HOW the structures and functioning of organizations are related to components of their institutional environments through processes of legitimation. Legitimacy is usefully conceived as not merely another resource to be possessed or exchanged but a condition reflecting the alignment of an organization to normative, regulatory, and cultural-cognitive rules and beliefs prevailing in its wider field and social environment (Scott 1995: chap. 3). The extent to which an organization is judged to conform to appropriate procedures, to legal rules and codes of ethics, and to taken-for-granted understandings about how things are done has critical implications for the amount of sanction and support conferred through its environment, and thus also for its survival. As chapter 6 illustrated, institutional environments can vary in complexity and over time. This being the case, we would expect the mosaic of environmental elements to which organizations become aligned—e.g., rules, beliefs, and associated field structures—to vary similarly. We provide evidence of such variation in this chapter and examine its implications for organizational survival.

GOVERNANCE STRUCTURES AND HEALTHCARE ORGANIZATIONS

Although organizations, such as hospitals, home health agencies, and health maintenance organizations, can be regarded as governance systems in that they coordinate and supervise various aspects of the provision of health services, here we focus on structural and cultural frameworks at the field level that guide and control hosts of organizations. Numerous types of broader governance systems exist in the healthcare arena. We believe that three of the most influential types of governance structures are professional associations, public agencies of various sorts, and corporate systems involving multiple organizational components. Generally speaking, we view the three eras as largely defined by the changing profile of governance structures—the dominance of medical professional controls during the first era, the rapid development of public, particularly federal, governance systems during the second era, and the emergence of corporate structures in the third era. But this portrait is certainly oversimplified. Many types of professional associations exist, and while medical societies were dominant during the early period and remain strong throughout all the eras, professional managerial associations have arisen and gained power during later periods. Similarly, while public regulatory bodies increased in power and prominence during the second era, they were not absent in the first, and continue to exercise great influence up to the current time. Multiunit corporate structures grew in size and numbers dramatically during the third era, but a number of multihospital systems, frequently operating under the umbrella of a religious order or denomination, have existed throughout all eras (see chap. 8).

In the current chapter, we concentrate on two of these governance systems, professional associations and governmental agencies, examining their effects on the legitimation of hospitals. Before describing our measures and analyses, we first discuss the concept of legitimacy, noting its general features and analytic subtypes.

LEGITIMACY AND ORGANIZATIONAL SURVIVAL

Organizations require more than material resources and technical information if they are to survive and thrive in their social environments. They also need social acceptability and credibility. Sociologists employ the concept of legitimacy to refer to these conditions. The importance of this ephemeral idea has seldom been doubted, but exactly what is meant by legitimacy has been the subject of much debate. Suchman (1995b: 574) provides a useful definition that will guide our own approach. He proposes that:

> *Legitimacy* is a generalized perception or assumption that the actions of an entity are desirable, proper, or appropriate within some socially constructed system of norms, values, beliefs, and definitions.

These "socially constructed systems" are, in our view, social institutions, and governance structures are a particularly important component of these institutions. Governance structures vary in terms of what institutional elements they emphasize and what types of control mechanisms they use. Employing Scott's (1995) analytic categories distinguishing regulative, normative, and cultural-cognitive elements, we can see that each provides a somewhat different basis for legitimacy. The *regulative* view stresses conformity to rules and, if necessary, the exercise of rewards and penalties: legitimacy as legally sanctioned behavior. The *normative* view stresses internalization of and compliance with collective values and norms: legitimacy as morally governed behavior. And the *cognitive* view stresses consistency with cultural-cognitive schemas and models: legitimacy as recognizable, taken-for-granted structures and behavior.

Professional associations are most likely to emphasize normative elements and controls. Governmental agencies and purchasing groups are most likely to emphasize regulative elements (including coercive power), exerting legal authority and rewards and sanctions in order to exercise control. Corporate organizations, such as healthcare systems, rely on both regulative and normative controls over their component units. And what are the sources of cognitive legitimacy? Cognitive rules (concepts, classifications, typifications, schemas) are promulgated and enforced by all of these legitimating agents as well as by broader frameworks of widely shared cultural beliefs.

In our empirical study of hospitals, we examine the normative controls exercised by professional associations over hospitals. To assess the effect of public agencies, we examine how participating in one regulatory program (the Hill-Burton hospital construction program) affects hospitals. Rather than assessing cognitive legitimacy at the level of the individual organization (since we lacked appropriate data for doing so), we follow the practice of organizational ecologists and examine the effect of this factor at the population level.

Normative Legitimacy

The approbation of professionals and their associations is a particularly crucial aspect of legitimacy for organizations functioning in sectors such as medical care. Over the years, professional assessments of organizations have become an increasingly formalized process as professional associations have established formal criteria and assessment regimes in order to evaluate conformity to their standards. In this manner, professional logics are instantiated in governance systems at both field and organizational levels. Whereas licensing is officially a governmental process, although typically conducted in association with the relevant professional interests, accreditation is a "nongovernmental, professional-sponsored process" aimed at promulgating high standards for the industry (Somers 1969: 101). Among other benefits, these standards help to insure that certain jobs and positions are reserved for persons with appropriate professional credentials (Freidson 1986).

In the United States, professional power over healthcare organizations began to be centered in hands of physicians in the early twentieth century when, following the publication of the Flexner report exposing deficiencies in medical education, the American Medical Association (AMA) sought to define and enforce standards of medical education in both schools and hospitals (Starr 1982). Hospitals were included because much of the clinical training of physicians occurs in these settings. The earliest attempts at professional accreditation of hospitals go back to 1913, when the AMA Council of Medical Education began inspecting hospitals with the cooperation of state and city hospital committees. In 1914, the AMA published its first list of hospitals approved for training interns (Somers 1969). In 1918, the American College of Surgeons, needing more adequate medical records on which to base its evaluation of fellows, formulated its "Minimum Standards for Hospitals."

In more recent decades, the dominance of physicians has declined somewhat, both because of internal divisions and external challenges (see chap. 6). As medical specialization increased, and as physicians' interests began to become more fragmented, the number of professional groups seeking to assess and influence hospital performance has grown apace. Thus, for organizations such as hospitals, professional normative legitimation is by no means a unitary process: different medical professional associations bring to bear not only different standards but focus on varying aspects of hospital structure and procedure. Not only hospitals, but all types of healthcare organizations are subject to multiple accreditation agencies (for HMOs and PPOs, see table 2.1). Fragmentation in professional authority affects the legitimation of healthcare organizations.

And it is not only medical professionals that attempt to exert influence on medical organizations. Professional managers have organized, formed their own associations, and increasingly become influential in the accreditation process. Foremost among these is the American Hospital Association (AHA). Initially called the Association of Hospital Superintendents, this association was formed in 1899 but did not become influential as a trade association until the post–World War II period (Starr 1982). Since that time, it has carried out accreditation reviews of hospitals focusing on conformity to administrative standards. Beginning in 1952, the AHA became a participant in the Joint Commission on the Accreditation of Hospitals, together with various physicians associations (see below).

Normative Legitimacy and Hospital Survival

Sources of legitimation. To examine these complex legitimation processes as they affect hospitals, we gathered data on accreditation activities conducted by seven rather diverse professional associations (see also Ruef and Scott 1998). The associations studied were the American Hospital Association (AHA), the California Hospital Association (CHA), the Blue Cross Association (BCA), the American College of Surgeons (ACS), the Joint Commission on the Accreditation of Healthcare Organizations (JCAHO), the Liaison Committee for Medical Education (LCME), and the Accreditation Council for Graduate Medical Education (ACGME) (see table 7.1).[1]

While some of these associations attempt to assess quite broad and general aspects of hospital functioning, others are clearly more specialized in their purview. Associations such as the AHA and the CHA are primarily concerned with the assessment of conformity to administrative or managerial standards while others—for example, the ACS and the ACGME—focus their attention primarily on professional or technical standards of medical education and care. Indeed, hospitals have long been recognized by medical sociologists as a remarkable example of a bifurcated organization characterized by a dual authority structure: the administrative structure, under the direction of a hospital manager, is responsible for the operation and maintenance of the hospital facilities and equipment and for oversight of

Table 7.1   Proportion of Bay Area Hospitals with Accreditations by Type, 1945–90

Form of Legitimacy	Accreditation or Membership	Mean Proportion of Hospitals in Sample
Managerial	American Hospital Association (AHA)	0.741
	Blue Cross Association (BCA)	0.729
	California Hospital Association (CHA)	0.833
Technical	American College of Surgeons (ACS)	0.267
	Medical School (LCME)	0.158
	Residents (ACGME)	0.316
Both	Joint Commission (JCAHO)	0.867

NOTE: All accreditations existed from 1945 to 1990, with the exception of CHA (1945–63) and JCAHO (1954–90).

1. The AHA, which is the source of our data, tracked a number of other hospital accreditations, memberships, and certifications during the period analyzed. Some of these, such as Medicare certification, were excluded from the present analysis because they are rooted primarily in regulatory institutional elements (see the discussion later of regulatory legitimacy). Others, such as internship approval by the ACGME, largely overlap with included indicators (in this case, ACGME residency approval) but are available for a more limited time frame and so were dropped from the analysis.

the nursing staff; and the medical structure, operating under the supervision of the medical staff, with its chief and various committees, is responsible for quality of care (Smith 1955; Scott 1982b).

We briefly describe three of these associations and the focus of their legitimating activities. The American Hospital Association became active following World War II, and currently provides standards for a wide range of managerial functions (AHA 1974–87). During the period 1974–87, the AHA released more than 90 standards to its member hospitals, classified into three broad groups: (1) policy strategies, representing the official position taken by the AHA on a variety of broad policy issues at the national level; (2) policies and policy statements, incorporating advice on general practices to be pursued by acute-care facilities (for example, a 1969 policy indicates that "philanthropy should be encouraged as a source of funding"); and (3) guidelines and technical advisories, which offer more specific recommendations (for example, steps for considering whether or not to engage in contracting and for evaluating contractor performance). Of the sixty AHA guidelines and advisories issued between 1974 and 1987, more than fifty were oriented toward managerial issues, including finance, governance and organization, and human resources management.

An example of an association focusing primarily on technical and medical standards is the Accreditation Council for Graduate Medical Education. The ACGME is sponsored by five other organizations, including the AMA, the American Board of Medical Specialties, and the AHA, for the purpose of accrediting hospital residency programs. While the ACGME guidelines incorporate a number of managerial standards concerning educational administration and procedures for assessing resident eligibility and selection, the great majority of them concentrate on more technical issues related to residency programs (AMA 1995). These medical standards are provided by residency review committees associated with the twenty-six medical specialty associations (see chap. 6). For example, the program specifications for residency education in anesthesiology include training requirements that expose residents to a variety of subspecialty disciplines, with one month rotations in obstetric anesthesia, pediatric anesthesia, neuroanesthesia, cardiothoracic anesthesia, and pain management, as well as a two-month rotation in critical care. Residents are also required to complete a specific inventory of clinical components, for example, 20 anesthetics for caesarean sections. It is noteworthy that such standards are not imposed directly on residents; rather, the residency review committees are charged with ensuring that the technical infrastructure of a hospital can support such activities.

The Joint Commission on the Accreditation of Healthcare Organizations exemplifies an agency that attempts a more comprehensive assessment, including both the administrative and technical, medical activities of hospitals. The JCAHO can claim such a broad mandate only because it represents a cooperative effort, joining together the AMA and AHA, as well as the American College of Physicians and the American College of Surgeons, in a joint venture. This conjoint agency was formally created in 1952 (originally called the Joint Commission on the Accreditation of Hospitals), taking over the review functions initiated by the ACS. A broad set of requirements for accreditation has been developed, with standards set for (1) administration, including governing board responsibilities, physical plant and services, record keeping, and support functions; (2) nursing, including personnel and supervision; and (3) medical staff organization, including review of clinical work (Somers 1969). Recently, the JCAHO has required hospitals to adopt total quality management structures and procedures to provide "documented evidence of certain quality improvement practices" (Westphal, Gulati, and Shortell 1997: 371).

The JCAHO is probably the most influential governance body operating in the realm of health care organizations. But it is important to emphasize that its influence is primarily normative, not regulative. It operates through the power of its moral authority rather than its coercive powers. Indeed, its influence upon hospitals is "self-imposed." A JCAHO review process is initiated only in response to a voluntary request from a healthcare provider.

The other sources of normative legitimation considered generate similar technical or managerial norms, although their concerns are often more limited than those of the AHA, ACGME, or the JCAHO. The Blue Cross Association (BCA) imposes standards of cost accountability on hospitals via contractual relationships with Blue Cross medical plans (Anderson 1975). The American College of Surgeons is primarily concerned with the standards and procedures employed in operating rooms and surgical wards, including the facilities required to conduct specialized procedures such as cancer care (ACS 1966). The functions of the CHA and the LCME are similar to those of the AHA and the ACGME, respectively, differing mainly in their geographic scope and the level of medical education targeted.

These seven sources of legitimation are not independent from one another but interrelated through a complex web of historical events and connections. For example, the Blue Cross concept of hospital prepayment was endorsed by the AHA in 1933 and, in 1941, regional Blue Cross plans gained institutional membership in the AHA (Anderson 1975). At the same time, the overlap among the norms espoused by each of the sources is partial at best, with divisive tensions characterizing many of their relations. For example, during the 1940s and 1950s, the AHA leadership was quite distrustful of Blue Cross methods despite their official endorsement (Anderson 1975).

Dimensions of legitimation. Rather than considering the legitimation of each of these associations in isolation or attempting to lump them into homogeneous groups, we employ a factor analysis in order to discern the extent to which there exist latent dimensions implicit in these assessments. Each accreditation was operationalized as a binary variable. Aside from those time periods when particular types of accreditation were not carried out, the data cover a 46-year range, from 1945 to 1990. Table 7.1 reports the years for which data were available for each accreditation body, the mean proportion of hospitals receiving approval from each legitimating source, and our intuitions regarding the focus of legitimation (managerial, technical, or both). To evaluate the extent to which more than one dimension was employed by professional associations in making these normative judgments, we conducted an exploratory factor analysis (Kim and Mueller 1978; see Appendix C for a full discussion of exploratory factor analysis methods and procedures).

Table 7.2 reports the results of the exploratory factor analysis. As expected, the accreditations cluster rather neatly into two groups, one corresponding to the normative legitimacy associated with technical medical functions and the other to the normative legitimacy associated with managerial functions. JCAHO accreditation contributes moderately to both dimensions. Similarly, the ACS accreditation contributes to both dimensions, although it is more strongly aligned with the technical dimension. ACS attention to both technical and administrative aspects of hospital functioning may reflect the historical circumstance that it was an important precursor of the Joint Commission as a general accreditation agent for hospitals.

A few negative values also appear in table 7.2 suggesting that hospitals seeking legitimacy may be required to make some trade-offs between the demands of technically oriented medical associations and those of professional bodies emphasizing managerial criteria. The requirements for state-of-the-art professional training and quality of medical care can conflict with those imposed on managers to improve efficiency and reduce costs of care.

Table 7.2   Rotated Factor Solution for Managerial and Technical Legitimacy

	Factor 1 Technical Legitimation	Factor 2 Managerial Legitimation
Residents	.8822	−.0332
Medical school	.8094	−.1630
College of Surgeons	.6170	.2306
Joint Commission	.3507	.2636
Blue Cross	−.0642	.7465
AHA	.1449	.6965
CHA	.0396	.6502
Eigenvalues	2.0208	1.5582
Cumulative variance explained	28.9%	51.1%

NOTE: Analysis includes 4004 cases (hospital-years); all federal hospitals have been excluded.

Since the two legitimacy factors account for over 50 percent of the variance in the accreditations, we employ the corresponding factor scores (computed via the Bartlett method) in analyses of hospital survival reported below. Our expectation is that both types of normative legitimation will be positively associated with organizational survival.

Varying salience of legitimation agents. Before commencing our empirical examination of the effects of the two types of normative legitimacy on hospital survival, we want to incorporate a central motif from our previous chapters. The medical care sector has been undergoing fundamental change in its institutional underpinnings: actors, logics, and governance systems have been transformed during the period of our study (chap. 6). If our arguments are correct, then we would expect to observe that the relative importance or salience of different classes of legitimating agents would also have experienced change. Not only are different actors and logics involved, but the actors and logics may have become more or less salient to the issue of organizational survival.

Effects on Hospital Survival

Several event history models of hospital survival were estimated (see Appendix C for a more detailed discussion of event history analysis methods and procedures). Prior to examining the effects of our measures of normative legitimacy, we first consider the effects of variables related to the organizational structure of hospitals and to aspects of their material-resource environment. Organizational characteristics include hospital age, size, market niche, and ownership status. Age is measured in years from time of founding.[2] Hospital size was operationalized in terms of bed capacity. Market niche was coded to distinguish general hospitals from specialist. And hospitals were grouped into three ownership types: for-profit, nonprofit (including both religious and secular facilities), and government hospitals (including city, county, district, and state-owned facilities). Finally, we included a binary variable for multihospital system membership, since interorganizational ties may affect both survival and legitimacy.

In order to capture effects of the material-resource environment, we include measures of urbanization (a rough proxy for both demand and competitive pressures) and physician-to-population ratios (indicating physician supply) assessed at the county level. The effects of these variables on hospital survival are reported in the baseline specification (model 1) of table 7.3.

In the baseline model, three variables were observed to affect hospital survival. Consistent with numerous studies of organizational mortality that document the "liability of smallness" (e.g., Barron, West, and Hannan 1994) and our results in chapter 5, larger hospitals had significantly lower failure rates. For-profit hospitals were also slightly more likely to fail than public or nonprofit forms. This result can be interpreted as a legitimacy effect: throughout most years of the period of our study, for-profit hospitals were relatively rare and were not considered by the general public to exhibit the appropriate archetype for this population. It may also reflect a relative lack of community support (or "embeddedness") for these organizations as compared with public and nonprofit forms (see Baum and Oliver 1992). Finally, organizations which were members of multihospital systems had markedly lower rates of exit. As we will review more extensively in chapter 8, systems can provide economic and non-economic (e.g., reputational) benefits to hospitals that serve to insulate them from environmental uncertainty and turbulence.

Model 2 adds the factor scores representing the extent to which each hospital has been accorded normative legitimacy, either technical or managerial. Adding these legitimacy measures improves model fit substantially (likelihood ratio $\chi^2 = 29.66$, df = 2, p < .001). Both forms of legitimacy play an important role in decreasing organizational mortality, taking into account the aforementioned organizational characteristics and aspects of the resource environment. In the case of technical legitimacy, top-rated hospitals such as Stanford University Hospital, which typically received

---

2. For those organizations undergoing equal-status mergers, the previous organizational event histories were coded as exits and the time clock of the new (merged) hospitals was set to zero in order to reflect a potential "liability of newness" effect (see Amburgey, Kelly and Barnett 1993).

Table 7.3 Effects of Normative and Cognitive Legitimacy on Exits from Bay Area Hospital Population, 1945–90

Variable	Model 1	Model 2	Model 3	Model 4
Intercept(s)	−3.298 (1.138)**	−5.329 (1.253)**	—	—
1945–65	—	—	−5.310 (1.351)**	20.961 (18.314)
1966–82	—	—	−4.403 (1.366)**	22.145 (18.547)
1983–90	—	—	−3.563 (1.370)**	22.957 (18.508)
Organizational Structure:				
Age	0.002 (0.005)	0.007 (0.005)#	0.008 (0.005)#	0.008 (0.005)#
Size (log beds)	−0.523 (0.148)**	−0.207 (0.164)	−0.179 (0.157)	−0.165 (0.158)
For-profit ownership	0.509 (0.316)#	0.394 (0.306)#	0.254 (0.318)	0.264 (0.320)
Government ownership	−0.022 (0.410)	−0.399 (0.426)	−0.896 (0.441)*	−0.849 (0.443)*
System member	−0.871 (0.389)*	−0.950 (0.391)**	−1.596 (0.411)**	−1.538 (0.416)**
Organizational Evaluation:				
Technical Legitimacy	—	−0.694 (0.218)**	—	—
1945–65	—	—	−0.560 (0.390)#	−0.685 (0.426)#
1966–82	—	—	−0.821 (0.313)**	−0.801 (0.308)**
1983–90	—	—	−0.695 (0.323)*	−0.725 (0.324)*
Managerial Legitimacy	—	−0.475 (0.105)**	—	—
1945–65	—	—	−0.566 (0.168)**	−0.561 (0.170)**
1966–82	—	—	−0.772 (0.208)**	−0.739 (0.209)**
1983–90	—	—	−1.008 (0.361)**	−0.999 (0.362)**
Environment:				
Physician ratio	0.136 (0.101)	0.230 (0.103)*	0.051 (0.111)	0.074 (0.112)
Urbanization	1.307 (1.044)	1.250 (1.063)	0.863 (1.138)	0.966 (1.131)
Organizational density[a]	—	—	—	−0.538 (0.374)#
Density^2/1000[a]	—	—	—	2.688 (1.846)#
Number of cases	4004	4004	4004	4004
Number of events[b]	64	64	64	64
−2 Log likelihood (d.f.)	619.16 (8)	589.50 (10)	564.04 (16)	562.00 (18)

NOTES: # $p < .10$; * $p < .05$; ** $p < .01$ (one-tailed tests)

a. Covariate is lagged by one year.

b. One exit event excluded because of missing covariate information.

factor scores between 2.0 and 2.4, are estimated to improve their survival chances on the order of five times that of hospitals receiving only average legitimacy scores. The effect on a hospital of being accorded managerial legitimacy was also significant but somewhat less pronounced: top-rated hospitals improved their survival chances on the order of twice that of their average counterparts.

In our third model specification, we allow the effects of the legitimacy coefficients to vary across the time periods associated with the three eras. The period-specific intercepts in model 3 suggest a secular increase in baseline rates of hospital mortality through the period, with an exit rate of 0.005 ($e^{-5.31}$) during the era of professional dominance and a rate of 0.028 ($e^{-3.56}$) during the era of market reform, all other factors held equal. But the results of particular interest are those that reflect the interaction of legitimacy factors and eras. These results reveal some small but interesting differences across the time periods. Technical legitimacy was only marginally associated (p < .10) with improved hospital survival during the first era—that of professional dominance— while managerial legitimacy exhibited an effect that was far more statistically significant (p < .01). Indeed, we find that managerial legitimacy demonstrably improved hospital survival chances in every era. We suspect that this result reflects the growing salience of administrative norms across the three eras. Historical studies taking a longer view have noted the early dominance of trustees, followed by the growing power of physicians. And only since World War II have hospital administrators begun to move hospitals into the world of modern business practice (Perrow 1963). Those hospitals moving more rapidly in this direction, as indicated by their managerial factor scores, exhibited an enhanced survival capacity.

Moreover, the importance of the managerial factor is seen to rise over time, as indicated by progressive increases in the coefficient's magnitude in each era. As funding systems become more complex and as the organizational systems become more elaborate and interconnected—with increasingly integrated systems and increased levels of alliance formation and contracting (see chap. 8)—managerial competencies (or at least managerial credentials) become more salient.

It may be surprising that technical legitimacy was only modestly associated with hospital survival during the era of professional dominance. We believe this is because hospitals during this period, while subject to strong professional pressures from physicians and their associations, were still primarily oriented to their immediate locality. Recall that this first era was characterized by a "voluntary ethos": most hospitals were independent and less connected to and influenced by broader systems and movements. Formalized professional connections and accreditations have lower salience under such circumstances. Not until funding decisions become more centralized and distant do formal credentials begin to have strong effects on hospital survival. Endorsement by professional agencies, for example, was often the basis for reimbursement eligibility under the government programs instituted during the era of federal involvement. The more formalized signifiers of professional competence and standing gained greater salience in the absence of immediate contacts and experience. And these symbols of legitimacy continue to foster hospital survival in the third, managerial era, although to a diminished degree.

Overall, the log likelihood χ^2 of model 3 versus model 2 is significant at the p < .001 level (likelihood ratio $\chi^2 = 25.46$, df = 6), verifying the improved fit of the model when previous equality constraints imposed on period parameters are removed.

Cognitive Legitimacy

The "new" institutionalism emphasizes cultural-cognitive forces at work in institutional environments. Social actors, both individual and collective, are seen to be socially constructed. A set of constitutive rules resides in each institutional complex, defining what types of social actors can exist, what their respective rights and capacities are, and what types of actions they can legitimately take (Meyer, Boli, and Thomas 1987; Krasner 1988). Thus, the cognitive view stresses conformity to templates and archetypes, which provide the models for structural design, but also to schemas and scripts, which provide menus for routines and actions. More recently, theorists have emphasized that institutional change can be studied by examining changes over time in these archetypes and scripts (Greenwood and Hinings 1996). While the conformity of individual hospitals to these archetypes and scripts can be assessed, we evaluate the effects of cognitive legitimacy at the population level of analysis.

Carroll and Hannan (1989) employ organizational density as an indirect indicator of legitimacy. They propose that the prevalence of a given organizational form—the numbers of organizations adopting a given form—provides a useful measure of the "taken-for-grantedness" of that form in a given arena. We adapted this assumption in chapter 3 to suggest that, in situations in which numerous populations of organizations represent competing models of service delivery, the relative prevalence of one or another organizational form may be viewed as indicating changes in the relative legitimacy of these providers. Underlying this assumption is the argument that legitimacy contributes to organizational survival, increasing founding and reducing failure rates.

We also suggested in previous chapters that the current period, which involves a diverse assortment of rapidly changing forms of managed care (including various types of HMOs, PPOs, POSs, and MSOs) may be seen as a period in which delivery systems are in transition and have not yet settled on one or a few models around which to organize the delivery of services. The lack of a clear, agreed-upon organizational archetype is expected to reduce the survival chances of these forms.

Carroll and Hannan suggest, first, that the legitimacy associated with an organizational form increases with its density but at a decreasing rate. As they note, "once a form becomes prevalent, further proliferation is unlikely to have much effect on its taken-for-grantedness" (1989: 525). They also argue that the relation between legitimation and survival rates is non-monotonic: increases in density enhance survival for members of the population up to some point (termed the carrying capacity of the environment) at which level further increases result in higher rates of failure, as legitimation processes are superseded by competition processes. In sum, "organizational density increases legitimacy at a decreasing rate and increases competition at an increasing rate" (Carroll and Hannan 1989: 526).[3] Note that these arguments are developed at the population rather than the organizational level. These forms of legitimacy and competition are measured as a characteristic of the population: density of organizations as they vary over time.

Effects on Hospital Survival

We test these arguments by examining the effects of density on hospital failures. It is important to point out, however, that this test of Carroll and Hannan's arguments is not definitive because our data set on hospitals is left-censored: our study begins in 1945, at a point when hospitals were already established as a "mature" population. Still, we can at least examine whether our findings regarding the effects of normative legitimacy on organizational survival hold after we take into account the effects of cognitive legitimacy. Cognitive legitimacy is operationalized as the first-order effect of population density; competition is operationalized as the second-order effect of density (the squared density term).

Model 4 in table 7.3 adds the two density measures: organizational density to measure the effect of cognitive legitimation and density-squared

---

3. Hannan and Carroll's argument has been criticized by Zucker (1989) and by Baum and Powell (1995) among others. Zucker's primary objection is that the concept of legitimacy is only indirectly measured—as an effect rather than a cause of organizational growth. We agree that this is the case but also concur with Hannan and Carroll's defense that this is a commonly employed scientific procedure in the measurement of concepts. Further, we believe that the correspondence of legitimacy with prevalence is a plausible interpretation. Baum and Powell do not take serious issue with employing density to assess legitimacy but suggest that there are other, perhaps more important, aspects of legitimacy. We agree with this comment and have attempted to define and operationalize measures of various facets of legitimacy.

to measure the effect of competition. We note that the estimated first-order (legitimation) effect and second-order (competition) effect are consistent with the predictions and with previous findings of population ecologists: population-level cognitive legitimacy significantly decreases the rate of hospital exits, while competitive dynamics increase exit rates. But the covariates are only significant at the p < .10 level and the overall increase in model fit (likelihood ratio $\chi^2 = 2.04$, df = 2) is not significant. Adding the measure of cognitive legitimacy and of competition does not improve the fit above that of model 3. The left-censored nature of our data keeps us from concluding that cognitive legitimation is any less important than normative legitimation for these hospitals; it is instructive to note, though, that the inclusion of the density specification does not undermine the previous results supporting the effects of normative legitimacy. We continue to observe a periodized pattern of changing salience by era that is very similar to the one displayed in model 3.

Regulative Legitimacy

The regulative component of institutions focuses on explicit rule-setting, monitoring, and sanctioning by an oversight body holding power and/or authority over relevant actors. For organizations, such powers are often lodged in a variety of public agencies, but they can also be exercised by private bodies in the form of, for example, trade associations that enforce fair trade agreements or corporate headquarters that exercise authority over subsidiary units. We discuss corporate control in greater detail in chapter 8, where we consider the structure of healthcare systems. Here we restrict attention to the activities of public authorities.

A wide range of regulatory programs exists, and different healthcare organizations are subject to various oversight authorities (for HMOs and PPOs, see table 2.1). Among the earliest public regulatory activities initiated in the medical care arena were those involved in the licensing of healthcare personnel at the state level. Other activities, involving both state and federal agencies, include health planning and rate setting, as discussed in chapter 6 (see also, tables 6.1 and 6.2). An important characteristic of the more recent market building actions by public organizations is that, increasingly, reimbursement formulas are designed to create incentives to encourage providers to restrict service provision. Thus, in programs such as prospective payment systems (PPS), funding and regulative functions are explicitly combined. Indeed, this is one of the difficulties involved in assessing the effects of public regulatory agencies, a point we amplify below.

Analysts confront two general difficulties in examining the effects of regulatory authorities on the survival of medical care organizations. First, in fields like healthcare, which are characterized by strong institutional pressures, the approval of public agencies holding general certifying authority controls the conditions of organizational existence. As a consequence, for such agencies, examining the relation between regulatory approval and organizational survival verges on being empirically tautological. Licensed home health agencies provide an instructive case. In a separate analysis not shown here, we find that those HHAs in the nine-county San Francisco Bay region that had their license suspended (or lost it outright) were 37 times more likely to exit the population than those that had maintained active licenses. While the effects of varying levels of cognitive and normative legitimation for these organizations is of empirical interest, the fateful character of regulative legitimacy seems more obvious and hence, to be of less interest.

Similar considerations often hold true at the population level of analysis. In some cases, the very definition of an organizational form hinges on an act of regulatory legitimation. For example, while HHAs have existed in one form or another since the late nineteenth century (see chap. 2), their modern incarnation as provider of medical services (as opposed to more social and assisted-living services) relies heavily on the HHA provisions in the 1965 Medicare Act (Salvatore 1985).

This suggests that a more prudent approach to examining the effects of regulatory legitimacy may be to move down from the population and organizational levels to the level of subunits or more specialized activities. Examining the effects of regulatory activities on organizational subunits or specialized functions can help us avoid the difficulties entailed in considering broader endorsements heavily enmeshed in issues of organizational survival. But to do so raises the second difficulty, namely, the conflation of institutional and resource dependence arguments. The support of regulatory bodies is often combined with the material benefits (or constraints) associated with the endorsement of these regulatory actors (Singh, Tucker, and House 1986). While in general this conflation is consistent with our view of regulatory institutions as exerting their effects via rewards and sanctions, it is still desirable, where possible, to attempt to distinguish between legitimation and funding effects.

In some cases, where reimbursement formulas are inadequate to support the costs of the services rendered, certification for program participation may be a mixed blessing, if not the kiss of death. Medicare certification for hospitals provides a useful example. In another separate analysis, survivor model estimates for the Bay Area suggest that hospitals that are certified to serve Medicare patients were three times more likely to exit the population than those that were not certified. We do not think, however, that this result implies that Medicare approval has a delegitimating effect on hospital organizations. Medicare approval does not involve direct certification by a federal agency but rather accreditation by the JCAHO. When we control for this legitimating effect (which is positively associated with hospital survival), the remaining negative impact of Medicare certification appears to result from the fact that some of these hospitals are serving patient markets that present very burdensome demands on the care system, such that the costs of providing necessary services are greater than those covered by the reimbursement formulas.

Participation in the Hill-Burton Program

To explore other effects of regulatory legitimacy and funding on hospital survival, we examine the participation of hospitals in the federal Hill-Burton program. Formally named the Hospital Survey and Construction Act, Titles VI and XVI of the Public Health Service Act of 1946, this program applied to particular organizational activities rather than to organizations as a whole (see also the previous discussion of this program in chap. 6). Between 1949 and 1990, Hill-Burton funded 110 construction projects in the San Francisco Bay Area, including 83 hospital projects (directed at general, specialty, and psychiatric hospitals) and 27 projects involving other types of facilities (for example, public health centers, rehabilitation centers, outpatient facilities, and nursing homes).[4]

As shown by the initial approval dates plotted in figure 7.1, the projects commenced a gradual buildup from the late 1940s through the mid-1970s, with the peak period of project approvals occurring in 1967–68, just following the passage of Medicare/Medicaid. With the decline of health planning paradigms during the 1970s (see chap. 6), Hill-Burton and other categorical grant programs were consolidated and few construction projects were supported by federal funds thereafter. The lion's share of funding was reserved for hospital projects. The average size of Hill-Burton grants for hospital construction in the San Francisco area was approximately $850,000

---

4. The Hospital Survey and Construction Act (Title VI), was passed in 1946, but no Bay Area project was funded until 1949. Disbursement of funds under this program ended in 1978. Thereafter, only smaller construction projects were funded under Title XVI.

compared with under $250,000 for other projects. Yet Hill-Burton funds covered a smaller proportion of total construction costs for hospital projects (24 percent) than for nonhospital projects (30 percent).

Our analysis focuses on funding events specific to acute-care hospitals, which involved 80 projects between 1949 and 1990 (the three other hospital projects were directed to psychiatric hospital facilities). Since some hospitals received approval for multiple projects simultaneously, we define a funding event to include all Hill-Burton projects approved for a given facility in a given year. This constraint yields 72 funding events for analysis. Funding events can involve the founding of a new facility (11 events); they can also involve the expansion of an existing facility or its relocation to a new plant (61 events). The reasons for participating (or not) in this program could differ greatly depending on an organization's location and standing within the healthcare field and its needs for various types of legitimacy and funding supports. Case Illustration 7.A describes a range of these experiences for three Bay Area facilities: San Jose Hospital, which received Hill-Burton funding, Stanford Hospital, which elected not to apply, and the Kaiser Permanente system, which found itself excluded.

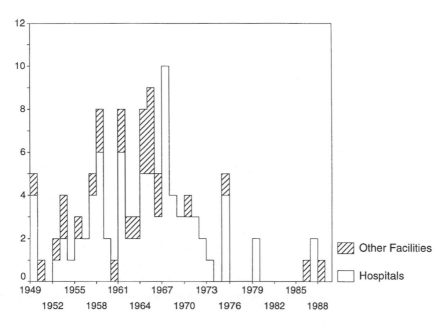

Figure 7.1 Bay Area Hill-Burton (Title VI and XVI) Projects, 1949–90

NOTE: The initial Hill-Burton program was established in 1946 as Title VI of the Public Health Services Act. It was extended on a smaller scale as Title XVI in 1975.

Case Illustration 7.A   **Hill-Burton Financing and Legitimacy: Program Effects on San Jose, Stanford, and Kaiser Permanente Hospitals**

In the late 1940s, several San Jose area hospitals planned expansions in response to a communitywide need for additional medical and hospital services. San Jose Hospital (SJH) began a philanthropic drive with the hope of collecting $1 million to fund its expansion but fell short of its target. Vying with other hospitals for charitable contributions limited donations, but, more important, potential donors were skeptical of the hospital's voluntary commitment, since it had only converted from for-profit ownership a few years earlier (see Case Illustration 4.B). This lack of credibility as a voluntary nonprofit hospital led SJH to change its name temporarily to the Community Service Hospital of Santa Clara Valley in an attempt to improve its public image (Visions 1984).

As a consequence, SJH was enticed to apply to the Hill-Burton program by the regulatory approval associated with participation as well as by the additional funds. Although its original proposal submitted in 1946 was rejected, a less ambitious version was approved in 1949. The $426,00 federal grant was used, along with community donations, for a 65-bed expansion (Visions 1984). Hill-Burton funds also enabled SJH to purchase new radiology and laboratory equipment and to construct open heart surgery facilities. Thus, both SJH's technical and regulatory legitimacy were enhanced as a result of its involvement with Hill-Burton.

Of our four focal organizations, only San Jose Hospital received Hill-Burton funding. Other organizations also built facilities around the same time, but did not partake of the program. In Stanford Hospital's case, this lack of participation was by choice, but this was not so for the Kaiser Permanente system.

In the late 1950s, Stanford's medical school planned to move its hospital from San Francisco to the Stanford University campus 40 miles to the south near Palo Alto. At the same time, the City of Palo Alto was preparing to expand and modernize its existing facility (Palo Alto–Stanford Hospital, 1967). Instead of building two new hospitals, Palo Alto and Stanford decided to invest their resources in one facility that would be shared by both Stanford medical school faculty and Palo Alto physicians. Funding was provided by a $4 million bond approved by residents of Palo Alto and $20 million from the university's endowments and gifts (Starkweather 1981). Completed in 1959, the university and the city jointly owned and operated the facility for nine years (Andreopoulos 1994).

Although Hill-Burton funds could have contributed to the construction of the Stanford–Palo Alto facility, the approval of the joint hospital would not have been assured, since its goals and services did not fit the standard voluntary hospital profile for program participants. The hospital combined both highly specialized tertiary services and general community medicine and was not especially targeted to uncompensated and indigent care.

In addition, the Stanford–Palo Alto hospital, unlike SJH, had less need for the regulatory sanction conferred by the Hill-Burton program. Stanford's standing as a nonprofit institution was well-established, and the City of Palo Alto's involvement in the project added an aura of local community service. Moreover, the shared hospital could also rely heavily on the clinical and technical reputation transferred from Stanford's former hospital in San Francisco to sustain its image, growth, and survival.

Like Stanford Hospital, Kaiser Permanente used sources other than Hill-Burton to construct its facilities, but for very different reasons. Because KP's principles of prepayment and group practice violated prevailing healthcare norms in the 1940s and 1950s, KP was constantly under attack from organized medicine (Foster 1989; Hendricks 1991, 1993). Although KP constructed several hospitals during the heyday of Hill-Burton funding, its trustees "realized it would be of no benefit to their program because AMA opponents would not admit the need for more hospital beds in the regions" it served (Hendricks 1993: 95). In addition, because KP did not offer services to the public at large, but only to its own members, KP hospitals "diverged from the 'charitable' purpose of the independent 'voluntary' hospital supported by Hill-Burton" (Hendricks 1993: 215). Thus excluded from participation in the Hill-Burton program, as well as from most sources of community funds, KP financed its hospitals with money from Henry J. Kaiser and loans from the Bank of America (KP 1969). Although the regulatory legitimacy conferred by Hill-Burton participation would have been welcomed by KP, it was too far outside the parameters of standard healthcare definitions to consider applying.

Summary

The Hill-Burton program was most salient for a subset of Bay Area hospitals: voluntary, community organizations that treated underserved populations and areas. For these hospitals, participating in Hill-Burton offered symbolic as well as financial value. For San Jose Hospital, Hill-Burton funding reinforced its nonprofit and local service orientations to a skeptical community. By contrast, other hospitals, like Stanford, which could rely on other sources for funding and legitimacy, did not participate. In the special case of Kaiser Permanente, which would have benefited from both Hill-Burton financing and regulatory approval, its deviance from field-level structure and financing norms and consequent persecution by organized medicine prevented its participation.

As suggested by our earlier discussion of regulatory processes, it is important to differentiate analytically between the effects of material resources obtained from some oversight group and the effects of regulatory legitimacy conferred by that group. Hospitals that were approved for Hill-Burton funding received a funding stream to support facility construction or expansion. What were the implications of this set of resources for organizational viability? On the one hand, increased resources might be expected to buffer hospitals from environmental pressures normally associated with organizational development or expansion (for example, time invested in soliciting funds from philanthropic sources). This would lead us to expect a decline in rates of hospital failings during periods of Hill-Burton funding. On the other hand, the ready availability of federal support might entice hospitals to risk undertaking foundings or expansions that might otherwise have been imprudent. Moreover, as organizational ecologists have pointed out, change can be dangerous to organizations, disrupting routine processes and undermining the reliability and accountability of an organization (Hannan and Freeman 1984). Thus, the direct effects of Hill-Burton funding on hospital survival were difficult to predict.

There are, however, other, symbolic benefits enjoyed by Hill-Burton hospitals. Being selected as worthy recipients of federal funding is often interpreted by observers as an important signal of credibility (DiMaggio 1983). Hospitals receiving Hill-Burton funds were formally required to provide a specified amount of care for uninsured or indigent patients and, more generally, to be responsive to the needs of patients within their service areas. But these mandates were never enforced (Starr 1982), and so Hill-Burton recipients could enjoy all the symbolic benefits accorded to organizations meeting the institutional standards of community service—the hallmark of the voluntary ethos logic—without necessarily suffering from all the implied costs and constraints. These considerations suggest two propositions regarding the impact of the Hill-Burton program on the viability of participating hospitals. First, hospitals participating in Hill-Burton projects will experience decreased exit rates during the period when they are associated with the program, an expected effect of regulatory legitimacy. Second, hospitals participating in Hill-Burton projects will not experience either increased or decreased failures during the period when they are involved in construction efforts, as federal funding acts to offset the risks associated with organizational change.

The propositions point to different time clocks for Hill-Burton effects. For regulatory legitimacy, the relevant time clock is the period when an organization is formally recognized as working under Hill-Burton obligations. This period of "obligation" extends far beyond the period of hospital construction or expansion—typically twenty years after project completion, according to the legislation. For funding effects, the relevant time clock is limited to the period of actual facility planning and construction, which averaged a little more than three years in the Bay Area during the time of our study.

Effects on Hospital Survival

A simple, constant-rate survivor model was estimated to explore the impact of Hill-Burton funding and regulatory legitimacy on hospital exit rates (see table 7.4). Organizational and environmental covariates correspond to those included in previous tests of normative legitimacy effects. The basic model, model 1, includes a binary dummy variable for the regulatory legitimacy conferred by Hill-Burton. We find, as expected, that the effect of regulatory legitimacy on exits is negative and significant. A hospital under Hill-Burton obligations is twelve times less likely to fail than one that has not received this regulatory legitimation. The log-likelihood statistic suggests a significant improvement in fit over earlier models, which included only technical and managerial indicators of legitimacy (see table 7.3, model 2; likelihood ratio $\chi^2 = 16.12$, df $= 1$, p $< .001$). Model 2 of table 7.4 adds a covariate for annual funding levels. While the corresponding parameter estimate is positive, suggesting an increase in exit rates during construction phases, it is not statistically significant. The absence of a significant effect of funding level on hospital failure rates supports our expectation that, although organizational change is always risky, the receipt of additional resources may act to buffer the organization from these disturbances.

To summarize, all three types of legitimation were found to be positively associated with hospital survival. Cognitive legitimacy, assessed by organizational density at the population level, was found to relate positively to hospital survival rates while competition effects, measured by a squared density term, were negatively associated with survival rates. Accreditation regimes established by professional associations to oversee their concerns and enforce their standards were employed to measure normative legitimacy at the organizational level. The extent of accreditation approvals received from two types of professional bodies—medical and managerial—were found to be positively associated with hospital survival. The legitimacy accorded by the medical associations was found to be particularly salient for hospital survival during the era of federal involvement because, we believe, more centralized funding agents relied heavily on accreditation bodies to help them decide which institutions to support. Managerial legitimacy was positively associated with hospital survival throughout our study, 1945–90, and its effects tended to increase during the later eras as managerial logics became more salient over time.

Regulatory legitimacy, as indicated by approval for receipt of Hill-Burton construction funds, was also positively associated with hospital

Table 7.4   Effects of Regulatory Legitimacy and Funding on Exits from Bay Area Hospital Population, 1945–90

Variable	Model 1	Model 2
Intercept	−5.418 (1.243)**	−5.451 (1.245)**
Organizational Structure:		
Age	0.007 (0.005)	0.007 (0.005)
Size (log beds)	−0.171 (0.163)	−0.170 (0.163)
For-profit ownership	0.321 (0.304)	0.325 (0.304)
Government ownership	−0.346 (0.431)	−0.338 (0.431)
System member	−1.051 (0.392)**	−1.043 (0.392)**
Organizational Evaluation:		
Technical legitimacy	−0.598 (0.218)**	−0.610 (0.220)**
Managerial legitimacy	−0.412 (0.105)**	−0.415 (0.105)**
Regulatory legitimacy	−2.661 (1.023)**	−2.935 (1.096)**
Hill-Burton funding ($ mil)	—	2.787 (1.997)
Environment:		
Physician ratio	0.286 (0.104)**	0.287 (0.104)**
Urbanization	1.323 (1.068)	1.326 (1.069)
Number of cases	4004	4004
Number of events[a]	64	64
−2 Log likelihood (d.f.)	573.38 (11)	572.40 (12)

NOTE: *p < .05; ** p < .01 (one-tailed tests)

a. One exit event excluded because of missing covariate information.

survival. We attempted to distinguish between the symbolic effects of being approved for funding and the effects of funding levels. Our findings suggest that the symbolic effects were more strongly associated with hospital viability.

LEGITIMACY, PERFORMANCE, AND HOSPITAL SURVIVAL

We have examined the effects of varying types of legitimacy regimes on hospital survival, after controlling for important structural and environmental features, but there remains the possibility that our results reflect differences in hospital performance—the quantity or quality of work performed—rather than differences in legitimacy. Both legitimacy and performance ratings involve assessments of organizational characteristics judged against some type of standard.[5] But, while legitimacy is rooted in institutionalized

5. A third type of assessment involves organizational reputation or status. Such assessments can be constructed on the basis of virtually any social attribute that seems relevant to the evaluating subject,

systems of legal, moral, and cognitive codes and often focuses on conformity to structural and procedural standards, performance focuses attention on outcomes or effects, and standards tend to be set in relation to competitors' or one's own past performance.

For some types of organizations, performance as reflected in quality of work or efficiency of production is of critical importance to survival. In these organizations performance standards are clear and performance values readily assessed by consumers. Such is not the case in healthcare organizations. Rigorous evaluation of performance—particularly, at the level of healthcare organizations—is difficult. There remains, up to the present day, a lack of consensus on success metrics and their operationalization (cf. Donabedian 1980–85; Aday et al. 1993). Variation in patient care mix makes comparisons in performance across facilities problematic, and the detailed data required to analyze performance (e.g., patient discharge reports) have become available only in recent decades (Pryor et al. 1985; Flood and Scott 1987).

It is partly for these reasons that much historical emphasis in the sector has been on legitimacy rather than performance.[6] The early accreditation regimes focused on conformity of hospital structures and processes to normative professional standards, not strict outcomes assessment. Systematic indicator-based performance assessment of healthcare organizations is a very recent feature of accreditation systems (Lohr 1990). The JCAHO began using such a system (the Indicator Measurement System) in 1994. In Case Illustration 7.B, we describe Kaiser Permanente's relatively recent implementation of performance-based assessment to address its traditional concern with quality of care.

Case Illustration 7.B   Quality and Performance at Kaiser Permanente

Whereas quality of care has always been an important emphasis of the Kaiser Permanente system, systematic measures of performance are a recent development. Because of the seemingly intangible nature of quality, understandings and meanings have differed considerably among actors and over time. As one observer wrote, "about the only indisputable point [about quality] is that doctors and patients see it differently" (Williams 1971: 44). Definitions of quality used in the system have ranged from highly

---

for example, aesthetics of the architecture or prestige of the members of the board of trustees. Such characteristics are often employed by observers as indirect indicators of performance (see Podolny 1993).

6. More generally, all professionals strongly prefer that evaluations of their performance be on the basis of their conformity to accepted practice rather than on the nature of the outcomes achieved (see Dornbusch and Scott 1975).

specific (e.g., Keene 1971) to extremely general, as revealed in this 1971 exchange between a Permanente physician and an interviewer: "Doctor, how do you define high quality care?" "The kind you want when you are sick" (Williams 1971: 44).

Although diffuse notions of quality appeared to satisfy physicians and patients for many years, increasing competition and concern for cost-effective medicine in the 1990s brought more methodical attention to matters of quality and performance. In 1993, KP's Northern California region became one of the first health plans in the nation to release a quality report card. The Permanente Medical Group's department of quality and utilization developed the report card in collaboration with Andersen Consulting, using more than 100 performance measures to indicate quality (KP 1994b). KP was also part of a consortium of health plans, large employers, and the National Committee for Quality Assurance that created the Health Plan Employer Data and Information Set (HEDIS). HEDIS was designed to rate performance levels of different health plans to help employers and consumers gauge more accurately the value received from their healthcare expenditures (KP 1994b).

KP implemented the HEDIS measures in 1994 as a way to communicate performance to both internal and external constituents. Previously, KP did not collect such data systematically, and regions frequently developed their own evaluation systems and methods. But faced with new demands in the era of managed care, Kaiser Foundation Hospital's CEO David Lawrence noted that

> purchasers and members will not wait for us to make slow, step-by-step progress in [the critical areas of reducing costs and improving members' care experience]. If we don't make improvements rapidly and exceed their expectations, they will take their health care needs to our competitors. Key to making necessary improvements is knowing how we measure up now. (KP 1994b: 1)

KP began comparing outcomes according to internal and external benchmarks, particularly the U.S. Public Health Service's Healthy People 2000 initiative, and set specific goals for improving child immunization rates, breast cancer screening, and prenatal care. A number of programs were established to encourage KP staff to monitor their own performance and share their experiences with others, such as Learning Link, an on-line bulletin board accessible to all employees. Regions also established directors of performance improvement, measurement, and quality assurance. In combination, the proliferation of these programs, policies, and structures within the KP system represent a dramatic departure from earlier concerns for quality and performance, which were important but vaguely conceived in terms of general medical and popular standards, toward highly systematic and measurable managerial definitions.

Given these limitations—controversies over criteria, measurement, and data availability issues—no satisfactory indicators of hospital performance in terms of producing desired medical outcomes are available for the entire period of our study. But one success metric with some merit is the occupancy rate, which reflects the average bed capacity utilization in a hospital (bed census divided by total number of beds). This measure has a number of advantages. It assesses a hospital's ability to attract patients; a high level of utilization is a goal sought by virtually all hospitals. It provides some indication of the reputation assessments made by physicians in determining what facilities to utilize in treating their patients. It can also be considered an indicator of hospital efficiency: existing resources and fixed capital are more fully exploited the higher the ratio of patients to beds. Finally, the measure provides a broad proxy of managerial savvy: administrators who properly anticipate the demand contours of their patient niche are better able to adjust operational scope accordingly. Thus, while the occupancy rate glosses over numerous detailed nuances of hospital efficacy, it does provide a general assessment of technical and managerial performance (albeit not necessarily professional quality of care). And this measure is available for all hospitals for the full study period.

Effects on Hospital Survival

Table 7.5 introduces occupancy rate as a performance measure together with the previously employed measures of the resource environment and normative and regulative legitimacy. As shown in model 1, controlling for performance does not change the impact of any of the legitimacy variables; in terms of both statistical significance and magnitude, these coefficient estimates remain quite comparable to previous specifications (cf. table 7.4, model 1). In this respect, it appears that the impact of legitimacy assessments on organizational survival is separable from performance effects. The occupancy rate itself is quite significant in this model, with full occupancy hospitals' exit rates estimated to be one-third ($\exp[-2.134 \times 0.5]$) that of hospitals with 50 percent occupancy. A likelihood ratio test suggests that the addition of the performance measure improves model fit over the first specification in table 7.4 (likelihood ratio $\chi^2 = 10.20$, df $= 1$, p $< .01$).

In our view, institutional environments affect not only the salience of "socially constructed" organizational assessments, such as those proxied by our legitimacy measures, but also the salience of more "objective" assessments tied to issues of performance. While quality assurance and return on investment have become buzzwords that place considerable pressures on healthcare facilities in the current era of market reform, such evaluation criteria are relative newcomers in this organizational field.

In order to provide some preliminary insights on this claim, we estimated a periodized model of performance impact, as shown in model

Table 7.5   Effects of Organizational Performance on Exits from Bay Area Hospital Population, 1945–90

Variable	Model 1	Model 2
Intercept(s)	−4.119 (1.308)**	—
1945–65	—	−4.869 (1.589)**
1966–82	—	−3.628 (1.493)**
1983–90	—	−2.682 (1.481)*
Organizational Structure:		
Age	0.005 (0.005)	0.007 (0.005)#
Size (log beds)	−0.034 (0.159)	−0.098 (0.153)
For-profit ownership	0.194 (0.308)	0.122 (0.317)
Government ownership	−0.522 (0.430)	−0.799 (0.432)
System member	−1.252 (0.394)**	−1.677 (0.406)**
Organizational Evaluation:		
Technical legitimacy	−0.554 (0.219)**	−0.526 (0.226)**
Managerial legitimacy	−0.421 (0.107)**	−0.594 (0.127)**
Regulatory legitimacy	−2.646 (1.024)**	−2.759 (1.026)**
Performance (occupancy)	−2.134 (0.653)**	—
1945–65	—	−0.943 (1.348)
1966–82	—	−0.879 (1.061)
1983–90	—	−2.091 (1.296)#
Environment:		
Physician ratio	0.228 (0.108)*	0.089 (0.113)
Urbanization	0.998 (1.082)	0.749 (1.157)
Number of cases	4004	4004
Number of events[a]	64	64
−2 Log likelihood (d.f.)	563.18 (12)	545.60 (16)

NOTE: # p < .10; * p < .05; ** p < .01 (one-tailed tests)

a. One exit event excluded because of missing covariate information.

2 (table 7.5). The results provide a more sobering image of the salience of performance for hospital survival than that intimated in the previous model. Occupancy rates do not have any significant impact on hospital mortality in the eras of professional dominance and federal involvement. During these two periods, full-occupancy hospitals experienced mortality rates that are 0.62 (for the first era) and 0.64 (for the second era) times those of hospitals with 50 percent occupancy. By contrast, in the era of market reform, a comparable full-occupancy hospital experienced a mortality rate that was 0.35 times that of a hospital with 50 percent occupancy.

In short, organizational performance—as measured by the material-resource criterion of utilizing a high proportion of available beds—has clearly become more important to hospital survival as the healthcare field has moved toward market-oriented logics. Whereas community hospitals with lower occupancy rates could previously survive on philanthropic sources of support, the new institutional environment increasingly favors the closure or acquisition of such facilities. A changed institutional environment has altered the criteria employed to assess organizational effectiveness and to determine which organizations will survive. The new context places greater weight on measures of performance than did previous eras. Accreditation bodies and the criteria they employ vary in their salience, and their activities and interests need to be viewed in a contextual and historical light.

CONCLUSION

Three facets of legitimacy—normative, regulative, and cognitive—have been examined as they affect hospital survival. Also, three different levels of analysis have been employed. Normative legitimacy was measured at the organizational (hospital) level; regulative at suborganizational (funded projects) level; and cognitive at the population level. Each of these measures was found to affect hospital survival rates in the expected direction: the higher the legitimacy, the greater the likelihood of survival.

We also examined the effect of the three institutional eras on the relative salience of normative legitimacy. While the results vary in statistical significance, the pattern of findings suggests that the physicians associations' normative support for hospitals was of most value to hospitals during the era of federal involvement when funding became more centralized, as federal agencies relied on formal accreditation indicators to assess the quality of hospitals. Managerial associations' normative support for hospitals was significantly associated with hospital survival throughout all periods, but was marginally stronger in the era of managerial logics and increased market pressures.

Hospitals receiving Hill-Burton funding for construction were more likely to survive independent of the financial revenues received in association with this program. Regulative legitimacy enhanced their survival chances. Hospital performance, measured by occupancy rate, was also found to be associated with hospital survival, with a particularly strong effect during the era of market competition. Legitimacy effects remained when performance levels were taken into account.

Our focus has been on hospitals, not because they are the only organization dependent on legitimacy, but because we were able to develop more and better indicators with which to explore the various facets of legitimacy. Many audiences exist for every organization, and their cognitive, normative, and regulatory assessments affect the survival chances of these organizations. Moreover, the salience of these assessments vary depending on the wider institutional context.

Eight

Horizontal, Vertical, and Virtual Integration of Healthcare Organizations

To this point in our study, we have mostly treated organizational actors involved in healthcare delivery in the San Francisco Bay Area as if they were independent and disconnected entities. Here we consider changes in the relations among these organizations and their connections to broader, more encompassing systems. These developments are important at three levels. First, at the level of the organization, they allow us to examine the manifold ways in which organizational members of the field relate to one another. Second, they constitute the emergence of a new, developing population of organizations: healthcare systems. Third, at the field level, they represent the development of a new type of governance structure that acts to coordinate and control the behavior of other actors—both individual and collective.

Beginning during the latter years of the nineteenth century, organizations in numerous sectors—principally manufacturing and distribution—came together to form larger, horizontally or vertically integrated systems (we define these terms below). With some notable exceptions, healthcare organizations trailed far behind other organizations in developing such systems. The same cannot be said for another, more recent general trend. During the past two decades, organizations in many sectors have formed looser, contractual connections that allow them to collaborate more effectively with similar or diverse organizations. Rather than lagging behind, healthcare organizations have been in the forefront in developing these types of virtual linkages.

The relations formed are of various types, but all have implications for organizational boundaries. Some connections, such as contracting for services, involve changes in the operational boundaries of the organization. For example, a hospital may contract with a home health agency to provide services following hospitalization. The hospital has expanded its service domain, becoming at least indirectly involved in providing new services, *265* for example, hospices. Other connections, such as becoming a member of a multihospital or healthcare system, may or may not entail large adjustments in the work performed but do involve major changes in the formal, ownership boundaries of the organization. As the operational and formal boundaries of organizations shift, the definition of the population to which they belong becomes less clear and the utility of this level of analysis for tracking change is impaired (see Thornton and Tuma 1995). It is under such circumstances that the organizational field becomes a useful, if not essential, level of analysis for tracking organizational dynamics.

This chapter is ordered to reflect the historical emergence of types of connections and associated reconfigurations of boundaries among health-care organizations. Shortell and colleagues (Shortell et al. 1996) describe these developments as occurring in three stages, which map closely on to the three institutional eras in American healthcare presented in previous chapters.[1] In the first stage, from early in this century until the late 1960s, the healthcare field was marked by the proliferation of local community hospitals and physicians in independent or small group practices. These provider arrangements were expanded, but left basically unaltered, by the post–World War II Hill-Burton program to fund hospital construction and medical school improvements. Although loose associations of hospitals formed to pursue limited mutual goals, individual service units remained predominantly independent and freestanding.

During the second stage, extending from the middle 1960s through the late 1970s (thus corresponding roughly to our era of federal responsibility), multihospital systems emerged and grew rapidly. Horizontal linkages were increasingly forged between hospital organizations, with the creation of both for-profit and nonprofit systems. In the third stage—corresponding to our era of managerial control and market mechanisms—connections were forged among a variety of players, including not only hospitals, but also physician groups, insurance companies, health plans, and more specialized providers. Some of these new healthcare systems have been structured according to principles of vertical integration—the creation of multifunction healthcare corporations. Others involve looser ties based on contracts or alliances. We attempt to sort out and illustrate these multiple types of linkages among healthcare organizations. In doing so, we introduce the last of our five focal populations: healthcare systems.

---

1. Shortell and colleagues describe a fourth stage (community healthcare management systems), but as it is their conception of the future of healthcare systems, it is less relevant to our historical examination of systems in the Bay Area.

Although this chapter is devoted to examining systems of healthcare organizations, it is important to emphasize at the outset that the word "system" applied to this context encompasses a great variety of organizational forms. The systems examined vary greatly in size, geographical spread, formal structure, type of ownership, degree of control, importance and permanence of connections, and, generally, in extent of "systemness." No one or small set of archetypes has developed to date to guide designers; there remains much creativity and improvisation in composition and form. As Shortell and colleagues (1996: 228) comment: "When you've seen one organized [healthcare] delivery system, you've seen one organized delivery system."

Our discussion is in two parts, the first of which examines the development of hospital associations and multihospital systems, the ways in which these arrangements affect governance structures, and factors affecting hospital affiliation with such systems. In the second part of this chapter, we consider the nature and variety of integrated healthcare systems—systems that also include components other than hospitals.

Multihospital Systems

The Development of Hospital Associations and Multihospital Systems

Associations

The earliest and most pervasive type of system connecting hospitals—the primary organizational provider of healthcare in this country—was the hospital association. Such loose, horizontal connections among similar types of providers developed both at national and local levels, providing a mechanism to allow its members to pursue common, but limited, objectives.

The American Hospital Association was originally organized as an assembly of individuals, the National Hospital Superintendents' Association, but in 1917 "changed from being a personal membership society to an organization of institutions" (Weeks and Berman 1985: 195). This organization along with others, such as the Catholic Hospital Association, worked to give expression to and defend the common interests of hospitals. As a political interest group, the AHA was not active at the national level until after World War II, when members became concerned about the government's policy of rapidly shuttering hospitals. Around this time (1944), the AHA established a permanent office in Washington, D.C., and soon thereafter helped to shape the influential federal Hill-Burton legislation (Weeks and Berman 1985).

Hospitals also frequently formed associations at the local level. For example, six hospitals in the eastern San Francisco region formed the Associated Hospitals of East Bay in 1958 in order to pool information and combine strength in their negotiations with labor groups (Michaels 1981). Some associations, like this one, were quite general in purpose, allowing members to share information and to take stands on the basis of common interests. Others were more focused, supporting the development and coordination of shared services, such as laundry or medical supplies and equipment. Unlike the networks and alliances developed later, these early forms were not intended to provide hospitals with competitive advantages over one another (Brown 1996). Rather, they typically included all local hospitals, exemplifying the shared community service ethic that pervaded the field during the first era.

Multihospital Systems

Although multihospital systems have existed since early in this century, they did not rise to national attention until the 1960s and failed to attract the interest of healthcare researchers until a decade later (Dranove and Shanley 1995; Brown and Lewis 1976; Money, Gilfillan, and Duncan 1976; Zuckerman and Weeks 1979). The AHA did not even define or systematically track their development until 1980 (AHA 1982). Recall from chapter 2 their definition of multihospital systems as "religious, investor-owned, or other organizations that own, lease, sponsor, or contract-manage two or more hospitals" (AHA 1983a: B3). We adopt this definition in our study.

Multihospital systems represent an organizational form created by the *horizontal integration* of two or more hospitals under one managerial hierarchy. That is, the basic units comprising the systems are similar to one another, commensalistic (literally, "eating from the same table") or occupying the same niche, rather than complementary in the functions performed. This type of system—often referred to as a "chain"—is argued to provide economies of scale, improved recruitment and retention of clinical and managerial personnel, greater access to capital, and expanded opportunities for growth and market share (Zuckerman 1979).[2]

2. Chains are even more common among specialized providers. For instance, three large ESRDC chains (Total Renal Care, Gambro Healthcare, and Fresenius) control 55 percent of the market in the U.S., and each have over 200 affiliated centers (Snow 1997).

The great majority of the roughly 200 hospitals in the United States that were part of a system in 1945 (excluding federal hospitals) were affiliated with the Catholic Church.[3] These "systems," however, primarily reflected the organizational structure of the church (in which various orders would create their own network of care facilities), not the operational relations among hospitals. Prior to 1965, only 5 percent of nonfederal hospitals belonged to systems, which were exclusively nonprofit (either religious or secular). No investor-owned systems existed (Alexander and Amburgey 1987; Ermann and Gabel 1986). In 1965, however, the arrival of the Medicare and Medicaid programs, while introducing a complex set of regulations and reimbursement procedures, also provided a new and more reliable stream of income to hospitals (Luke et al. 1989; Dranove and Shanley 1995). These conditions spawned the development of the first investor-owned systems, which grew rapidly. Brown (1996: 24) observes: "As the promise of cost-plus reimbursement for hospitals and universal coverage came into play, entrepreneurial physicians and others were able to convince equity market players that the industry would be a gold mine for investor capital."

As early as 1970, 29 investor-owned systems had been formed, incorporating some 207 hospitals (Ermann and Gabel 1986). The major for-profit systems, such as Hospital Corporation of America (HCA), Humana, and American Medical International, sought administrative economies of scale by purchasing large numbers of hospitals and selling their managerial services (contract management) to others (Dranove and Shanley 1995). These systems or hospital chains grew largely by acquiring financially troubled hospitals—not those in inner cities serving minority populations and uninsured patients but "poorly managed hospitals in communities with young, growing, well-insured populations" (Ermann and Gabel 1986: 476). In some cases, investor-owned systems bought floundering hospitals only to close them, shifting patients to the system's remaining facilities in the same locality (Schiller 1995).

Investor-owned systems expanded rapidly through the 1970s, and nonprofit secular and Catholic systems also increased, although more slowly.

---

3. Consistent with our practice throughout this volume, we omit federal hospitals and systems from analytic study. The five federal systems constitute 2 percent of hospital systems in the United States, operating under the auspices of the Departments of the Army, Navy, and Air Force, the Veterans Administration, and the Department of Health and Human Services. In the Bay Area, two federal systems were present at the termination of our study: the Veterans Administration with two hospitals (one in San Francisco and one in Palo Alto), and the Department of the Air Force with one hospital (at Travis Air Force Base in Solano County).

By 1980, at the threshold of the era of market mechanisms, 25 percent of nonfederal hospitals in the United States belonged to systems of all types (Alexander and Amburgey 1987). Analysts argued that systems allowed hospitals to cope more successfully with elaborated regulatory systems and centralized funding, encouraged cost savings through economies of scale and managerial controls, and provided access to new bases of capital and revenues (Starr 1982). The nationally operated systems initiated the process of vertical integration in healthcare (see below). Corporate organizations such as HCA and Humana acquired and built psychiatric hospitals and nursing homes, as well as acute-care hospitals. Many entered the related fields of alcohol and drug dependence treatment, home health, and extended care (Ermann and Gabel 1986).

More generally, hospital systems—both for-profit and nonprofit— grew rapidly in this period as an organizational response to the increased complexity of the institutional environment. Organizations, as open systems, react to environmental complexity by developing structural components—usually administrative offices and departments—that "map" the new challenges posed by the environment (Alexander and Scott 1984; Fennell and Alexander 1987). For example, as the funding environment became more complex and highly regulated, financial officers were added to the administrative structure of hospitals. Systems provide one means for individual hospitals to share the costs of additional administrative components.

With the third era underway in the early 1980s, prospective payment legislation and additional selective contracting by Medicare/Medicaid and private insurers brought new challenges to the healthcare field and new motivations to form systems (Dranove and Shanley 1995). Both secular nonprofit and investor-owned systems proliferated swiftly during the period 1984–88. By contrast, Catholic systems, which had experienced an extended period of gradual growth until 1980, commenced a steady decline that has continued up to the present. Other church hospital systems show little change throughout the period of our study.

Because of the diverse rates of growth among ownership types, the overall ownership profile of the nation's hospital systems has changed substantially in the last fifty years. In 1945, approximately 80 percent of systems were Catholic, the remainder being related to other churches or secular nonprofits. By 1995, Catholic systems made up only 20 percent of the systems; secular nonprofits had increased to 60 percent and investor-owned systems had increased to 15 percent. Throughout the study period, the number of other, non-Catholic, church systems remained relatively constant, rising slightly from a few systems in 1945 to under 10 percent in 1995.

A rather different picture emerges, however, when we shift the focus from systems to hospital membership in systems. This occurs because systems, particularly the two largest types—investor-owned and nonprofit—tend to differ in a number of ways, including system size. Investor-owned systems tend to be larger than nonprofit systems. In addition, they are less geographically concentrated, spreading across several states, although especially encamped in the southern and western portions of the country, which are growing rapidly and contain younger populations (Ermann and Gabel 1984). As of 1995, investor-owned systems included about 1,100 hospitals, while nonprofit systems (both church-related and secular) included about 1,400 members.

More generally, multihospital and healthcare systems constitute an important and prevalent new type of organizational population. They have transfigured the landscape of this field from one in which virtually all hospitals—the most visible and influential type of organizational player—were independent and freestanding in 1945 to a situation in 1995 in which more than 270 systems exist, incorporating more than 2,500 facilities (federal and nonfederal) or approximately 50 percent of all acute-care hospitals in the United States.

Trends in Bay Area Systems

Multihospital systems were established among Bay Area facilities long before the organizational form gained national prominence in the 1960s.[4] Seven systems operated in the Bay Area in 1945 (see fig. 8.1). While their number did not grow substantially until 1968, there is little doubt that the presence of an expanding Kaiser Permanente (KP) system affected the development of others in the Bay Area (Burda, Gardner, and Greene 1992). The population reached a peak of 25 systems in 1986. Since that time, it has contracted to its present level of approximately seventeen systems as a result of a wave of mergers at the national and local levels. For example, Catholic Healthcare West and Daughters of Charity National Health System–West merged in 1995 (Kertesz 1995). The secular nonprofit system, Good Samaritan Healthcare (formerly Health Dimensions), merged with the investor-owned system Columbia/HCA in 1995 (see Case Illustrations 4.A

4. Data for multihospital systems for the period 1945–79 in the Bay Area were obtained from case histories of hospitals and hospital systems. See Appendix A.

and 4.B). And, at the national level, Columbia acquired several investor-owned systems, including HCA, Epic, Healthtrust, and Humana (Lutz 1995, 1996).

Although the number of systems in the Bay Area has declined since 1986, the proportion of Bay Area hospitals that belong to systems has increased fairly steadily over the period of our study. In 1945 only 12 percent of Bay Area hospitals, or about 10 out of 82, were members of systems (fig. 8.1). System membership grew along with the size of the hospital population in the region, albeit more slowly. When the total number of hospitals in the Bay Area achieved its zenith of about 115 in 1964, nearly 20 percent were system members. During the next three decades, however, the proportion of hospitals in systems continued to rise as the total population fell. About 30 percent of hospitals were system members in the 1970s, with a dramatic increase after 1984, rising to almost 70 percent by 1995.

Figure 8.2 shows the number of Bay Area systems by ownership type. In 1945, there were three Catholic systems, three secular nonprofit systems, and one non-Catholic church system in the Bay Area. Until investor-owned systems entered the region in 1965, the growth in number of total systems was entirely accounted for by the entrance of new Catholic systems. Currently, the distribution by ownership type in the Bay Area is roughly

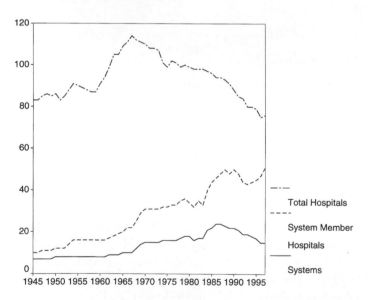

Figure 8.1   Bay Area Hospitals, Member Hospitals, and Systems, 1945–97
NOTE: Excludes federal facilities.

equivalent to that in the rest of the country, except that the proportion of federal hospital systems (not shown in fig. 8.1) is higher and the proportion of secular nonprofit systems is somewhat lower.[5]

In order to give a sense of the early types of systems, we provide a summary and brief description of the nonfederal systems operating in the Bay Area in 1945 (see Case Illustration 8.A). The resulting profile portrays the influence of the dominant professional and community-oriented ethos of that era on the kinds of hospital systems that were formed.

Case Illustration 8.A **Multihospital Systems in the Era of Professional Dominance**

The rise of multihospital systems in the United States is generally associated with increases in the environmental complexity and turbulence of the healthcare field, changes in the federal government's role in funding and governing healthcare, and competition among hospitals in over-bedded communities. But some multihospital systems long predated the first noticeable appearance of these trends in the 1960s. In many ways, these systems were (and are) distinct from those founded today. For example, of the seven systems that had member hospitals in the Bay Area in 1945, all were nonprofit and had constructed their own facilities and all but one provided charitable care as part of a social mission. Although at the time most hospitals were freestanding, these systems and their member hospitals were compatible with the prevailing norms of professional dominance and a voluntary ethos. Thus, although different, they were not considered deviant from other healthcare organizations—with the exception of Kaiser Permanente, as discussed below.

The three Catholic systems present in the Bay Area in 1945 emerged during the 1800s. One, the Daughters of Charity, St. Vincent de Paul, was originally founded in France in 1633 and established in the United States by St. Elizabeth Seton in 1809. The Daughters began providing health services nineteen years later (Daughters of Charity 1998) and in 1945 owned two hospitals in the Bay Area: Mary's Help in Daly City and O'Connor Hospital in San Jose. A second Catholic system, the Sisters of Providence, was founded in 1856 in Seattle, Washington. The sisters established hospitals in Washington, Oregon, and California during the early 1900s and owned Providence Hospital in Oakland in 1945 (Shortell et al. 1996). A third system, the Sisters of Mercy, was founded in Ireland in 1831 and established in the United States in 1854 by Mother Baptist Russell. St. Mary's Hospital in San Francisco was founded by the Sisters of Mercy in 1857 (Montgomery 1990) and was still operating in 1945. The order also

---

5. In 1997 a comparison of the numbers of systems operating in the United States and in the Bay Area shows nationwide: Catholic 55 (20 percent), other church 13 (5 percent), nonprofit 163 (58 percent), for-profit 44 (16 percent), federal 5 (2 percent), total 280 (100 percent); and areawide: Catholic 4 (24 percent), other church 1 (6 percent), nonprofit 7 (41 percent), for-profit 3 (17 percent), federal 2 (12 percent), total 17 (100 percent).

owned five other hospitals in California and Arizona in the 1940s (Topham 1950). All three systems provided charitable care and built their facilities in underserved areas, consistent with the mission of the Catholic church.

A fourth church-related system was sponsored by the Seventh-Day Adventist church. The national Adventist health system began in 1860, when Dr. John Kellogg (creator of Corn Flakes) founded the Western Health Reform Institute in Battle Creek, Michigan (Adventist Health 1998). The institute emphasized "wellness"—a holistic model of health care including exercise, diet improvement, and stress reduction. This model was brought to the Bay Area by Dr. John Kellogg's brother, Dr. Merritt Kellogg, who founded the Rural Health Retreat and St. Helena Hospital in 1878, the only Adventist hospital in the Bay Area in 1945 (St. Helena 1998).

The three Bay Area secular, nonprofit systems shared several characteristics with the religious organizations. A nonprofit, charitable system, Shriners Hospitals was founded in 1919, when the Shrine of North America (part of an international fraternity) voted to open a network of hospitals throughout the United States to treat crippled children. Shriners Hospital in San Francisco, opened in 1923, was the fourth facility founded in the States. As with all Shriners hospitals, it treated children with orthopedic birth defects, injuries, and diseases, free of charge (Shriners 1998).

A second secular system, the University of California (UC), established hospitals in the Bay Area during the early 1900s. The UC medical school in San Francisco, established in 1873, built its first hospital in 1907. The hospital provided services to the community, including charitable care for the city's indigent population, as well as training opportunities for medical students (UCSF 1994). In 1945, UC also operated a hospital at the Berkeley campus to serve its student population.

Kaiser Permanente (KP), the third secular system, established its presence in the Bay Area in the 1940s. Kaiser Industries imported its health plan, initiated at construction sites for aqueduct and dam projects of the 1930s, to Bay Area naval shipyards during World War II. To serve shipyard workers, KP built hospitals in Oakland and Richmond (Hendricks 1991). In 1945, the Kaiser health plan opened to the public and, because of its use of prepaid practice plans and employment of physicians, immediately faced opposition and persecution from the AMA. Permanente physicians were barred from practicing in community hospitals, making it necessary for KP to maintain its wartime hospitals to serve its new members (see Case Illustration 5.A). As a consequence, unlike the other cases, KP developed as a system under duress.

Summary

Most early systems were motivated by the desire to increase access to general (in the case of Catholic systems) or specialized (in the case of the Adventists and Shriners) medical care. Their nonprofit status reflected charitable and educational missions consistent with norms in the era of professional dominance. KP, which treated only plan members at its facilities, challenged conventional models of hospital organization, not because it operated as a system, but primarily because of the nature of its financing and its emphasis on preventive care.

After the mid-1960s, secular nonprofit systems and investor-owned systems provided the primary source of growth in the size of the population (see fig. 8.2). Catholic systems have declined in numbers after 1990. The first investor-owned system entered the Bay Area in 1965 to be rapidly followed by many more up to a peak in 1986. Secular nonprofit systems, while present in the area from the beginning of our study, did not commence their period of robust growth until 1982 but have declined again in numbers during the early 1990s because of mergers.

The proportion of Bay Area systems of different ownership types changed dramatically since the entrance of investor-owned systems, as indicated in figure 8.3. Before 1965, and until about 1984, Catholic systems constituted the majority of all nonprofit systems. Investor-owned systems quickly rivaled secular nonprofit systems starting from the late 1960s. After 1984, the secular category accounted for the majority of nonprofit systems, edging out the Catholic systems, and after about 1990, comprised the largest proportion of any system type, including investor-owned. As of 1997, two systems in the Bay Area operating four hospitals were locally owned, six systems operating 30 hospitals were regional (western United States) in ownership and breadth of operations, and nine systems operating 20 hospitals were national in scope.

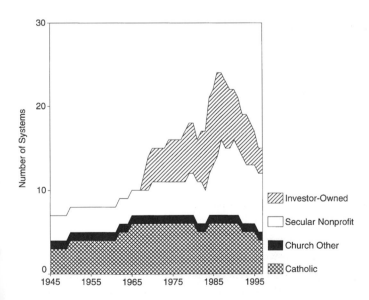

Figure 8.2   Bay Area Systems by Ownership Type, 1945–97

NOTE: Excludes federal facilities.

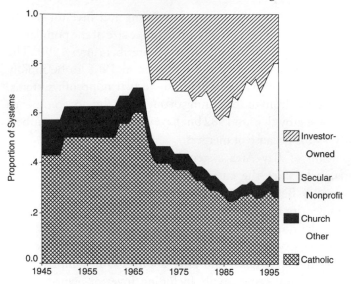

Figure 8.3   Proportion of Bay Area Systems by Ownership Type, 1945–97
NOTE: Excludes federal facilities.

Based on the number of facilities belonging to each system type (see fig. 8.1), secular nonprofits have always maintained the largest share of hospitals in the Bay Area, in part because of the pervasiveness of Kaiser Permanente. Throughout the period of our study, secular nonprofits have accounted for more than 50 percent of hospitals in systems. The proportion of Catholic hospitals has slowly decreased from 40 percent in 1945 to 20 percent in 1995. And the proportion of investor-owned hospitals in Bay Area systems has fluctuated around 20 percent from 1966 to 1995. In general, however, the overall proportions of member hospitals by ownership type parallels the proportions of systems of these types.

Governance Structures in Systems

During the era of professional dominance, heavy reliance was placed on professional systems, both formal associations and informal networks, to exercise control over activities within the healthcare field. These primarily normative mechanisms were supplemented during the era of federal involvement with regulatory controls exercised by governmental agencies at both state and national levels. Many of these governmental controls operated in close conjunction with professional systems. Administrative and managerial controls within individual healthcare organizations were present throughout all eras but were relatively weak until the era of federal responsibility. Healthcare administrators lacked legitimate power over physicians and were greatly restricted in their area of influence.

The degree and scope of administrative controls began to expand and evolve during the late 1960s. We have already noted that healthcare administrators were increasingly becoming professionalized (see fig. 6.5), and the size of organizational units—both individual organizations and systems of organizations—began to swell. Moreover, a larger fraction of medical staffs functioned as organizational employees, rather than as "free agents" (Kletke, Emmons, and Gillis 1996). During the past three decades, professional and public governance mechanisms have been increasingly supplemented—and challenged—by administrative, bureaucratic control systems.

What happens when an independent hospital joins a multihospital system? At the very least, new players and interests enter the scene. No longer is the exclusive focus on the locality in which the hospital resides. Some attention and energy must be devoted to dealing with a more distant and different set of interests, which may sometimes supersede those of any component unit. But, as we have emphasized, systems vary greatly in the extent of their "systemness," and how much multihospital system membership intrudes on affiliated facilities depends very much on the characteristics of the parent system and its governance structure.

As with every aspect of healthcare systems, there is considerable variety in governance arrangements, but empirical research by Morlock and Alexander (1986) reports that three governance models predominate among multihospital systems. They are (1) the *parent holding company,* characterized by a systemwide governing board and separate hospital governing boards; (2) a *modified parent holding company,* also containing a systemwide governing board but substituting advisory boards for governing boards at the local hospital level; and (3) a *corporate model,* in which only one board exists, at the system level. Clearly, these three models vary from low to high in degree of centralization of decision making.[6] Even more centralized are those corporate systems that focus decision making in its management structure rather than the systemwide board (Alexander and Fennell 1986).

6. In the same study, a factor analysis disclosed that the types of decisions made at the two levels also varied systematically. System-level decisions were more likely to concern the transfer or sale of assets and the formation of new companies. Hospital-level decisions were more likely to pertain to service additions and deletions at the local level, development of hospital operating budgets, and medical staff privileges (Morlock and Alexander 1986: 1124).

In their 1983 survey of all 247 U.S. hospital systems existing at that time, Morlock and Alexander found that 40 percent of the sampled systems followed the parent holding company model, 22 percent followed the modified model, and 23 percent the corporate model. Remaining systems (15 percent) followed some composite model. Contrary to expectations, empirical studies conducted in the mid-1980s revealed that secular non-profit systems tend to exhibit more highly centralized governance structure than either Catholic nonprofit or for-profit systems. Catholic and for-profit systems were more likely to manifest either a holding or modified holding company model (Morlock and Alexander 1986; Alexander and Fennell 1986). Investor-owned hospitals, however, also tend to combine decentralized governance structures—the use of local hospital boards—with strong central management structures exercising control over system budgets and administrative appointments (Starr 1982).

These differences can be interpreted in the light of the varying missions or goals of the three types of systems. Catholic hospitals are content to express their religious mission of service through the acquisition of hospitals that are expected, in turn, to embed themselves in local communities. A holding company model suffices for this purpose. Investor-owned hospitals, aimed at increasing profits, establish stronger centralized managerial controls to insure attention to profit-making goals but permit a more decentralized board structure, allowing individual hospitals to retain some autonomy in their service offerings so long as they meet financial objectives. By contrast, nonprofit systems pursue missions that emphasize the importance of service or functional integration (see below). They are more likely to embrace a "corporate" structure that seats authority in a single systemwide board in order to facilitate more unified planning of services and facility development. Exemplars of each of the system governance structures can be found in the Bay Area (see Case Illustration 8.B).

Case Illustration 8.B   **Diversity of Governance Structures in Bay Area Healthcare Systems**

Parent Holding Company

Catholic Healthcare West (CHW), the largest Catholic nonprofit system with hospitals in the Bay region, operates 33 hospitals in three Western states, seven of which are in the Bay Area (Scott 1997). Its governance structure is best characterized as a parent holding company. At the system level there is a 17-member board of directors responsible for systemwide vision, approving capital expenditures over $5 million, and appointing regional boards. In addition, at this level there is a 10-member board of nuns from the sponsoring organization. At an intermediate level, regional boards comprising 15 to 20 members, frequently including physicians and community leaders, are responsible for regional oversight and planning. At the local level, each hospital is overseen by a board of a hybrid structure, which consists of equal numbers of members from the local level and CHW representatives.

Modified Parent Holding Company

Sutter Health, a secular nonprofit system with eight hospitals in the Bay Area, employs a modified parent holding company model of governance. Governing boards exist at the system and the local unit level, but the amount of discretion accorded local decision making units is curtailed. In 1992, Sutter created a regional structure in which each of its three regions includes aligned physician organizations, hospitals, outpatient facilities, and related services. Each region is coordinated by a planning committee comprised of trustees, physicians, and system managers. These bodies report to a systemwide resource planning committee, made up of representatives from the three regional committees and the parent board, which makes resource allocation decisions for the system as a whole (Shortell et al. 1996).

Corporate Model

The major secular nonprofit system in the Bay Area, Kaiser Permanente, employs a corporate model. KP utilizes a single systemwide board having a degree of authority over resource allocation. Board members include executives from the Kaiser Health Plan and member hospitals, as well as outside representatives, including lawyers, academics, and business executives. There is no physician representation. The system is organized into regions that are managed by executive offices. Substantial control is exercised at this level, with powers over appointment of regional officers, budgets, planning, and operations of hospitals within the region. There are no local hospital boards. On the other hand, the system's Permanente Medical Group is overseen by a board of directors, all of whom are physicians, and has in place a set of local boards.

Most investor-owned systems, such as Columbia/HCA, employ a corporate model with a highly centralized management structure. Prior to its reorganization in January 1998, Columbia/HCA was headquartered in Nashville, Tennessee, and owned 340 hospitals, six of which are in the Bay Area. The corporation also includes many other types of holdings in the healthcare area, as described in Case Illustration 8.D. The system has been governed by a 10-member board of directors and 20 senior management officers who exercise either functional direction or oversight of one of the six geographical divisions (HCA Annual Report 1996). Individual hospital boards are permitted to remain in existence but govern under confined parameters established by the corporation.

Regardless of the specific configuration of governance developed, the emergence and widespread diffusion of systems dramatically alters the political economy of the local hospital (and other types of healthcare) units. A hospital lacking a separate governance or advisory body will necessarily be severed from attention to many localized community influences and responsive primarily to system-level concerns. But even hospitals retaining their own local governance units must now attend to a new center of power and authority having significant control over their operations and fate. The type of integration involved is conventionally described as "horizontal," but the critical new element introduced by these systems is a set of hierarchical relations.

Determinants of System Membership

We turn now to examine factors affecting hospitals' decisions to become system members. Previous empirical studies of this decision have emphasized a number of advantages associated with system membership, including (1) economic, such as cost savings from economies of scale or increased revenues from expanded market share (Zuckerman 1979; Luke, Begun, and Pointer 1989; Alexander and Fennell 1986; Alexander and Morrisey 1988; Dranove and Shanley 1995); (2) organizational, such as better planning, strategic positioning, a higher-caliber staff, and an increased capacity to cope with the regulatory environment (Zuckerman 1979; Alexander and Fennell 1986; Ermann and Gabel 1986; Alexander and Morrisey 1988; Dranove and Shanley 1995); (3) technological, including increased complexity of services and equipment and associated specialization (Luke, Begun, and Pointer 1989; Herzlinger 1992); and (4) community orientation, including improved access, convenience, and consumer sensitivity (Alexander and Morrisey 1988; Herzlinger 1992).

No doubt all of these factors are important, but in our own approach we emphasize three considerations. First, continuing the practice employed in previous chapters, we distinguish analytically between factors stemming primarily from the material-resource environment as compared with those arising from the institutional environment. The former factors include technological and competitive pressures and attempts to increase market share and client base. The latter include changes in the normative, regulatory, and belief systems governing healthcare institutions. These environments pose different kinds of challenges for organizations and require differing kinds of responses.

Second, we believe that too much of previous research emphasizes the perspective of the organization considering affiliation to the neglect of the perspective of the acquiring system. A hospital's entry into a multihospital system depends on choices made by both parties: the system and the hospital itself. Systems acquire hospitals either by building their own facilities or buying existing facilities (quite different strategies and situations can motivate buying as opposed to building hospitals). Hospitals make choices to remain independent or join systems, but being built by a system, while certainly a type of system entry, is obviously not a decision made by an individual hospital. In some instances, the factors that cause a hospital to desire system membership make that hospital attractive to systems acquiring facilities. By contrast, in other instances, the factors that cause a hospital to seek system membership may make the hospital unattractive to a system. We incorporate the potential incongruities between hospital and system choices and strategies in the arguments developed below.

A third consideration is the nature of the match between the hospital and system. Both hospitals and systems are usually motivated to attempt to maximize compatibility between the interests of the two parties. Many nonprofit hospitals, for example, are reluctant to join for-profit systems because of perceived incompatibilities in their management style and mission. Similarly, systems may seek to acquire members they believe to be more congruent with their philosophy and operational style. In short, matches between systems and members are not governed simply by economic rationales but also reflect institutional considerations at both the local organizational and system levels. To illustrate these three sets of processes and forces, Case Illustration 8.C provides a brief history of the factors leading to San Jose Hospital's decision to join a multihospital system.

Case Illustration 8.C **San Jose Hospital Joins a System**

In the mid-1980s, hospitals in the San Jose area faced many changes and challenges: an oversupply of hospital beds in the community, increased competition from HMOs— in particular, Kaiser Permanente in Santa Clara—and new, more restrictive rules for Medicaid financing. In the midst of this uncertain and turbulent environment, San Jose Hospital "found itself a 'classic inner-city hospital', [plagued by an] older physical plant, [a] large indigent population, [the] flight of the affluent patients to the suburbs, and an aging medical staff" (Starkweather 1990: 34). Hospital administrators pursued numerous adaptive strategies to deal with this situation, leading to a merger with a small, local multihospital system.

SJH's leaders were particularly concerned about its older, downtown image and unfavorable comparisons to the county hospital. They made substantial financial investments to improve their facilities, including a $2 million face-lift of the building's entrance and lobby, in an attempt to attract private patients (Starkweather 1990). And although SJH had one of the largest Medicaid populations in the state for a nongovernment hospital, in 1984 it decided not to submit a bid for the continued care of Medicaid recipients. An immediate drop in hospital utilization from 340 to 200 census patients following that decision led to the dismissal of 25 percent of the staff. Leaders felt these results made the hospital "leaner and stronger" and anticipated long-term financial benefits (Starkweather 1990).

In the short-term, however, SJH had one of the lowest occupancy rates in the San Jose area (57 percent in 1985, compared with an average rate for hospitals of about 70 percent) and a relatively weak position in the local market. Concerned that it would lose even more market share as the area became increasingly competitive, in 1985 SJH began to consider possible merger partners. The most obvious candidate was Good Samaritan, a large, relatively new community hospital located in a fast-growing San Jose suburb.

SJH's focus on Good Samaritan was based, in part, on the prior merger of Good Samaritan and Wheeler Hospital, a small, nonprofit facility in Gilroy, south of San Jose. SJH had served as a consultant to Wheeler in the mid-1980s and had previously proposed a consolidation with the smaller, rural hospital. But Wheeler chose to affiliate with Good Samaritan, which could fund its planned renovations. Because of their past relationships, SJH viewed both Wheeler and Good Samaritan as amenable partners. SJH also recognized that the combined market share of the three hospitals would rival that of Kaiser Permanente's in the South Bay and far supersede that of any other facility or system in the vicinity. Good Samaritan "saw the merger as essential to survival," and all parties expected short-term advantages, such as economies of scale, elimination of duplicate services, and the ability to improve borrowing capacity (Starkweather 1990: 36). In 1986, the three hospitals formed the Health Dimensions multihospital system, a nonprofit parent corporation with minimum holding company powers (Starkweather 1990). Although Health Dimensions struggled with financial difficulties in the 1990s and was eventually sold to Columbia/HCA (see Case Illustration 4.B), the initial 1986 merger of the three local hospitals was considered a success for several years.

Influences on System Membership

We identify three categories of factors that may influence a hospital to join a system: aspects of a hospital's structure, environmental characteristics, and evaluative criteria used by and imposed on organizations (e.g., legitimacy and performance). In discussing these influences and interpreting the results of our analyses, we consider the effects of these variables on both hospitals' decisions to join systems and systems' decisions to acquire hospitals.

Organizational structure. A hospital's age, size, and ownership status may influence system membership. We expect that younger hospitals will be more likely to join systems than older hospitals. Newer hospitals tend to have a less-established reputation and weaker legitimacy claims than older hospitals and thus experience problems attracting capital and physician referrals. Faced with the liability of newness (Stinchcombe 1965), they will affiliate with other hospitals in order to increase their chances of survival. Younger hospitals may also be more attractive acquisition targets to systems (in particular, investor-owned) than older hospitals, for they have less firmly established missions and governance structures.

We expect that smaller hospitals—hospitals with fewer beds—will have a greater need to join a system than larger hospitals because of their smaller market share, more limited access to equipment and capital, and vulnerability to competition and resource constraints (Goodstein, Murmann, and Boeker 1993; Alexander and Morrisey 1988). Although smaller hospitals may be more desirous of joining systems than larger hospitals, some systems may prefer to acquire larger hospitals to boost their overall capacity and market share. On the other hand, smaller systems may represent easier targets and pose fewer problems of assimilation.

We expect a for-profit hospital to be more likely to join a system than a nonprofit hospital, because systems can help a hospital increase profits and market share (Goodstein, Murmann, and Boeker 1993; Alexander and Morrisey 1988). Moreover, the growth of large for-profit systems, especially in their early years, was driven by aggressive acquisition of independent proprietary hospitals (Starr 1982); most nonprofit systems did not attempt to match the for-profits in the magnitude and scope of growth, for they did not regard this as an appropriate strategy. Thus, investor-owned hospitals were more likely than nonprofits to be bought out by systems, resulting in a greater number of investor-owned hospitals joining systems than nonprofit hospitals.

Evaluative measures. Measures of legitimacy and performance, which represent the criteria widely accepted in an organization's environment for assessing its efficacy, could have additional effects on system membership.[7] We expect that hospitals with weak managerial legitimacy will be motivated to join systems because systems can strengthen and augment a hospital's managerial resources (see Alexander and Morrisey 1988). Different types of systems may, however, be attracted to different levels of managerial competence. Some nonprofit systems may prefer to acquire strongly managed

---

7. See chapter 7 for a discussion of the types of legitimacy we employ, as well as the nature of legitimacy and performance as evaluative criteria used by and imposed on organizations. As noted, the salience of these criteria has changed over time with the institutional development of the healthcare field.

hospitals in order to take advantage of these strengths. Investor-owned systems are more likely to seek out hospitals experiencing administrative difficulties in order to impose their own management structures.

In our view, systems are more oriented to affecting and improving managerial than technical standards—particularly for those systems focusing on horizontal integration. Thus, it is less clear what effect, if any, technical legitimacy would have on system membership. As with managerial legitimacy, there may well be differences among systems in how they value this hospital feature. Since our measure of technical legitimacy (see chap. 7) strongly reflects the professional teaching and training programs conducted by a hospital, we would expect hospitals with higher technical legitimacy to be less inclined to join investor-owned systems. Teaching programs, as presently constituted, reflect an orientation to goals other than efficiency, cost cutting, and corporate profits. By contrast, nonprofit systems, given their broader goals, would be more likely to value technical legitimacy as an indicator of strong professional credentials and standing.

One of the most frequently cited reasons for system membership is performance deficiency. Whether the hospital is losing money, patients, or market share, affiliation with a system can provide an influx of resources and expertise to turn a failing hospital around. Thus we expect struggling hospitals to be more likely to join systems than solvent ones. For their part, systems may be attracted to struggling hospitals in order to acquire facilities at bargain rates. On the other hand, systems may be reluctant to acquire hospitals that they perceive as having performance problems. Perhaps it is for this reason that previous researchers have not found a significant relation between occupancy rate, one of the most prevalent measures of hospital performance,[8] and likelihood of joining a system (see Alexander and Morrisey 1988; Gamm et al. 1996).

Environmental characteristics. In addition to structural characteristics and evaluative measures, changes in the environment can influence system membership. Competition for market share and resources can encourage hospitals to join systems, whether large, national systems or smaller, local ones (Luke, Ozcan, and Olden 1995; Starkweather 1990). For their part, although systems may not seek out higher degrees of competition, they recognize that hospitals confronting these conditions are likely to be more willing partners.

---

8. For reasons described in chapter 7, good data are not available on quality of performance as measured by patient outcomes, and financial data pose problems of comparability. Hence, we again employ occupancy rate as an indicator of hospital performance.

We would also expect hospitals to be influenced by the models provided by other hospitals in their area (DiMaggio and Powell 1983; Fligstein 1985; Davis 1991). Hospitals may form or join systems in competitive response to the system formation of their rivals (Starkweather 1990) or to "keep up" with other hospitals in their area that are already members. Likewise, systems may be more likely to acquire or build hospitals in communities that already have system member hospitals. The legitimacy gained by a presence of systems would make it easier for systems, especially the investor-owned, to enter a community and attract hospitals.

Analysis of System Membership

We begin by comparing differences in selected variables by system type. The differences observed tended to be consistent with our predictions, although they must be interpreted cautiously because of the small sample size for systems of each type. To allow for statistically stronger evaluation of our hypotheses, we conducted event-history analyses of the likelihood of hospital entry into systems during the years 1945–91 using a Cox semiparametric model (see Appendix C). System entries were treated as repeatable events; we counted multiple entries for hospitals with serial memberships in a number of different systems. We considered an entry event as an existing hospital joining a system and excluded those hospitals built by systems (e.g., some Kaiser Permanente hospitals).

Note that, unlike many other analyses in this book, we do not include any period effects—representing the time periods or eras—in the analyses of system entry. Since most of these events have occurred during the latest two periods, we lack sufficient cases to pursue variation in these processes by era.

First we review selected descriptive differences among member hospitals by system type. Table 8.1 reports average differences of hospital characteristics (at the time of joining) among Catholic, secular nonprofits and investor-owned systems in the Bay Area. As expected, hospitals that join investor-owned systems tend to be younger than hospitals joining nonprofits, and larger hospitals are more likely to join secular nonprofits than the other two system types. Hospital members of secular nonprofit systems were more likely to have high technical legitimacy than hospitals in either of the other types, and hospitals that join investor-owned systems were most likely to have low managerial legitimacy. Investor-owned systems appear to seek out the more poorly managed hospitals in order either to attempt to turn them around or sell them off.

Table 8.1   Selected Differences among Bay Area Multihospital System Types, 1945–91

System Type	Age	Size	Hospital Characteristics at Time of System Entry	
			Technical Legitimacy	Managerial Legitimacy
Catholic (N = 3)	57	135	−0.19	0.90
Secular nonprofit (N = 23)	53	221	0.25	0.24
Investor-owned (N = 16)	39	104	−0.46	−0.31

NOTE: N = number of entries.

Table 8.2 shows the results of three models of system entry employing the event history data. Model 1, which is a significant improvement in fit compared with the baseline specification (likelihood ratio $\chi^2 = 72.10$, df $= 4$, p < .001), examines the impact of organizational structure on entry into multihospital systems. As expected, younger hospitals were more likely to enter systems than older ones, age having a significant negative effect on entry. Ownership differences were in the expected direction as well: for-profit hospitals were more likely to enter systems than nonprofits. Although we had made no predictions with respect to governmental facilities, the data indicate that municipal, county, and district hospitals were less likely to join systems than nonprofits. The only structural variable that ran counter to our hypotheses was hospital size, which was found to have a significant positive effect on system entry. The heightened visibility of large hospitals may make them more attractive acquisition targets to multihospital chains.

Adding legitimacy and performance variables in model 2 does not noticeably improve the fit of the model. Although the effects of technical legitimacy, managerial legitimacy, and performance are in the expected direction (increases in all three decrease the likelihood of system entry), they are not statistically significant. The relatively large standard errors are not surprising, given that the model glosses over heterogeneity in the impact of evaluative criteria by hospital ownership type (see table 8.1).

Model 3 adds environmental variables to the specification. The effect of competition is positive (with higher hospital competition increasing the likelihood of system entry, as predicted) but not significant. Some contagion was observed to occur among Bay Area hospitals. As the number

Table 8.2   Cox Models of Bay Area Hospital Entry into Multihospital Systems, 1946–91

Variable	Model 1	Model 2	Model 3
Organizational Structure:			
Age	−0.020 (0.007)**	−0.018 (0.007)**	−0.018 (0.007)**
Size (log beds)	0.311 (0.200)#	0.431 (0.213)*	0.385 (0.215)*
For-profit ownership	2.554 (0.396)**	2.390 (0.396)**	2.429 (0.399)**
Government ownership	−0.752 (0.495)#	−0.978 (0.517)*	−0.914 (0.518)*
Organizational Evaluation:			
Technical legitimacy	—	−0.224 (0.195)	−0.225 (0.197)
Managerial legitimacy	—	−0.190 (0.199)	−0.179 (0.208)
Performance (occupancy)	—	−0.729 (0.798)	−0.358 (0.862)
Environment:			
Competition (hospital density)[a,b]	—	—	0.009 (0.046)
Contagion (system density)[a]	—	—	0.031 (0.024)#
Number of cases	4008	4008	4008
Number of events	52	52	52
−2 Log likelihood (d.f.)	638.09 (4)	635.06 (7)	633.25 (9)

NOTES: # $p < .10$; * $p < .05$; ** $p < .01$ (one-tailed tests)

a. Covariate is lagged by one year.

b. Covariate is computed on a per capita basis (per 100,000 inhabitants).

of multihospital systems active in the region has increased, autonomous facilities have been more inclined to seek entry.

INTEGRATED HEALTHCARE SYSTEMS

Many of the healthcare systems created since the 1970s have expanded beyond the horizontal integration of similar organizational components, such as hospitals, by building linkages among a diverse set of organizations and actors. These more complex integrated systems were included in our descriptive overview of the growth of systems in the United States and the Bay Area in the first part of this chapter—many grew out of the earlier multihospital systems—but we have not yet considered the ways in which these newer types of systems differ from the earlier forms. Here, we describe differences across systems, including their centers of control, modes of integration, and types of integration.

Loci of Integration

The complexity of contemporary systems is reflected by a diversity of principal organizing units. Three contenders have emerged in the healthcare arena as competing centers of control. First, and most obviously, *hospitals* have served this role. They have been, as we know, the traditional centers of healthcare services, and, more than any other player, they are probably best equipped with expertise and leadership experience. On the other hand, hospitals have been primarily interested in keeping their beds at or near full capacity, and this criterion may not serve the best interests of a more diversified system. Shortell and colleagues (1996: 66) report that many systems are inhibited in their development "by the inability of the system to overcome the hospital paradigm."

A second possible locus of integration is the *medical group*. Physicians have long acted as the primary decision makers in the healthcare sector. However, there are many variants of physician groups. Clearly preferable in the current context are groups of primary care providers rather than multispecialty groups. The former are better positioned, in terms of temperament and training, to play the role of guide, broker, and gatekeeper, mediating between the patient and more specialized providers within the healthcare arena.

Insurance companies constitute the third possible locus of integration. Late entrants to the healthcare sector and long kept at arm's length by physicians, insurance companies are beginning to assume a more proactive role in packaging services, physicians, and facilities so as to appeal to consumer interests. Their limitations stem from their lack of experience in managing professional systems and their tendency to focus primary attention on financial considerations.

Modes of Integration and Interdependence

In addition to competing centers of control, contemporary systems exhibit differences in their degree of coupling and type of interdependence.

Loose versus Tight Coupling

A major change occurring in the nature of organizational systems in all sectors during the past 30 years is a shift from an emphasis on assembling system components under a single, unified ownership regime to one relying on looser types of control mechanisms that allow concerted action but preserve considerable autonomy among the participating units. These alternative arrangements are diverse and have received various labels including: contractual connections, relational contracting, quasi-firms, virtually integrated firms, strategic alliances, and networks (see Luke, Begun and Pointer

1989; Powell 1990; Kaluzny, Zuckerman, and Ricketts 1995). Healthcare organizations, compared with organizations in other industries, have been relatively quick to adopt these newer and, presumably, more flexible forms.

These new forms have developed in recognition of several hard-won truths. First, ownership and conventional authority structures often do not insure control over participants or activities. Second, the attempt to acquire valuable resources by purchasing them and asserting central managerial control over them may result in destroying their distinctiveness and value. Third, organizations that become too diversified have been found to function less effectively and efficiently than more focused firms. And fourth, alternative mechanisms exist whereby, in the absence of ownership ties, an organization does not have to resort to simple market exchange mechanisms in conducting its business. Alternative governance mechanisms to hierarchies and markets do exist. More generally, organization theorists have come to recognize the significance and increasing prevalence of *loose coupling* in both intra- and inter-organizational relations (see Weick 1976; Orton and Weick 1990).

The specific mechanisms used to forge looser ties among organizations differ widely from one another depending on the extent to which assets and resources are shared, the narrowness or breadth of linkages established, the elaboration of contracts to include broader rights such as review and profit-sharing, and the intended duration of the relation. What unites all of these various connections is that they preserve a substantial degree of organizational autonomy but at the same time are based on shared interests that are mutually beneficial to the parties concerned. The intent is to achieve the benefits deriving from scale along with those associated with specialization and flexibility (see Harrison 1994; Womack, Jones, and Roos 1990).

Symbiotic versus Mutualistic Interdependence

We also distinguish between two broad types of relations that are particularly significant in the healthcare context: symbiotic and mutualistic.[9] *Symbiotic* relations are more conventional, contractual ties between dissimilar organizations in which the parties agree to cooperate in specific and limited ways. The type of interdependence involved, in Thompson's (1967) terms, is more likely to be "pooled" or "sequential." The activities involved

---

9. A third type of interdependence—commensalistic—involving interdependence between similar units was discussed above. Commensalistic interdependence gives rise to horizontal integration.

either contribute to a common outcome (pooled) or must be performed in a given order (sequential). For example, a physician-hospital organization may contract with a physician group to reimburse them for all patients referred to a specific hospital based on a discounted fee-for-service rate.

By contrast, the *mutualistic* arrangement is one in which the interdependence between the cooperating parties is heightened by the fact that the contracts involved are risk-bearing. For example, a management service organization may negotiate capitation-based contracts with a medical group and hospital in which these entities agree to provide all necessary medical care to a specified group of patients for a fixed amount per patient. The providers in this arrangement are put financially at risk if the costs of care exceed the negotiated amount. Their outcomes are more highly interdependent than in a simple symbiotic relation and, hence, more attention must be devoted to the sharing of information and coordination of decisions and activities. In Thompson's (1967) terms, mutualistic interdependence is more likely to involve "reciprocal" ties, in which each party is obliged to take into account the other's actions in selecting their own.

Types of Integration

Just as the possible centers of control and modes of integration have become more complex, contemporary healthcare systems exhibit many types of integration, including vertical, physician-system, and functional. Diversification outside healthcare services is also prevalent.

Vertical Integration

The concept of *vertical integration* was developed in connection with the industrial firm and refers to the attempt to link within a unified control system two or more stages of the production and distribution of a product. To integrate "backward" is to extend control to earlier stages of production (e.g., acquisition of raw materials); to integrate "forward" is to extend control to later stages, including distribution facilities (see Chandler 1977). Applied to healthcare organizations, a vertically integrated system might incorporate, for example, outpatient or emergency room services, inpatient services, and extended care arrangements (see Starkweather and Carman 1987). As traditionally organized, these services are provided by independent units. A vertically integrated system brings them together under the same unified hierarchy.

The notion of integrating medical services around various stages gives rise to clinical integration, since it is possible to identify various stages of illness. Although this is the most commonly used application of the concept of vertical integration in healthcare organizations, it is somewhat problematic. Clement (1988) has observed that, viewed from the consumer (patient's) perspective, these stages do not routinely occur in a linear sequence: patients may enter the system at any stage, may return to an earlier stage of illness, and may leave the system at any stage in a given episode of illness. In short, the concept of "stages" refers to the stylized division of labor that has emerged around different types of care varying in intensity and duration. These, however, are not necessarily ordered in a one-directional time sequence for the specific patient undergoing treatment. To the extent that patients enter at divergent points and follow different sequences, the traditional mechanisms proposed by management theorists for coordination and control in integrated systems (e.g., Galbraith 1973) may not apply.

In addition, many of the recently emerging large system providers include among their holdings emergency and urgent care units, hospitals, home health agencies, and nursing homes. In numerous instances, the seemingly clinically integrated units of large healthcare systems are not within the same community or geographical locale, but scattered across diverse areas. Thus the same patients are not moving from one to another stage of service within the same system. Indeed, the fact that component units within a given community may be owned by and responsive to different corporate interests can prove to be a new obstacle to clinical integration of services. Providing a continuum of services for specific patients is not a goal for these systems. Rather, the system is simply pursuing a strategy of developing a portfolio of differentiated, related services. Such strategies are more likely to be pursued by investor-owned systems than by nonprofits, as suggested above.

Physician-System Integration

A second type of integration identified by students of healthcare organizations is *physician-system integration:* "the extent to which physicians are economically linked to a system; use its facilities and services; and actively participate in its planning, management and governance" (Gillies et al. 1996: 469). While this may seem a strange form of integration, recall that for most of this century physicians, although the most powerful figures in hospitals with the most control over the services to be dispensed, have operated as independent agents, many having staff privileges in multiple hospitals. As cost-containment pressures and competition have heightened in intensity, attempts to link hospitals and physicians in closer and more collaborative partnerships have become more common.

Morrisey and colleagues (1996) have identified four types of physician-system integration currently in use in the United States: physician-hospital organizations, management services organizations, medical foundations, and integrated healthcare organizations (see also Shortell et al. 1996). The systems vary principally in terms of extent or "tightness" of integrative mechanisms. The loosest form, the physician-hospital organization, allows for a variety of joint ventures, including freestanding ambulatory care centers or physician office buildings. More stringent are the ties involved in management services organizations and medical foundations. In these forms, the system buys the physical assets of its physicians, provides administrative services, and negotiates contracts with managed care plans. The strongest ties are to be found in integrated healthcare organizations that combine physician, hospital, and insurance services into a single entity.

These various forms for better integrating physicians and systems are much discussed in the healthcare literature but are not yet much in evidence in the healthcare field. A random survey of hospitals conducted in 1993 by Morrisey and colleagues (1996) reported that the great majority, over 75 percent, of responding hospitals were involved in none of these arrangements. Of all responding hospitals, about 15 percent reported involvement in a physician-hospital organization, 7 percent in a management services organization, 4 percent in a medical foundation, and 3 percent in an integrated healthcare organization. Note that the stronger the form of system integration involved, the smaller the number of hospitals reporting involvement.

Most observers believe that California hospitals are further along in these developments than are hospitals in other states (Enthoven and Singer 1996). The physician-hospital arrangements currently under development are, however, not easily categorized. Robinson and Casalino (1996) describe three approaches, each somewhat different from the models identified by Morrisey and colleagues. In the first approach, which most closely conforms to a management services organization model, hospital systems are investing in both integrated medical groups and independent practice associations (IPAs) as a means of "acquiring managed care expertise and of having a primary care base" (1996: 16). Among systems operating in the Bay Area, Sutter and Catholic Healthcare West (CHW) fit this pattern. In a second model, hospitals purchase minority ownership shares in medical groups and IPAs. Their intent is to develop long-term contractual relations while at the same time maintaining organizational independence. CHW, for example, owns part of the organization that manages the Hill Physicians Medical Group. A third set of hospitals neither own nor are owned by medical groups but perform as subcontractors to medical groups or HMOs. These latter arrangements are instances of the new types of loosely coupled relations.

Functional Integration

The third and most complex form of integration that has been described in the healthcare area is *functional integration:* "the extent to which key support functions and activities (such as financial management, human resources, strategic planning, information management, marketing, and quality improvement) are coordinated across operating units so as to add the greatest overall value to the system" (Gillies et al. 1996: 468). The functions enumerated are those long associated with modern management practices, but practices only recently adopted by administrators of hospital and other healthcare organizations (Shortell and Zajac 1990). But the important differentiating element in the present context is that these functions are carried out at a systemwide level and involve attempts to integrate all component operating units more fully into the system. Ideally, but not always in practice, functional integration provides "the foundation upon which physician-system and clinical integration are built" (Shortell et al. 1996: 48).

In the healthcare arena, functional integration often involves horizontal integration, since multiple, similar units, such as urgent care centers, are necessary if services are to be made available to geographically dispersed patient populations. Functional integration always involves diversification beyond the narrow range of acute-care, inpatient services offered by traditional hospitals. A wider range of related services—home health care, extended care—is required if clinical integration is to be provided; and a wider range of nonrelated services—physicians' services, insurance functions—is also needed if the critical functions involved in healthcare provision are to be managed.

Functional integration may involve symbiotic or mutualistic interdependence in varying degrees and combinations. Integration in such systems may be achieved either by means of vertical or virtual mechanisms: the services provided by the system may be either "made" (produced by component units owned by the system) or "bought" (purchased either through service contracting or risk-bearing arrangements). Functional integration is often achieved not by ownership of the components involved but the building of relational contracts and alliances among formally independent units. Most contemporary functionally integrated healthcare systems are based on both ownership and contractual relations.

Diversification

While vertical integration focuses on connecting stages in the process of producing a given product or service and/or players providing these services, diversification refers to the incorporation of diverse products or services under the same hierarchical structure. As Clement (1988) points out, the diversity may refer to production technologies, consumer groups, or consumer functions—that is, it may involve diversification in either production technologies or markets. The critical feature linking all of these variations is that "when a firm does diversify, it must acquire new assets and develop new skills" (1988: 106).

Diversification may be either related or unrelated to the core competence of the organization. *Related* diversification for an acute-care hospital might involve a movement into mental health or home health care (different production technology) or into school or occupational health (a different consumer group or function). *Nonrelated* diversification might involve, for example, the operation of a retirement center or management of an insurance company.

In Case Illustration 8.D, we examine the diversification of two systems connected to San Jose Hospital. Soon after its founding by SJH and two other local hospitals (see Case Illustration 8.C), the small, local Health Dimensions system became involved in a wide variety of healthcare services and financing plans. When Health Dimensions (then known as Good Samaritan) was sold to Columbia/HCA in 1996, its entities became part of a highly diversified healthcare system in its own right. The diversification of both of these systems involved three types: (1) elaboration of acute-care services (in non-hospital–based facilities); (2) development of services closely related to acute care; and (3) development of services unrelated to acute care.

Case Illustration 8.D   **Diversification in Bay Area Healthcare Systems: Health Dimensions and Columbia/HCA**

Health Dimensions

After its founding in 1986, Health Dimensions pursued a strategy to become "more than just a hospital—a diverse, full health care system" by branching out into nonhospital services, creating new types of formal linkages with physicians, and integrating healthcare financing with service provision (*Business Journal* 1986). It created two subsidiary corporations—one for-profit, the other nonprofit—that extended the scope of its services substantially. The for-profit venture formed ties with Health Advantage, a diversified organization that concentrated on providing alternative healthcare in nonhospital settings. Health Advantage also founded the Northern California Heart Center (a freestanding outpatient catheterization clinic) and the Northern California Kidney Stone Center. The nonprofit subsidiary merged with the Santa Clara County Visiting Nurses Association in order to integrate home health care into the hospital-based system. In addition, Health Dimensions created a network of for-profit primary and urgent care facilities in a joint venture with physicians and created a physician group practice, the Medical Group of Santa Clara County.

The system was not content simply to extend its reach and scope as a provider. As a part of his overall strategy, CEO Robert Kirk recognized the need for the system to become a "major player" in the financing of health care. In 1986, Health Dimensions, along with 13 other area hospitals, purchased the Bay Pacific Health Corporation, the fourth largest HMO in Northern California. The system also acquired part ownership in TakeCare and Lifeguard, two nonprofit HMOs, and formed an IPA-HMO (Stark-weather 1990).

Columbia/HCA

Investor-owned Columbia Hospital Corporation was formed in 1988 when founder, Richard L. Scott, attempted to acquire Hospital Corporation of America (HCA). After his takeover bid failed, Scott purchased two hospitals in El Paso, Texas. By 1992, Columbia owned 24 hospitals, and by 1995, in part because of a merger with HCA and the acquisition of HealthTrust, had accumulated 332 hospitals in 37 states. Columbia/HCA currently owns 6 hospitals in the Bay Area.

During the 1990s, Columbia/HCA diversified its holdings. It purchased two orthopedic products laboratories in 1990 (Lumsdon and Hagland 1994), as well as Medical Care America, a network of 96 ambulatory surgical centers, in 1994. In 1995, Columbia/HCA formed the Columbia Homecare Group, and by 1997, had acquired 570 home health agencies. In 1997, Columbia/HCA's holdings also included 60 rehabilitation units, 17 outpatient rehabilitation facilities, and 117 psychiatric units. And, by 1997, Columbia/HCA had alliances with over 1,400 physician practices, including joint ventures, Columbia/HCA-owned medical groups, and enrollment in its PPO, the Health Advantage Network. Most of these alliances arose from the acquisition of other systems rather than from new ventures (Kuttner 1996).

After a rash of lawsuits and investigations concerning possible Medicare fraud, illegal insider trading, and inappropriate financial bonuses for physicians, Columbia/HCA's CEO and founder, Richard L. Scott, and several other top executives resigned in 1997 (Limbacher 1997). The new system executives instituted a restructuring plan, including selling the Columbia Homecare Group and 20 percent of its outpatient surgical centers, and spinning off 108 hospitals into three new companies with separate boards and their own names (Limbacher 1997). Columbia/HCA also acquired a cable television channel, America's Health Network, in order to build Columbia/HCA's brand recognition (Jaspen 1997). But, in 1997, the system decided to let hospitals drop the Columbia moniker, and the system even removed the name Columbia from its headquarters building in Nashville, Tennessee. How this giant healthcare system negotiates its future and which pieces of its diversified system will be kept or divested remains to be seen.

COMBINING FORMS OF INTERDEPENDENCE AND MODES OF INTEGRATION

Table 8.3 summarizes some of the principal distinctions made in our review of types of interdependence and mechanisms for managing these connections. Examples are provided of these integrating mechanisms in the healthcare arena.

Table 8.3 is created by a simple cross-classification of two dimensions: (1) the type of interdependence involved between care units and (2) the mode of integration mechanism employed to achieve better coordination. The logic of the table is based on the insight by Pfeffer and Salancik (1978: 43) that "the typical solution to problems of interdependence and uncertainty involves increasing coordination, which means increasing the mutual control over each others' activities." In short, organizations deal with interdependence by creating governance structures. Interdependence is subdivided into three categories: (1) commensalistic, involving relations between similar units; (2) symbiotic, involving relations among dissimilar units in which the level of interdependence is relatively low or circumscribed; and (3) mutualistic, involving relations among dissimilar units that are more highly interdependent. Governance mechanisms are classified by degree of coupling into those that are looser versus those that are more tightly integrated. As the examples suggest, there is a rich array of governance mechanisms currently being employed in the healthcare arena.

Evidence of Rising Integration in the Bay Area

We turn now to examine evidence regarding the increasing levels of connections among healthcare organizations in the San Francisco Bay Area. We focus primarily on the developing connections among our principal organizational populations: hospitals, health maintenance organizations, home health agencies, and renal disease centers. Systematic data enabling us to track these changes were not available before 1976, and so the period of

Table 8.3 Typology of Interdependence and Coordinating Mechanisms

Type of Interdependence	Coordinating Mechanisms *With examples of hospital-based mechanisms* Loosely coupled ⟵———————⟶ Tightly coupled	
Commensalistic	Associations *Membership in AHA*	Horizontal integration *Entry into Multihospital systems*
Symbiotic	Service contracting *Contract with HHA or ESRDC*	Vertical integration *Own HHA or ESRDC*
Mutualistic	Risk-bearer contracting *Capitation agreement with HMO*	Functional integration *Entry into integrated system*

time covered is much shorter than in our earlier analyses. The effects of this limitation are reduced, however, since much of the action in the integration among organizational forms has been concentrated in the past two decades.

Growth of Contracting

Figures 8.4 and 8.5 provide data on changes over time in the proportion of hospitals that own or hold contracts with HHAs and with ESRDCs, respectively.[10] The plots reveal that an expanding proportion of hospitals are providing home health and kidney dialysis services and, moreover, that a rising proportion of the organizations that choose to provide these services are relying on contractual mechanisms to do so. Hospitals increasingly favor virtual over vertical integration, particularly in the case of kidney treatments.

The proportion of home health contracts was almost negligible in the late 1970s, with less than 10 percent of nonfederal Bay Area hospitals holding such contracts. By the early 1990s, that proportion had more than doubled to around 20 percent. Much of this development seems to have occurred after the beginning of the era of market mechanisms, marked by the passage of PPS legislation in 1983. The shift toward contracting is even more dramatic in the domain of renal disease treatment, where service contract adoption rose from a low of 2 percent of the organizational population in 1978 to 58 percent in 1991.[11] By the early 1990s, the relative

10. The definition of HHAs and ESRDCs for this analysis is broader than that employed in defining the organizational populations in chapter 2. In particular, we include here contractual and ownership relations between hospitals and *all* HHAs and ESRDCs in the area, not just those that are Medicare-certified.

11. For those few cases in which a hospital contracted for some subset of services in a domain and also owned others, we have coded that facility in the "contracting" category for analytical purposes.

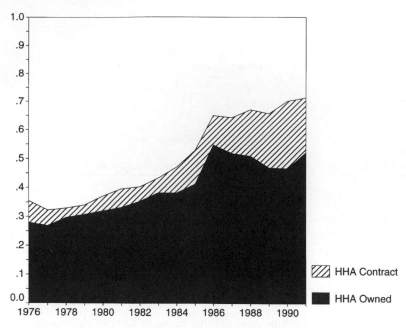

Figure 8.4   Proportion of Bay Area Hospitals with HHA Contracts and Ownership
Relations, 1976–91

proportion of hospitals that contracted for ESRD services, as opposed to
those that maintained their own kidney dialysis facilities, had reversed itself,
with contracting being favored by a two-to-one ratio.

This relatively large difference in the mode of provision of two important services raises an interesting theoretical question: why have evolutionary processes—whether ecological or adaptive—favored higher rates
of contracting in the ESRD than in the HHA domain? A possible answer
is suggested by our earlier discussion of niche specialization (see chap. 5).
Home health service provision involves a generalist niche, where many of
its activities enjoy a "spillover" effect from traditional hospital services and
routines. For example, a hospital could rely to some extent on its existing
nursing staff as a labor pool for home nursing personnel. By contrast, kidney
dialysis services involve a much more specialized niche, which may or may
not be able to draw on existing hospital capabilities. These arguments are
closely related to those developed by institutional economists, as discussed
in the next section.

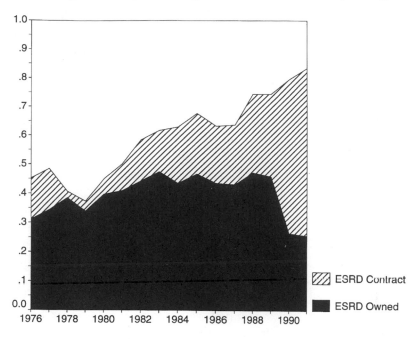

Figure 8.5 Proportion of Bay Area Hospitals with ESRDC Contracts and Ownership Relations, 1976–91

"Make" or "Buy" Decisions in Service Contracting

We can examine what sorts of factors affect a hospital's decision to provide a service within the framework of its own organizational structure ("make") or to contract for that service to be provided by some external organization ("buy").[12] These are the kinds of strategic decisions that have been addressed by the "new" institutional economics—in particular, transaction cost economics (see Williamson 1975, 1985). This perspective has been frequently employed by healthcare analysts to attempt to account for specific governance structures at the organizational level (e.g., Hurley and Fennell 1990; Mick 1990a; Robinson and Casalino 1996). As noted in chapter 1, transaction cost economists argue that organizational managers attempt to design governance structures in order to reduce the transaction

12. Yet a third alternative involves the development of a shared service arrangement with other hospitals. For analytical purposes, we include this choice in the category of external contracting.

(economic exchange) costs in which they are involved. This theoretical approach compares the relative costs and benefits associated with various possible structural arrangements. For example, external contracting affords the hospital greater flexibility in adding or eliminating services without large-scale resource investment, but at the same time it may introduce costs resulting from the need to monitor "opportunism" (the possibility that a partner may be dishonest) and the quality of service provision from the vendor. By contrast, in-house provision avoids these transaction costs but entails different costs in the form of capital expenditures, training, and coordination costs. It may also inhibit long-term adaptiveness on account of the sunk costs in personnel and equipment.

The transaction cost literature points to a number of environmental conditions under which hospitals might favor ownership ("make" decisions) over contracting ("buy" decisions). One involves the number of alternative vendors available to a hospital within a given service region. When the number of possible partners is large, the hospital gains leverage in choosing vendors and may refrain from contracting with partners thought to be overly opportunistic. In less competitive markets, on the other hand, the choice may be quite restricted so that leverage shifts to the vendors. Hospitals are expected to be more favorable to contracting under the former than the latter conditions. In short, we expect that hospitals will have a greater propensity to own, rather than contract for, services when the number of alternative vendors is small.

A second environmental condition affecting the make-or-buy decision involves the uncertainty and complexity surrounding contractual transactions. Institutional economists have pointed to the problem of uncertainty in contingent claims contracting, when the delivery of some product or service is tied to unknown future developments. According to this argument, service ownership will be favored in more turbulent environments (Williamson 1975). Our earlier arguments, however, suggest reasons for challenging this conclusion. Service ownership on the part of hospitals entails a sunk investment in a set of therapeutic modalities and can be undesirable in uncertain environments where adaptivity is a primary concern. Moreover, a more sociological version of institutionalism emphasizes the salience of changing logics. We note that the recent turbulence in the healthcare field has been accompanied by a market-oriented logic that carries with it a normative commitment to market (e.g., contracting) as opposed to hierarchical (ownership) governance structures to manage exchange relations. Considering the era of market mechanisms (1983–present) as a period of heightened turbulence and increased market orientation, we expect that hospitals will have a lower propensity to own services (and a greater likelihood of entering into contractual agreements) during this most recent era than during the earlier period of federal involvement.

We have already pointed out, in our discussion of figures 8.4 and 8.5, that there is an apparent difference between hospitals' propensity to acquire HHAs as compared with ESRD units. We argued that this is a function of the niche specificity of the service category: home health being the more generalist form and kidney disease treatment the more specialist. Hospitals are expected to be more likely to own HHAs than ESRDCs because they can more easily and efficiently incorporate the generalist services. The same prediction can be made employing the language and logic of institutional economists. Whether an organization makes or buys a specific service appears to depend in part on the specificity of the assets involved: the more specific the assets, the more likely that the service will be contracted out (Williamson 1981). These arguments support our expectation that hospitals will be more likely to contract for kidney treatment than for home health services.

Structural features of hospitals may also affect make-or-buy decisions. Our earlier historical review noted a progressive evolution of hospital structures, from autonomous acute-care facilities during the era of professional dominance, to the emergence of multihospital systems and chains during the era of federal involvement, to the current period in which we witness the creation of integrated delivery systems. Given this stylized evolutionary path, we anticipate that hospitals that are members of integrated systems will be more likely to expand their portfolio of services beyond conventional boundaries to incorporate less traditional but related services such as home health and kidney disease treatment. We treat other structural variables, such as age, size, and ownership, as controls in this analysis.

We also examine the influence of hospital performance on contracting decisions. When hospitals have historically maintained high occupancy rates, they are more likely to add new services in-house, believing that patient demand will be able to sustain those services. Hospitals that have experienced low occupancy rates will be more inclined to contract out for the new services, believing that the sunk costs associated with service addition cannot be justified by demand.

Analysis of "Make" or "Buy" Decisions

Our analyses of service contracting employed a pooled sample of hospital make-or-buy decisions for home health and renal disease services. The pooled cases included 280 contracting decisions by hospitals in the Bay Area between 1976 and 1991. Of these decisions, 110 resulted in an outcome that favored service contracting with an external vendor, while the remaining 170 cases favored in-house service provision. A series of logit models was estimated to consider the impact of structural, evaluative, and environmental characteristics on the decision outcomes. For purposes of these analyses, the dichotomous dependent variable was coded as a 0 for a contracting (buy) decision and a 1 for a service ownership decision (see table 8.4).

As shown in the first model specification, structural characteristics generally had a limited impact on the make-or-buy decision. Although a likelihood ratio test reveals that this model is a significant improvement over a specification including only the intercept ($\chi^2 = 34.80$, df $= 6$, p $< .001$), most of the variance is explained by a single variable: service niche specialization. Make-or-buy decisions involving ESRD services are treated as specialized, and decisions involving home health services are treated as reflecting a more generalist niche. The observed negative parameter estimate is consistent with our expectation that asset specialization leads to a lower probability of a "make" decision and greater probability of a "buy" decision.

The effect of multihospital system membership, the other structural variable of theoretical interest, was not statistically significant. Contrary to our prediction, system hospitals in the Bay Area had a slightly greater tendency to engage in contracting than nonsystem hospitals. Control variables such as organizational age, size, and ownership had no notable impact on make-or-buy decisions.

The introduction of evaluative characteristics (model 2) improves the model fit only slightly (likelihood ratio $\chi^2 = 4.11$, df $= 3$, ns). Consistent with our theorizing, the most significant impact is witnessed for hospital performance. Those facilities with high occupancy rates are more likely to add new services in-house than facilities with low occupancy rates. The latter hospitals are inclined to experience greater anxiety about patient demand and are therefore "risk-averse" with respect to make-or-buy decisions. Other evaluative characteristics, such as technical and managerial legitimacy, do not have any notable effect on the decision-making process.

A final model adds environmental characteristics to the specification (likelihood ratio $\chi^2 = 7.69$, df $= 2$, p $< .05$). As predicted, the heightened turbulence during the era of market reform markedly decreases the probability of service ownership. When hospitals confront a more complex and competitive environment, they are less willing to invest resources in acquiring new services and more apt to invoke contractual arrangements.

Table 8.4   Logit Models of "Make" or "Buy" Decisions for Bay Area Hospital
Services, 1976–91[a]

Variable	Model 1	Model 2	Model 3
Intercept	1.416 (1.126)	− 0.224 (1.527)	0.760 (1.649)
Organizational Structure:			
Age	−0.001 (0.004)	0.001 (0.005)	0.003 (0.005)
Size (log beds)	−0.020 (0.224)	0.082 (0.269)	−0.049 (0.282)
For-profit ownership	0.110 (0.466)	0.326 (0.483)	0.382 (0.495)
Government ownership	−0.267 (0.345)	−0.225 (0.365)	−0.020 (0.378)
System membership	−0.280 (0.295)	−0.357 (0.323)	−0.221 (0.332)
Service niche specialism	−1.465 (0.265)**	−1.460 (0.271)**	−1.231 (0.335)**
Organizational Evaluation:			
Technical legitimacy	—	−0.118 (0.196)	−0.092 (0.201)
Managerial legitimacy	—	0.019 (0.248)	0.063 (0.253)
Performance (occupancy)	—	1.751 (0.909)*	1.482 (0.940)#
Environment:			
Turbulence[b]	—	—	−0.966 (0.363)**
Competition (vendor density)	—	—	0.050 (0.038)#
Number of cases [c]	278	278	278
Number of ("make") events	169	169	169
−2 Log likelihood (d.f.)	337.54 (6)	333.43 (9)	325.74 (11)

NOTES: # $p < .10$; * $p < .05$; ** $p < .01$ (one-tailed tests)

a. The dependent variable is dichotomous, coded 0 for contracting ("buy") and 1 for service ownership
("make").

b. Period effect for era of managerial-market orientation (1983–91).

c. Two cases excluded because of missing covariate information.

We also expected the number of vendors in the same county as a hospital
to increase the likelihood of contracting. The empirical results, however,
showed the opposite result: the density of vendors in the county increased
the probability of service ownership rather than contracting out. This result
may be more reflective of the extent of patient demand for home health
and ESRD services (which is unmeasured in these models) than vendor
competition per se.

Purchaser and Provider Agreements in Risk-Bearing Contracting

We shift now to consider a set of relations involving hospitals that are
more likely to entail higher levels of interdependence. While the HHA
and ESRDC linkages discussed in the previous section more often involve
symbiotic interdependence, the purchaser agreements, in which hospitals
enter into contracts with increasingly powerful purchasers and medical

providers of healthcare services, are more likely to involve mutualistic interdependence (refer to table 8.3).

Figure 8.6 shows the changing proportion of hospitals entering into contracts with a wide range of providers of physicians' services, on the one hand, and purchasers of services for "covered lives," on the other. As we have argued throughout this volume, healthcare organizations increasingly find themselves at the center of a nexus of contracts involving both payors (and their intermediaries) and providers (see fig. 2.2). In constructing figure 8.6, we construe purchaser-provider agreements broadly to include a wide variety of capitated, direct service, and discounted fee-for-service contracts between hospitals, on the one hand, and insurance carriers, insurance pools, HMOs, PPOs, labor unions, corporations, and governmental entities, on the other. Excluded from this definition are simple fee-for-service agreements and standard Medicare/Medicaid contracts. The data show a quite dramatic increase in both the proportion of hospitals with purchaser-provider agreements and in the numbers of contracts entered into by hospitals. In the short period between 1980 and 1990, the proportion of hospitals with no agreements dropped from over 70 percent to under 30 percent. At the same time, the proportion of hospitals entering into six or more contracts increased from zero percent in 1980 to over 40 percent in 1990.

Factors affecting mutualistic contracting. The rate of occurrence of contracting events may be affected by several sets of variables, again including structural characteristics of hospitals, evaluative dimensions of hospital organizations, and environmental characteristics. Among the structural features, organizational age is likely to play an especially important role. Older hospitals are expected to be less likely to engage in risk-bearing contracting because of increased conservatism and structural inertia. By its very nature, risk-bearing contracting threatens the reliability of such venerable institutions, forcing the adoption of new organizational patterns, new types of relations, and new monitoring mechanisms. Younger hospitals are expected to be better able to cope with such extensive changes. Conversely, we assume that once hospitals have adopted a number of purchaser-provider contracts, this will provide encouragement for those facilities to engage in further mutualistic affiliations. According to this logic, the barriers posed by structural inertia against risk-bearing contracts should decrease with previous change events.

Apart from the role played by structural inertia, the decision on whether to engage in purchaser-provider contracting presents possible threats to

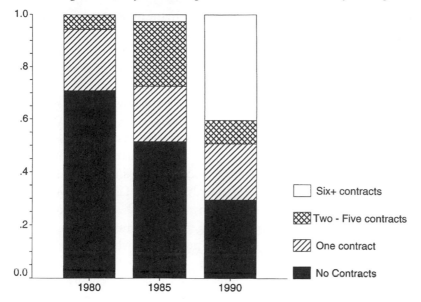

Figure 8.6 Proportion of Bay Area Hospitals with Purchaser and Provider Contracts, 1980–90

the identity of a hospital organization. Facilities that have long viewed themselves as fairly autonomous entities (though embedded in community networks) may be hesitant to become too entangled in a web linking them with large insurance carriers and HMOs. Purchaser contracts bring stable revenue flows, but they also invite incursions from the purchasers, who seek to put in place new oversight mechanisms for monitoring efficiency, patient satisfaction, and quality of care (Robinson 1995). By contrast, hospitals that have become system members are more likely to adopt purchaser agreements, in part because the corporate offices of systems encourage if not require them to do so. We also expect for-profit facilities to be more likely to embrace these newer, risk-bearing relations.

Just as system membership is not a decision made exclusively by the hospital member, so we must also consider the attractiveness of the hospital from the point of view of the prospective partners—the purchasers and providers who enter into the contracts with hospitals. In order to seek out contracts with a given hospital, purchasers must first of all recognize the organization as a potential target of affiliation. Other things being equal, the larger the hospital, the more likely it is to be visible to prospective partners. Size may also be regarded as, in some ways, an indicator of cultural-cognitive legitimacy (see chap. 7), indicating the greater acceptance and recognition of the hospital in its service area. On the other hand, population ecologists argue that size also increases structural inertia (see Hannan and Freeman 1984), and this effect might serve to dampen propensities toward mutualistic affiliation. Empirically, then, it is unclear what effects may be associated with hospital size and provider contracting.

Another potential antecedent of a hospital's capacity to attract mutualistic exchange partners is its normative legitimacy—the extent to which it receives the endorsement of appropriate managerial and technical professional associations. As discussed at length in the previous chapter, normative legitimacy is assessed in terms of scores based on accreditations and certifications received from meeting the standards set by professional governance structures. Given that our interest is in contractual ties, we would expect the receipt of normative approval from managerial associations to be especially significant in garnering affiliations with purchasers, who are expected to use such signals as a means of identifying opportunistic or incompetent administrative staffs in hospitals. The technical legitimacy of a hospital may also be a consideration in selecting contracting partners, but we would expect it to be less salient in this regard.

Analysis of purchaser-provider agreements. Our event history models of provider and purchaser contracting treated these affiliations as events to which a hospital may be subject repeatedly. Data for this analysis are available for the period 1981–87 only. The primary "clock" of the contracting events is based on the time that has elapsed since the last observed event or entry into the set of hospitals at risk of engaging in such agreements. Two other time clocks are accommodated indirectly. One, organizational age, is incorporated into the models as a covariate. Heterogeneity of event rates affected by another clock, historical time, is treated as an underlying "nuisance" function (see Appendix C, Organizational Adaptation).

Model 1 in table 8.5 considers the effects of organizational structure on hospital contracting with purchasers and providers. Hospital age significantly reduces the likelihood that a hospital will enter into (or be selected for) a contract. The increased conservatism (structural inertia) of some venerable facilities leads them to avoid the relatively novel practice of purchaser contracting. This conservatism can be overcome insofar as an organization has previous involvement in provider-purchaser contracting. Such previous experience is significantly ($p < .01$) associated with entering into additional contracts.

Two other structural variables are not consistent with our predictions. Both for-profit status and system membership are found to decrease con-

Table 8.5 Cox Models of Bay Area Hospital Purchaser-Provider Contracting, 1981–87

Variable	Model 1	Model 2	Model 3
Organizational Structure:			
Age	−0.010 (0.003)**	−0.008 (0.003)**	−0.008 (0.003)**
Size (log beds)	0.196 (0.133)#	0.132 (0.160)	0.184 (0.163)
For-profit ownership	−1.095 (0.358)**	−0.905 (0.379)**	−0.843 (0.382)*
Government ownership	−0.204 (0.218)	0.002 (0.239)	0.008 (0.239)
System membership	−0.608 (0.203)**	−0.472 (0.218)*	−0.463 (0.216)*
Existing contracts[a]	0.160 (0.016)**	0.158 (0.016)**	0.157 (0.016)**
Organizational Evaluation:			
Technical legitimacy	—	0.036 (0.122)	0.075 (0.126)
Managerial legitimacy	—	0.505 (0.208)**	0.507 (0.206)**
Performance (occupancy)	—	1.034 (0.608)*	1.020 (0.613)*
Environment:			
Competition (hospital density)[a,b]	—	—	−0.167 (0.113)#
Number of cases	551	551	551
Number of events	127	127	127
−2 Log likelihood (d.f.)	1308.62 (6)	1298.63 (9)	1296.52 (10)

NOTES: # $p < .10$; * $p < .05$; ** $p < .01$ (one-tailed tests)

a. Covariate is lagged by one year.

b. Log-transformation applied to covariate.

tracting rates markedly. In the latter case, in particular, we had expected that autonomous hospitals would be less likely to engage in risk-bearer contracting because of the threats posed by this practice to organizational independence and identity. A specific counterargument can be offered, however, from the perspective of resource dependency (Pfeffer and Salancik 1978). According to this line of reasoning, autonomous hospitals are *especially* susceptible to mutualistic contracting because they lack the broader network of resources available to multihospital system members.[13]

Turning to the effects of organizational evaluation (model 2), we find that managerial legitimacy has a positive and significant effect on purchaser-provider contracting, as expected. This finding concurs with the widespread opinion in the field that professional accreditation is an important precondition for purchaser contracts (Bergman 1994). Organizational performance (as proxied by the occupancy rate) also encourages contracting ($p < .05$).

13. The case of Kaiser Permanente also poses problems for the analysis. KP system hospitals primarily serve KP's enrollment population and therefore have relatively few contracts with outside purchasers. When KP hospitals are removed from the analysis, the significance of the system membership covariate drops to the $p < .05$ level in model 1.

In both these respects, then, the ability of a hospital to attract purchasers by signaling managerial competency and patient demand for its services seems to be more important than the functional need of a poorly run hospital to gain access to purchaser funding streams. The final evaluative criteria, technical legitimacy, shows a positive effect on contracting but is not statistically significant.

A third model adds environmental conditions to the specification. The number of hospitals operating in a given county tends to lower the rate of contracting for each individual hospital because of heightened competition among the facilities (although the result is only marginally significant at the p < .10 level).

Conclusion: The Changing Structure of Linkages among Healthcare Organizations

This chapter has reviewed the changing levels and types of connections among healthcare organization. We have examined how individual organizations, principally hospitals, have been transformed during the period of our study. They began life operating primarily as independent, locally embedded organizations that occasionally formed loose associational ties with other hospitals to pursue common interests. Next, predominantly in the second era of federal involvement, hospitals began to become affiliated with other hospitals, forming multihospital systems or chains. These horizontal connections based on commensalistic relations provided a precursor form to developments now underway. During the third era, fueled by competitive pressures and a rapidly developing corporate logic, hospitals have increasingly become submerged in integrated health systems—systems that vertically or virtually connect multiple types of providers together with insurance functions and medical group participants.

These manifold developments are summarized as they have affected selected providers in the San Francisco Bay Area during the more recent period, between the years 1980 and 1990. Figure 8.7 displays some of the many types of linkages that have developed among healthcare units. Horizontal ties between, for example, chains of home health agencies or between hospitals involved in multihospital systems, are distinguished from vertical or functionally integrated ties linking different kinds of providers. As noted, horizontal ties are even more common among specialized providers such as ESRDCs and HHAs, than between hospitals: large primarily for-profit chains have proliferated in the past two decades (Gray 1986; Snow 1997).

We also differentiate between vertical ties that are based on ownership and virtual ties based on relational contracting. We have not attempted to represent the further distinctions made earlier between symbiotic and mutualistic relations.

Two percentages are provided for each relation, the first pertaining to 1980, the second to 1990. In both cases, the reference unit is the organizational form toward which the arrow is pointed. For example,

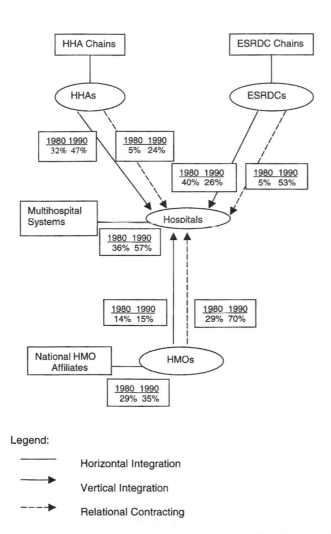

Figure 8.7 Comparison of Linkages among Organizational Populations in the Bay Area, 1980 and 1990

32 percent of the hospitals in our population owned HHAs in 1980 compared with 47 percent in 1990. In all instances save one, we observe an increase in these linkages. Some of these changes are rather modest. For example, there have not been large increases in vertical ties between HMOs and hospitals but, by contrast, contractual linkages between these forms have increased from 29 to 70 percent. The percent of hospitals both owning and contracting with HHAs has risen during the 10-year period. The only case in which a reduction in ties occurs involves the case of vertical (ownership) ties between hospitals and ESRDCs. In 1980, 40 percent of the hospitals owned such facilities, whereas in 1990 only 26 percent did so. What we observe, however, is not a reduction in the frequency of this relation but a change in its form: during the same period the number of hospitals contracting for ESRD services increased from 5 percent in 1980 to 53 percent in 1990. Virtual ties are replacing vertical connections in this linkage. Similarly, horizontal ties between providers continued to increase during this period. The numbers of hospitals involved in multihospital systems or integrated healthcare systems increased from 36 percent in 1980 to 57 percent in 1990. Likewise, the proportion of HMOs affiliated with national bodies increased during the decade from 29 percent to 35 percent. Vertical linkages are not replacing horizontal ties: both types are on the rise in the healthcare field.

Although figure 8.7 is a useful vehicle for representing changes over time in the numbers and types of relations between selected components of the healthcare field in the Bay Area, it does distort one important facet of the changes underway. It depicts the various organizational components as though they all were retaining their independence—their status as autonomous entities. This is largely the case when the linkages involved are horizontal, although participants involved in such ties find some constraints on their actions. This is less the case when the linkages involved are virtual, for example, relational contracting. Here, there is greater interdependence and higher constraints on activities jointly undertaken, requiring varying degrees of mutuality and reciprocal adjustments. Still, however, the organizational entities involved maintain their formal independence. In the case of vertical integration, however, organizational components lose their independent identity, being subsumed and submerged into a broader enterprise. Organizational boundaries, both functional and formal, are redefined by vertical integration.

Viewed at a higher level, the developing ties between organizational populations not only link these players into complex networks and alliances. Some of them result in the erosion of the boundaries between organizational populations and the creation of new types of populations. One of our populations, healthcare systems, contains organizational forms that have developed by encompassing—and eliminating as independent entities—other, more specialized organizations. But note also that some of the healthcare systems described—those based on virtual rather than vertical relations—create systems that preserve the formal boundaries and identity of participating units. Such systems appear to be particularly well suited to the logics of the healthcare field, since they maintain autonomy but facilitate flexibility.

This means, however, that some "new" populations of organizations, such as integrated healthcare systems, are comprised of radically different kinds of structural forms. Some are tightly coupled, vertically integrated forms, while others are loosely coupled network forms.[14] Catholic Healthcare West and Columbia/HCA are both regarded as healthcare systems, but are they appropriately considered to be members of the same organizational population? If the answer is yes, then the conventional definition of population, which rests on the use of similar structural archetypes, will need to be revised.

14. The same kind of wide variation in organizational forms now exists in the automobile industry, among others. Toyota's network structure of relational contracts represents a quite different mode of organizing from General Motor's more vertically integrated structure (see Womack, Jones and Roos 1990).

Nine

INSTITUTIONAL ENVIRONMENTS AND THE ORGANIZATIONAL FIELD

FROM THE BEGINNING OF THIS STUDY, we have characterized the transformation of the U.S. healthcare field over the past half century as an instance of "profound institutional change." Change has occurred, often abruptly, in the fundamental constitutive logics and governance structures that undergird the field, ultimately reaching across levels and types of actors, albeit at varying rates. Belief systems and governance arrangements have incorporated novel logics and rules; new types of providers, intermediaries, and field-level organizations have appeared on the scene alongside traditional players; and relations and boundaries among virtually all actors have been substantially reconfigured.

In previous chapters, especially chapters 5 and 6, we provided a dense depiction of these changes. Using our conceptual framework of institutional and material-resource environments, we identified trends along several dimensions. Still, our theme has been that the multiple variables exhibit an underlying coherence reflecting large-scale, latent phenomena. In this chapter, we sort through the thicket of forces at work in transforming the American healthcare sector in order to discern these fundamental influences and describe their trajectory and timing. We then analyze the relationships among these fieldwide forces to provide some understanding of the mechanisms that have produced these profound institutional shifts. We conclude by examining the effects of changes in institutional logics and material-resource conditions on our organizational populations.

DEPICTING PROFOUND INSTITUTIONAL CHANGE

Institutional Logics

312   Table 9.1 displays three groups of indicators selected to represent the primary logics we have identified in the U.S. healthcare field. The variables

comprise a diverse array of measures of logics as reflected in governance structures, funding sources, and professional affiliations.[1] Employing a confirmatory factor analysis, we use these multiple indicators to model the existence of latent phenomena, or factors—in this case, the dominant field logics—and to estimate their magnitude over time in standardized metrics, or factor scores (see Appendix C for a description of factor analysis methods and computation of factor scores).

Professional dominance is represented by a combination of both professional association and voluntary ethos indicators that are most closely linked to the first era identified in our study. The factor for *federal involvement* includes measures of the federal government's expanding role as a source of overall health expenditures, as well as of health insurance and medical research funding in particular.[2] The *managerial-market orientation* factor incorporates variables related to shifts in physician perspectives embracing (or co-opting) managerial initiatives and in health insurance trends toward market reforms and managed care plans.

The standardized coefficients, or loadings, which signify the strength of each indicator's correlation and contribution to the latent factor, range from .820 to .996. The comparative fit index (CFI) measures the degree of overall association and coherence among the indicators. Although such measures of fit are not especially important in evaluating confirmatory factor models, this index is very strong for each factor, ranging from .949 to .998.[3]

Figure 9.1 presents the factor scores calculated for the three primary logics, with each standardized for comparability. The trends graphically capture several important aspects of the institutional transformations in U.S. healthcare discussed in earlier chapters. First, the graph demonstrates the relative pacing of change, with both abrupt and more gradual turns. Professional dominance, ascendant at the beginning of the study period, gradually dwindles in force, slowly at first and then much more rapidly after 1963. Experiencing a brief resurgence in 1970, the score declines

1. Unfortunately, our data from discourse coding and policy mapping (see chap. 6) could not be included because of methodological issues of sampling, data consistency, and coverage.

2. Other measures of federal involvement (e.g., federal expenditures for hospital construction and federally employed physicians) take a shift downward during the mid-1970s, reflecting a change in the nature of federal intervention rather than its absence (away from provision of infrastructure or direct services and their planning, in favor of funding for private delivery of services or research activities and the structuring of private incentives). Consequently, these measures were not incorporated into the federal involvement factor.

3. The CFI (Bentler 1990) ranges from 0 to 1 and indicates a better fit as it approaches 1. Values over .90 are generally considered very strong. Three CFI scores are reported since each factor was estimated separately (see note 4 for a description of a joint factor model of the three primary logics).

Table 9.1 Confirmatory Factor Models of Primary Logics in U.S. Healthcare, 1948–94

Latent Factor	Indicators	Descriptions	Standardized Coefficient	Model Fit
Professional dominance	AMA membership	Proportion of active physicians	0.969	CFI = 0.949
	Blue Cross/Blue Shield benefit expenditures	Proportion of civilian health plan benefits	0.966	N = 47
				$\chi^2 = 15.243$
	Blue Cross/Blue Shield enrollees	Proportion of civilian insured	0.956	
				df = 2
	Philanthropy for health and hospitals	Proportion of national private health expenditures	0.846	
Federal involvement	Medicare & Medicaid enrollees	Proportion of civilian insured	0.996	CFI = 0.998
	Medicare & Medicaid benefit expenditures	Proportion of civilian health plan benefits	0.992	N = 46
				$\chi^2 = 2.574$
	Federal health expenditures	Proportion of national health expenditures	0.983	df = 2
	Public medical research funding[a]	Proportion of national medical research expenditures	0.820	
Managerial-market orientation	Physician executives	ACPE membership as proportion of active physicians	0.987	CFI = 0.967
	HMO & independent plan[b] enrollees	Proportion of civilian insured	0.977	N = 47
	HMO & independent plan[b] benefit expenditures	Proportion of civilian health plan benefits	0.934	$\chi^2 = 21.074$
				df = 5
	Medicaid enrollees in HMOs	Proportion of Medicaid enrollees	0.983	
	Medicare enrollees in HMOs	Proportion of Medicare enrollees	0.974	

NOTES: a. Includes negligible amounts of nonfederal funds. Does not include research and development expenditures of pharmaceutical companies (see fig. 6.6).

b. HMO, employer self-insured, and other independent health plans not underwritten by insurance companies or Blue Cross/Blue Shield (see figs. 5.2 and 6.2).

again from that point to the end of the study period. The striking bolt in federal involvement in 1965 represents the strongest instance of profound change observed throughout the length of the study. This dramatic increase in federal involvement is observed to coincide with a substantial drop in the professional dominance score. Following the initial shock of federal involvement, we observe a relatively gradual and incremental change process, marked by increases for federal involvement and decreases for professional dominance logics. Managerial-market logics are present at modest levels throughout the entire period of study but do not begin their challenge to unseat existing logics until the late 1970s. The managerial-market logics sharply accelerate their rate of increase during the early 1980s, marking the onset of the third era. It is important to observe, however, that this development occurs with little correspondingly abrupt change in the other two logics.[4]

Second, the trends depicted demonstrate that although the three periods are marked by the rise in prominence of a particular logic and accompanying governance arrangements, the eras are not tightly configured containers. While professional dominance logics and structures loom large in the first era before the passage of the Medicare and Medicaid programs, both federal involvement and managerial-market logics are evident but weak during this period. Federal actors were providing infrastructural support throughout this period in the form of research, facilities, and manpower expenditures; similarly, HMO and prepaid health insurance plans, now a major component of the managed care movement, have a long history, with some early forms even predating the beginning of our study period.

The later two eras display even more institutional heterogeneity. The second era of federal involvement is marked by the ascendance of this logic, which then coexists along with the continuing—albeit diminished—logic of professional dominance. As Starr (1982) notes, an "accommodation" was made between public and professional interests during this period. Although professionals suffer a marked decline in dominance with the expansion of federal involvement, they are not replaced, but rather, joined by public agencies and interests during the second era.

---

4. All factors in these analyses were estimated separately. But in order to explore the relationship between the primary logic factors, we also estimated a joint model that included covariation among the three latent variables. As expected, the professional dominance factor is negatively correlated with federal responsibility and managerial-market orientation, strongly in the former case and moderately in the latter (-0.99 and -0.67, respectively). The federal responsibility and managerial-market orientation factors are positively correlated with each other at 0.58 (all covariations significant at $p < .01$). Once standardized, factor score trends generated from the joint model were virtually identical with those from the separately estimated factor models.

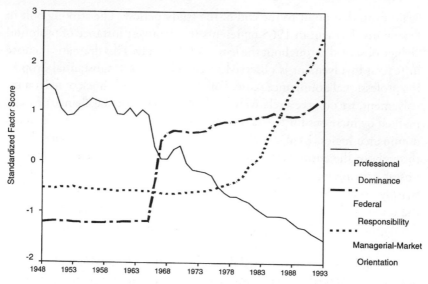

Figure 9.1   Primary Logics in U.S. Healthcare, Factor Score Trends, 1948–93

The forces depicted in figure 9.1 dramatically demonstrate the complexity of the current, third era. Three logics—professional, public, corporate—are all present, active, and contending with one another. While the managerial-market logics experience rapid ascendance, federal involvement also increases during this period. The logic of professional dominance continues to decline throughout this period, but by no means has it been eliminated.[5] More generally, all three logics retain considerable salience, leaving the field far from its uncontested configuration of the late 1940s.

This situation appears to reflect what Scott (1994: 211) has characterized as a shift from a condition in which one institutionalized belief system dominates a field, as illustrated by the position of the medical establishment in 1945, to one in which there exist two or more "strong, competing or conflicting belief systems" that contend for supremacy. The move from the former to the latter state has been shown to be fateful

5. It should also be noted that the declining trend in figure 9.1 represents a weakening of organized medicine's institutional domination of decisions, policies, and perspectives in the healthcare field, rather than the demise of the medical profession per se. For example, the quality of medical care—a core value of the medical profession—remains an important concern in healthcare delivery, although it now also becomes defined increasingly in managerial terms (Westphal, Gulati and Shortell 1997). Despite sharing discretion over aspects of medical treatment with other paraprofessionals, alternative providers, and even managers (see chap. 6), physicians have remained in control of critical knowledge and expertise, which affords them powerful structural positions within healthcare organizations and systems (Hickson et al. 1971, Crozier 1964).

for organizational populations, which are expected to exhibit more variety of forms, greater complexity of structure, and reduced legitimacy—the consequences of multiple, sometimes conflicting expectations and logics (Meyer, Scott, and Strang 1987; Meyer and Scott 1983).

Institutional Fragmentation

The relative unity (or, conversely, fragmentation) of governance is an important dimension of field structuration, reflecting the degree to which participants in a sector confront a coherent institutional environment. Similar to conflict among competing logics, fragmentation of regulatory, funding, and coordinating structures confronts organizations with multiple and often incompatible demands and expectations. Indeed, there is a close relationship, since governance structures are major carriers of (often several, inconsistent) institutionalized belief systems (see chap. 6). Thus, we expect that their fragmentation will both affect and be affected by institutional logics.

Hospital Accreditation Regimes

In chapter 7, we examined the effects of hospital accreditation regimes, viewed as normative governance systems exercising control over member hospitals. Our focus was on the extent to which different accreditation agents provided endorsement for hospitals and, in turn, what implications these assessments had for hospital survival. Implicit in our discussion was a recognition of the multiplicity of sources offering normative support to hospitals. It is clearly the case that the numbers of alternative sources attempting to exercise normative influence over the structure and operation of hospital organizations has increased since 1945.

From a field governance perspective, however, the more relevant question is whether there has been an increased tendency for hospitals to seek accreditation from a specific subset of these sources rather than from a broader spectrum. This would serve as an indicator of the certainty with which organizations seek normative legitimacy and construct their portfolios of institutional linkages. We can ask, then, if there has been historical variation in the unanimity (or conversely, entropy) of realized institutional linkages in the healthcare field, when holding the number of possible linkage types constant. Suppose that we find that in one period 70 percent of all hospitals have AHA memberships while only 20 percent have JCAHO accreditation. Then, at a second time period, suppose that 70 percent still retain their

AHA endorsement but now 60 percent have JCAHO accreditations. Even though the number of types of institutional sources has not increased, there has been increased fragmentation in the unity of governance insofar as a higher proportion of hospitals administrators now feel compelled to respond to two sets of normative standards rather than only one.

The extent to which fragmentation of governance exists along this dimension can be measured in terms of an entropy index proposed by Shannon and Weaver (1963).[6] Applied to the fragmentation of accreditation regimes, the measure compares the proportion of all linkages that involve each particular governance structure, taking into account the number of possible institutional linkages. The metric ranges from 0 (for a field in which all organizations are linked to a single governance structure) to 1 (for a field in which organizations are equally likely to be linked to any governance structure).

The entropy of institutional linkages for Bay Area hospitals was computed for the period from 1954, the first year that JCAHO accreditation was offered, to 1991. All of the legitimacy sources used in the previous analyses, presented in chapter 7, were included (with the exception of the California Hospital Association because the data were not available for the entire period).[7] The plot of the entropy measure reveals a gradual upward trend over time, indicating that there has been an increase in the entropy of linkages and, correspondingly, a modest increase in the fragmentation of hospital governance regimes employing normative authority (see fig. 9.2). The years before the passage of Medicare/Medicaid reveal considerable fluctuation in the entropy metric, suggesting that the importance of various institutional linkages was still under debate by field participants. After 1965, there is a leveling off of the measure, reflecting increased consensus during the era of federal involvement. Following the mid-1970s, and continuing into the early 1990s, however, hospitals seem to evidence greater uncertainty about the importance of linkages with oversight associations, resulting in a gradual increase in the diversification of their portfolios of institutional linkages.

6. The entropy measure is calculated as:

$$-\sum_{i=1}^{n} \frac{\log y_i}{\log n} \, y_i$$

where n is the number of institutional linkages and y_i is the proportion of Bay Area hospitals with the ith institutional linkage.

7. The institutional linkages included the following accreditations and memberships: American Hospital Association, Blue Cross Association, American College of Surgeons, Joint Commission on Accreditation of Healthcare Organizations, Liaison Committee for Medical Education, and Accreditation Council for Graduate Medical Education.

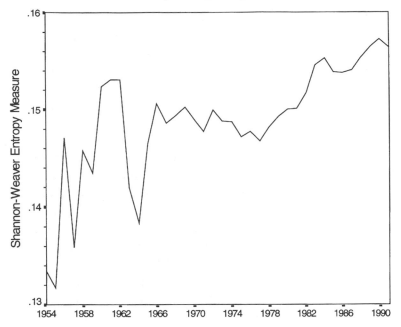

Figure 9.2   Fragmentation of Governance in Bay Area Hospital Accreditations, 1954–92

In short, during the past half century, hospitals have not only been confronted by an increasing number of professional bodies attempting to exercise normative control over their activities, personnel, and structural arrangements (as discussed in chap. 7). Our entropy index indicates that hospitals also increasingly relate to differing combinations of normative authorities. This, in turn, suggests either growing differentiation among hospitals in the work they do and the bodies providing oversight of that work or a lack of consensus among field participants about which bodies hospitals can turn to for legitimation. In either case, governance structures exercising normative oversight over hospitals have become increasingly fragmented.

Fieldwide Fragmentation

Hospitals are an important organizational population but only one of several collective actors in the healthcare sector. In order to develop more general measures of these trends in field-level structures, we combined several indicators to derive factors for the fragmentation of governance structures and funding mechanisms throughout the study period. Funding arrangements are certainly dependent on the existence of regulatory and coordinating structures and are often analytically subsumed under them. But the configuration of funding can itself fatefully shape the construction of organizational fields (DiMaggio 1991), and it has certainly been a consequential feature of governance structures in American healthcare (Starr 1982). In these analyses, we separate funding from more general indicators of governance to discern if its fragmentation has a distinct effect.[8]

Table 9.2 lists the indicators selected to represent these field-level dimensions. *Fragmentation of governance* is estimated at three separate levels with indicators reflecting the expansion of governmental regulatory functions in healthcare and the splintering of professional governing structures and normative systems. The standardized coefficients for the national and state levels are again very strong (from .914 to .999). The loadings for the Bay Area factor are slightly weaker (with one coefficient estimate of .733), but still substantial.[9]

Figure 9.3 displays the factor scores over time for each level of governance, standardized for comparability. It is obvious that the amount of fragmentation has increased at all three levels from 1950 to the early 1990s. At the local level, fragmentation of governance structures appears to have occurred earlier than at the state or national levels, increasing most rapidly during the period 1950 through the early 1960s. The splintering of local governance structures outpaced state and national developments up until 1960, especially as indicated by the specialization of physicians. Since 1960, fragmentation at this level has increased more slowly, but relentlessly, up to the present, with the additional proliferation of local planning and coordination agencies (see fig. 6.10 and Case Illustration 6.A). At the state level, fragmentation has steadily risen from the beginning of the period, the rate of increase accelerating somewhat after 1970. And at the national level, fragmentation in governance structures increased quite rapidly between 1950 and 1955 and again between 1970 and 1975. Declining slightly between 1975 and 1980, fragmentation is again on the increase, rapidly so since 1985. Except for short periods between 1950–55 and 1980–85,

8. Although the notion of centralization (the converse of fragmentation) often connotes concentration of programmatic decision-making and authority, in addition to the expansion of governance and concentration of funding sources (Scott and Meyer 1991), we use the latter two constructs as proxies for the more inclusive concept.

9. The CFI value of .837 for fragmentation of governance at the national level, although below .90, still reflects a moderate degree of factor cohesiveness. The CFI values of 1.00 for the fragmentation of governance factors at the other two levels are an artifact of the factor models being saturated (i.e., they have just enough data to estimate all parameters but no degrees of freedom left to provide a meaningful estimate of fit).

Table 9.2 Confirmatory Factor Models of Field Fragmentation in U.S. Healthcare, 1945–94

Latent Factor	Indicators	Descriptions	Standardized Coefficient	Model Fit
Fragmentation of Governance	Federal government agencies	Health-related federal government agencies	0.999	CFI = 0.837
National	U.S. statutory code	Proportion of index pages related to "Health" and "Medicine"	0.914	N = 44
				$\chi^2 = 99.657$
	Physician specialists	Proportion of private practice, active non-federal physicians	0.933	df = 5
	Board-certified medical specialties	Certified specialty boards, and general & sub-specialty certificates	0.935	
State	California government agencies	Health-related California government agencies	0.994	CFI = 1.00
	California statutory code	Proportion of index pages related to "Health" and "Medicine"	0.995	N = 50
				$\chi^2 = 0.000$
	Licensed health occupations	California state-regulated health occupations and professions	0.991	df = 0
Local	Physician specialists	Proportion of active nonfederal physicians in the Bay Area	0.923	CFI = 1.00
	Hospital accreditations[a]	Entropy measure of Bay Area hospital institutional affiliations	0.870	N = 47
				$\chi^2 = 0.000$
	Local health planning bodies	Health planning bodies with jurisdiction in the Bay Area	0.733	df = 0
Fragmentation of Funding	Insurance type[b]	Entropy measure of health benefit expenditures by insurance type	0.977	CFI = 1.00
National	Sector source[c]	Entropy measure of national health expenditures by sector	0.987	N = 46
				$\chi^2 = 0.000$
	Public level[d]	Entropy measure of public health expenditures by level of government	−0.927	df = 0

NOTES: a. Accreditations and memberships: American Hospital Association (AHA), Blue Cross Association (BCA), American College of Surgeons (ACS), Joint Commission (JCAHO), medical school (LCME), and residents (ACGME). JCAHO proportions are coded as 0 prior to 1954.

b. Insurance types: Blue Cross/Blue Shield, commercial insurance companies, HMO and independent plans, and government (Medicare and Medicaid) programs (see fig. 6.6).

c. Sectors: public or private.

d. Levels of government: federal, state, and local.

state governance structures closely mirror national structures in extent of fragmentation. This occurs largely because federal programs mandate or provide incentives for states to create oversight authorities.

The *fragmentation of funding* factor was calculated at the national level using the Shannon-Weaver entropy measure described previously (varying from 0 [fully concentrated] to 1 [fully fragmented]) for three dimensions of funding: type of insurance (employing four categories), sector source (whether from private or public sources), and public level of expenditures (whether local, state, or federal).[10] The standardized loadings for this factor are all well above .90 in absolute terms.[11]

Fragmentation of funding is juxtaposed with that of governance at the national level in figure 9.4. National funding sources experience modest decreases in unity from the early part of the study period to the advent of

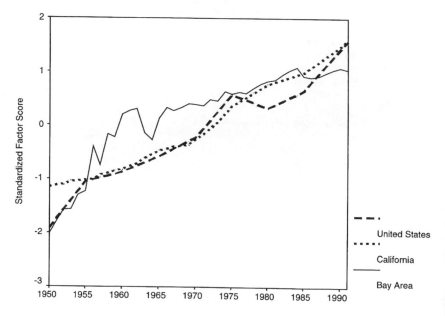

Figure 9.3   Fragmentation of Governance Structures in U.S., California, and Bay Area, Factor Score Trends, 1950–91

10. The entropy measure is the same as that used for hospital accreditations and memberships (see note 6), except that n represents the number of categories in each funding dimension and y_i is the fraction of total funds in the ith category (see table 9.2 notes for the composition of categories in each dimension).

11. Although the CFI is at its maximum of 1.00, this is an artifact of the degrees of freedom equalling 0 (see note 9).

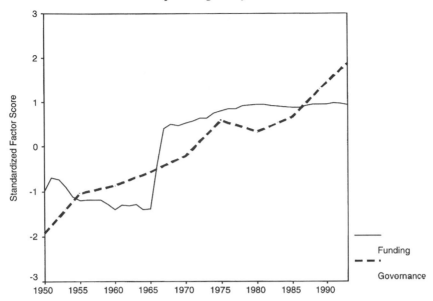

Figure 9.4   Field Fragmentation in U.S. Healthcare, Factor Score Trends, 1950–93

the second era. The implementation of the Medicare/Medicaid programs served to increase rapidly and substantially the fragmentation of funding in the field, with a relative leveling off from the mid-1970s onward.[12] However, as described above for the national level, fragmentation of governance structures rises continually through the early part of the study period, at a comparatively constant pace through the beginning of the era of federal responsibility. Only after the mid-1970s is there a slight move toward increased unification of regulatory structures (corresponding to the trend for federal health-related agencies), with a second wave of fragmentation beginning in the era of managerial-market orientation in the early 1980s and continuing into the 1990s. Since governance structures are an important source of unity and order in any institutional field, their heightened fragmentation cannot help but undermine the stability of field actors, both individual and collective.

12. The entropy measure of public level funding shifts downward with the start of Medicare and Medicaid, becoming less fragmented after 1965. Since, however, this concentration of public funding at the federal level is strongly related to the overall fragmentation of funding in the field, it is employed with the other two measures and contributes to the funding fragmentation factor with a significant negative loading; see table 9.2.

Dynamics of Institutional Change

Having developed composite measures of field-level logics and the coherence of governance structures, we next develop empirical models to explore the relationships among these measures and to provide insights into the processes of institutional formation and decline. We are witnessing the transformation of a relatively mature sector, with established logics and stable organizational forms, into a field in the throes of destructuration— including the breakdown of forms, the dislodging of belief systems, and the dismantling of governance structures. Moreover, there is also evidence of field restructuration, as we observe attempts to put into place new organizational players, logics, and systems of governance. How do these two processes unfold? Which influences are most crucial in dislodging existing logics and in generating new alternatives? And how and to what extent do they relate to each other?

In the following analyses, as in previous chapters, we distinguish institutional factors—logics, governance structures, and their level of coherence— from material influences—resources important to healthcare organizations as technical, production systems providing services. Both sets of variables are assessed at the level of the organizational field. Moreover, as before, we attempt to discern the interrelationships between the two: institutions define in basic ways the nature, meaning, and use of material resources, and material conditions may impinge on and stimulate the rethinking of institutional arrangements.

In terms of material explanations for the profound institutional changes in the healthcare sector, we rely on fairly conventional arguments. The most prominent is, of course, the impact of the dramatic rise in medical care costs (see discussions in chaps. 5 and 6), which has stimulated various efforts to restrain the inefficient utilization of medical resources and encouraged the rationalization of healthcare organizations through modern management and financial techniques. These increases in costs are assessed using the medical price index.

To capture a second material variable, focusing on advances in medical technology, we used the number of newly issued medical and drug patents. The effects exerted by technological advances, however, are controversial. Many observers view medical technology—in the form of unrestricted use of sophisticated medical innovations—as helping to fuel the escalation of healthcare costs. Others herald new technology as one of healthcare's potential saviors, making possible the use of less expensive treatment options, the provision of services in less costly settings (such as the clinic and home, instead of hospital), and improved information processing capabilities (see chap. 5).

Our discussion of institutional environments and processes has suggested several implications of logics and field fragmentation for the rise and decline of institutional configurations. At first glance, it might be tempting to assume that the decline of an existing integrated complex of logics, such as the traditional professional dominance and voluntary ethos in American medical care, would be directly related to the rapid ascendance of a contentious challenger, such as the recent embracing of managerial and market-oriented logics. However, the factors and contexts influencing the construction of a new institutional regime may not be the same as those leading to the demise of an earlier framework (Strang 1990). Similarly, the factors resulting in the decline of one institutional logic may differ substantially from those affecting the diffusion of a new challenger.

With respect to the healthcare field, figure 9.1 shows little direct correspondence in the timing in decline of the logics of professional dominance (occurring in the mid-1960s) with the rise in managerial-market logics (beginning in the early 1980s). Rather, visual inspection of the trend lines suggests that the weakening of professional dominance is most strongly associated with the advent of the era of federal involvement initiated by Medicare/Medicaid in 1965—programs initially formulated so as to be respectful of the interests of physicians and other traditional medical care interests. To accommodate this apparent separation, we conducted independent analyses of factors influencing the deinstitutionalization of professional dominance and of those affecting the institutional advancement of a managerial-market orientation.

In addition to the federal involvement logics, which emphasized equity and access to healthcare services and a strong role for the federal government in ensuring these values, our previous discussions have also highlighted the role of secondary logics in catalyzing change in the traditional constitution of the field. The consumer health movement, an offshoot of a more general human rights movement arising during the 1960s, created waves in the healthcare field, most noticeably in the early 1970s. At about the same time, the alternative health movement, stressing wellness and prevention over the established medical profession's bias toward acute health care, rose to prominence by offering treatment modalities outside of orthodox medical practice (see chap. 6).

Up to this point, however, we have been agnostic as to whether these secondary logics served primarily to destabilize traditional medical care, encourage the entrance of other contesting logics prevailing in the broader society, or both. We attempt to address these questions in our analysis. Unfortunately, we have been able to devise only limited indicators for the consumer and alternative health movements at the national level, precluding the construction of more reliable factor measures. We use only single indicator measures—the number of health-related titles in the *Periodical Guide to Literature* for consumer health and the number of licensed chiropractors in the United States as a measure of alternative providers.[13] Hence, our conclusions regarding the effects of these two movements on our primary logics can only be suggestive.

Lastly, we are interested in the effects of field-level structuration—that is, the coherence of structures and interactions among sector participants—on deinstitutionalizing prevailing logics and promoting new ones. Also at issue is how institutional logics effect change—whether by a direct stimulation of new actors and behaviors or through the reconfiguration of governance structures, material resources, and the level of field structuration (see chap. 5). For example, the era of federal involvement introduced not only logics of equity and access (which were not wholly antithetical to the principles of professional dominance) but also a plethora of governance structures penetrating all levels of the healthcare field, causing fragmentation and providing conduits for subsequent logics to enter (see chap. 6).

Decline of Professional Dominance

We examine the influence of these material and institutional forces with a set of time series regression models. Because of significant multicollinearity in the raw data, all variables were calculated as annual difference scores (i.e., the increase or decrease from the previous year).[14] Table 9.3 includes two models of factors affecting the annual change in the trend for professional dominance. The first includes indicators of material-resource influences and institutional logics. The second adds the effects of field-level fragmentation.

In model 1 and model 2, neither the coefficient for medical technology nor for medical costs has a statistically significant effect on the trend for professional dominance. Although physicians' traditional pursuit of an

13. Compared to other practitioners, chiropractors represent a more reliable measure of the alternative health movement over time since, as described in chapter 6, they have maintained a relatively strong identity and distinct professional organization in relation to mainstream American medicine. Data for licensed chiropractors at the national level come from the Federation of Chiropractic Licensing Boards (1963–98) and the National Chiropractic Association (1952). The data may include practitioners with licenses in more than one state.

14. In addition, because of significant serial autocorrelation (i.e., correlation between values of a variable and any calculated residual errors, from one time point to the next), a Prais-Winsten generalized least-squares method (with a first order, one-period autoregressive correction) was used for the models in table 9.3.

Table 9.3 Decline of Professional Dominance: Indicators Affecting Factor Score Measure of Professional Dominance in U.S. Healthcare, 1951–93

	Variable	Model 1	Model 2
Constant		−0.046	−0.037
		(0.038)	(0.034)
Material Indicators			
Medical technology	Medical & drug patents	0.033	0.116
	(Δ1000s)	(0.092)	(0.078)
Medical costs	Medical price index	0.022	−0.022
		(0.027)	(0.020)
Institutional Indicators			
Primary logics			
Federal involvement	4-indicator factor score	−0.451**	0.533*
		(0.136)	(0.232)
Managerial-market orientation	5-indicator factor score	−0.148	−0.058
		(0.416)	(0.316)
Secondary logics			
Alternative health	Licensed chiropractors	0.001	0.001
	(Δ1000s)	(0.016)	(0.013)
Consumer health	Health-related periodicals	−1.647	2.461
		(4.830)	(4.332)
Field fragmentation			
Governance	4-indicator factor score		−0.171
			(0.287)
Funding	3-indicator factor score		−0.898**
			(0.191)
Number of cases		43	43
Log likelihood		28.95	39.53
Durbin-Watson statistic		2.16	2.07

# p < .10; * p < .05; ** p < .01 (one-tailed test)

increasingly high quality of medical care has been associated with the development of medical technology, technological expansion does not appear to be directly related to the decline of the medical profession's dominance. Similarly, the models indicate that the rise in medical costs per se did not weaken the institutional position of the medical profession within the healthcare field.

Contrary to our predictions, the two secondary logics, alternative health and consumer health (which we argued mounted some of the first substantial challenges to professional dominance), also do not exhibit significant effects. Recall, however, that we were able to devise only single-indicator measures of these logics. The absence of a detectable relation may result from inadequate measurement not fully reflective of the early onset of these movements.

Of the primary logics, only federal responsibility significantly influences professional dominance. In model 1, as might initially be expected, it undermines professional dominance. The introduction of the field fragmentation variables in model 2, however, depicts a somewhat different and more interesting pattern of effects. First, as predicted, both governance and funding fragmentation decreases professional dominance, although the effect is statistically significant only for the latter variable. The legitimacy of prevailing logics is undercut by the development of diverse and potentially conflicting sources dispensing resources and exercising authority.

Second, the inclusion of the field fragmentation measures also produces a dramatic reversal in the effect of the federal involvement logic on professional dominance. This shift in the direct relation between professional dominance and federal responsibility suggests that the apparently negative influence of federal intervention in the first model derives primarily from its indirect effect of increasing the fragmentation of field-level governance and funding, rather than from a more direct confrontation of logics. When field fragmentation is taken into account, the remaining positive and significant influence of the federal involvement factor implies that substantive aspects of the logic fundamentally upheld professional prerogatives and sought to accommodate, not challenge, professional dominance. The content of the logic was supportive, but its effects on the texture of governance regimes was such as to subvert the hegemony of the medical establishment.

The coefficients for managerial-market logics, although in the negative direction, do not have a significant effect on professional dominance. This suggests that the rising support for managerial and market approaches to healthcare issues was not itself the force that brought about the decline in professional power. Managers appear to have been the beneficiaries, not the agents, of deinstitutionalization.

Advance of Managerial-Market Orientation

Table 9.4 examines the same complex of measures but now evaluates their effects on the rise of managerial-market logics. Again, two models are estimated, the first including the variables for material-resource conditions and institutional logics, and the second adding measures of field fragmentation.

In model 1, medical costs exhibit a positive effect on managerial-market oriented logics. Clearly, escalating medical costs have played an important role in encouraging the development and acceptance of market strategies and managerial logics (see chap. 6). Advances in medical technology also support managerial logics. It is not clear from these models, however, whether this results from technologies that increase differentiation of work and managerial control, that appeal to the cost-saving rhetoric of the new logics, or that exacerbate medical cost inflation (and thus encourage market reforms).

Interestingly, the models do not provide evidence of a direct relationship between the managerial-market orientation and the other two primary logics, professional dominance and federal involvement. The primary logics associated with the first and second eras appear neither to support nor to inhibit the rise of managerial-market logics. Instead, secondary logics seem to play more of a role in advancing the managerial-market trend, as is evidenced, in particular, by the effect of the indicator for alternative health. Although there is no straightforward connection between the content of the managerial-market orientation and the alternative health movement, the increased receptivity to alternative providers may have served as a "foot in the door," priming the institutional terrain for subsequent contesting logics. The absence of an effect of our measure for the consumer health movement does not support our imagery of an evolution from client to consumer to customer ideologies, although, as mentioned above, the use of a single indicator precludes a definitive conclusion.

Lastly, while the fragmentation factors, especially for funding, helped predict the decline of professional dominance, they do not significantly affect the rise of managerial-market logics. It appears that the fragmentation of the healthcare field has been more important in cultivating the institutional landscape, clearing the ground rather than sowing the particular seeds that would grow.

FIELD-LEVEL FORCES AND ORGANIZATIONAL POPULATIONS

Throughout this volume, our central concern has been to account for changes in the characteristics of populations of organizations—density, ownership features, subtypes, linkages—in response to changes in material-resource and institutional environments. We pursue this theme here, but with a difference. To this point, our analyses have been conducted primarily at the level of the organization, the organizational population, and the local environment (sometimes with interaction effects from our broader institutional eras). Now we focus on field-level forces. We turn our attention

Table 9.4   Advance of Managerial-Market Orientation: Indicators Affecting Factor Score Measure of Managerial-Market Logics in U.S. Healthcare, 1951–93

	Variable	Model 1	Model 2
Constant		−0.022	−0.017
		(0.014)	(0.019)
Material indicators			
Medical technology	Medical & drug patents	0.090[*]	0.095[*]
	(Δ1000s)	(0.034)	(0.040)
Medical costs	Medical price index	0.035[**]	0.035[**]
		(0.008)	(0.009)
Institutional Indicators			
Primary logics			
Professional dominance	4-indicator factor score	−0.019	−0.015
		(0.069)	(0.091)
Federal involvement	4-indicator factor score	−0.068	−0.086
		(0.060)	(0.133)
Secondary logics			
Alternative health	Licensed chiropractors	0.017[**]	0.017[*]
	(Δ1000s)	(0.006)	(0.006)
Consumer health	Health-related periodicals	−0.142	−0.621
		(1.982)	(2.314)
Field fragmentation			
Governance	4-indicator factor score		−0.066
			(0.158)
Funding	3-indicator factor score		0.017
			(0.130)
Number of cases		43	43
Log likelihood		66.58	66.71
Durbin-Watson statistic		1.41	1.41

[#] p < .10; [*] p < .05; [**] p < .01 (one-tailed test)

to more macrolevel characteristics that can affect the fitness of various populations of healthcare providers. Unlike the regional demographic, geographic, and funding dimensions previously examined (see chap. 5), these characteristics typically operate at higher levels of analysis.

Field-level Forces and Fitness of Forms

The macrolevel environment confronting Bay Area providers, such as hospitals, HHAs, and ESRDCs, incorporates both material and institutional factors. Material resource considerations, including demands for cost effectiveness or technological innovation, are likely to play a critical role in dictating whether members of an organizational population thrive or fail. Indeed, the very existence of some populations appears to depend on medical innovations (such as the development of kidney transplantation and dialysis procedures for ESRDCs) or cost-effectiveness concerns (which provide the rationale for HMOs). Aside from such focused causal factors, however, it may be possible to identify more diffuse effects of material resource characteristics that favor one or another organizational population. Accordingly, we will briefly consider the impact of two material characteristics: complexity of technology and cost effectiveness.

Forms with complex technical cores, such as ESRDCs, are expected to thrive in environments where there is an emphasis on medical innovation, often regardless of whether such innovations have a direct bearing on the form's effectiveness or performance. Seen as technical production systems, these organizations are able to maximize their survival chances insofar as their day-to-day operations are congruent with a wider environment that encourages (or even demands) technological sophistication. Other forms, such as HHAs, that are less strongly associated with advanced technologies are expected to fare less well in technology-driven environments.[15]

The costs associated with the provision of healthcare by particular provider forms constitute another material consideration likely to influence organizational viability. In environments where concerns about cost effectiveness and medical inflation ride high, provider forms associated with relatively high operational costs (for example, hospitals and ESRDCs) will suffer reduced organizational entries and increased exits. Conversely, those forms popularly linked to low-cost treatments (for example, HHAs) are likely to thrive in such environments.

In considering these diffuse effects of cost effectiveness and technological complexity, two complications can be anticipated—one pertaining to the interrelationship of the two characteristics themselves and the other pertaining to their relationship with institutional dynamics. With regard to the first point, one might anticipate that the cost effectiveness and technological complexity of an organizational form will often be inversely correlated—with high complexity being linked to low cost effectiveness and vice versa. It is clear, however, that this association need not necessarily be the case. For instance, a provider may invest heavily in capital equipment so that worker skills would be reduced and salary savings effected. It is

---

15. This does not imply that HHA services, such as IV or chemotherapy administered in the home, involve no technological breakthroughs. Rather, we suggest that traditional versions of home health care—for example, when a visiting nurse attends to a patient—are relatively simple in terms of technological complexity compared to hospitals or ESRDCs.

important to consider these two factors separately in order to evaluate their possibly independent effects on providers and their specific contributions to the survival of these organizational forms.

One should also note that although these particular variables clearly involve material factors (technologies and costs), the arguments made are not necessarily restricted to materialist considerations. Technologies may lead to superior performances, and cost effectiveness may contribute directly to survival in a competitive environment. But in addition, when wider cultural beliefs favor technology and a concern with cost savings, those organizations embracing these approaches and ideologies may be advantaged, regardless of any specific contribution made to their effectiveness. Organizations that incorporate these ingredients into their structural archetypes may align themselves with dominant cultural logics and thereby improve their life chances.

The salience of institutional logics during each of the three eras is also expected to influence the life chances of our organizational populations. With the deinstitutionalization of professional dominance as a principal logic, we can analyze the viability of each form in terms of a simple dichotomy of alternative primary logics: those favoring *state-oriented* forms versus those favoring *market-oriented* forms.[16] State-oriented forms are those organizational populations that thrive under conditions involving strong support and active involvement of the federal government. Market-oriented forms are those populations that perform best under competitive, profit-driven conditions. Given the peculiarities of many organizational fields—healthcare, in particular—it is important to emphasize that these logics are not necessarily mutually exclusive and can be viewed as independent factors (like technological complexity and cost effectiveness). ESRDCs, for example, are simultaneously state-oriented, emerging in response to the 1972 Medicare amendment, which secured federal reimbursement for end-stage renal disease services, and market-oriented, attracting large numbers of investor-owned enterprises to this lucrative niche.

Data limitations are such that we can only use three of our five organizational populations in evaluating the effects of field-level dynamics. The Bay Area contains too few HMOs and healthcare systems to include these populations in our analysis. Employing our general knowledge of

16. All three primary logics cannot be included in models simultaneously because of issues of multicollinearity. In addition, attention is restricted to primary logics because secondary logics (consumer health and alternative medicine) have more limited construct validity. We do not include fragmentation indicators because to do so would eliminate additional years from the analyses, given the limited availability of fragmentation data prior to 1950.

the characteristics of the remaining populations, we propose a set of predictions in table 9.5 concerning the fitness of each population along the material-resource and institutional dimensions described. In general, we anticipate that forms that rank high along a particular dimension will exhibit increased entry rates and reduced exit rates when material or institutional environmental conditions provide support for that dimension. Conversely, forms ranking low will experience reduced entry and increased exit rates under the same conditions.

Briefly, our predictions can be summarized as follows. Hospitals have generally fared well in aligning themselves with technological complexity, but have been slow to embrace cost-effectiveness techniques. Because of the specifics of Medicare/Medicaid legislation, they have received moderate support from state programs (moderate, because Medicaid reimbursement formulae and prospective payment system requirements place severe financial restrictions on hospitals). Hospitals have been slow to adopt market-oriented practices and to embrace for-profit structures.

Home health agencies do not rely heavily nor are they associated in the pubic mind with high-tech services. They position themselves as providing alternatives to technologically intensive approaches. Moreover, because they help to postpone or substitute for hospitalization, they are generally regarded as highly cost effective. Since state policies have embraced these assumptions, legislation has been crafted to favor HHA providers. In spite of their primarily nonprofit heritage stemming from their roots in visiting nursing associations, market-oriented entrepreneurs have been widely attracted to this form in recent decades.

End-stage renal disease centers were created by a combination of technological innovation and state-level subsidies. The technology breakthroughs were necessary but not sufficient to encourage the development of this form, because patients could not afford treatments without federal assistance. Because of the high cost of treatment, the cost effectiveness of this form is not necessarily high. But given the substantial level of state support since 1972, the possibility of large profits has attracted proprietary firms to the ESRD niche.

Empirical Evidence

Population Entries

The separate factors derived earlier for logics of federal involvement and managerial-market orientations were again calculated as a series of annual

Table 9.5   Predicted Fitness of Organizational Forms in Material-Resource and
Institutional Environments

Form	Material Considerations		Institutional Considerations	
	Technological Complexity	Cost Effectiveness	State-Orientation	Market-Orientation
Hospitals	Moderate-high	Low-moderate	Moderate	Low
HHAs	Low	High	Moderate-high	Moderate
ESRDCs	High	Low	High	High

difference scores. This transformation allows us to evaluate the impact of relative changes in institutional logics on population entry and exit rates. For example, our hypotheses suggest that hospitals will experience a low level of fitness in market-oriented environments. Operationally, the prediction tested is that there will be a negative relation between year-to-year increases in the managerial-market factor score and hospital entries (and a positive relation for exits). For the sake of consistency, the same differencing procedure was applied to measures of costs (medical price index) and technology (number of medical and drug patents issued). Models of entries into the organizational populations are presented first, then models of exits.

The models of organizational entries within the Bay Area suggest a statistical pattern that is largely consistent with our predictions (see table 9.6). Growing medical inflation and calls for greater cost effectiveness have reduced entries of high-cost providers such as hospitals and increased entries of low-cost alternatives such as HHAs over the past few decades. Like hospitals, ESRDCs suffer lower entry rates in environments characterized by medical inflation and favoring cost effectiveness, but the effect is not statistically significant. Technological developments have operated to support the addition of ESRDCs and to reduce the addition of HHAs, as predicted. Kidney disease centers have capitalized on the strong support for technological solutions.

With respect to institutional considerations, the overall pattern of results is also supportive of our hypotheses. We find that hospitals and HHAs are advantaged by the development of federal involvement logics. ESRDCs also exhibit higher entries under these conditions, although this result is not statistically significant. The pattern associated with managerial-market logics is just as expected, but only the estimate for HHAs reach statistical significance. HHAs are more likely to thrive with increases in managerial-market logics, and ESRDCs also show a slight tendency to do

Table 9.6 Impact of Field-Level Forces on Entries into Bay Area Hospital, HHA, and ESRDC Populations

Variable	Hospitals		HHAs		ESRDCs	
	Model 1 (1948–92)	Model 2 (1948–92)	Model 1 (1967–92)	Model 2 (1967–92)	Model 1 (1970–91)	Model 2 (1970–91)
Intercept	−1.332 (0.169)**	−1.546 (0.209)**	−0.869 (0.207)**	−1.051 (0.218)**	−1.507 (0.311)**	−1.501 (0.324)**
Material Environment						
Medical technology	0.138 (0.688)	0.383 (0.754)	−0.573 (0.284)*	−0.953 (0.341)**	0.730 (0.425)*	0.572 (0.464)
Medical costs	−0.054 (0.017)**	−0.035 (0.026)#	0.043 (0.008)**	0.033 (0.008)**	−0.009 (0.013)	−0.018 (0.018)
Institutional Environment						
Federal involvement	—	0.968 (0.512)*	—	0.950 (0.627)#	—	0.949 (4.775)
Market orientation	—	−3.884 (4.231)	—	3.602 (1.338)**	—	1.927 (1.905)
Overdispersion (ϕ)	n/a	n/a	0.699 (0.199)**	0.611 (0.183)**	n/a	n/a
Number of cases	396	396	234	234	198	198
Number of events	62	62	235	235	48	48
−2 Log likelihood (d.f.)	351.44 (3)	345.98 (5)	636.12 (4)	624.98 (6)	245.92 (3)	244.90 (5)

# p < .10; * p < .05; ** p < .01 (one-tailed test)

better under these logics. The entry rate of hospitals has been slightly lower when market logics are on the rise.

An examination of the fit statistics for the Poisson regressions of organizational entries reveals that the addition of institutional logics improves model fit for two of the three populations. The likelihood ratio test comparing models 1 and 2 for hospitals (likelihood ratio $\chi^2 = 5.46$) is significant at the $p < .10$ level, while the same test for HHAs (likelihood ratio $\chi^2 = 11.14$) is significant at the $p < .01$ level. However, no substantial improvement is observed for ESRDCs ($\chi^2 = 1.02$). This result may reflect the relatively small number of entry events for this population.

Population Exits

Corresponding results for organizational exits are presented in table 9.7 for two of the three populations. ESRDCs could not be included in these analyses because the number of exit events observed was too small to support statistical analysis. Baseline models (not shown in the table) included organizational characteristics such as age, size (for hospitals), and integration (model 1, table 5.3). Subsequent models, presented in table 9.7, added institutional parameters and material-resource indicators in a nested fashion. Nested models allow us to investigate the extent that institutional logics and material-resource indicators explain more variance in outcomes than organizational attributes alone.

For both HHAs and hospitals, model 1 represents a significant improvement over the baseline model containing organization-level attributes only (likelihood ratio $\chi^2 = 11.98$; $p < .01$ for HHAs; $\chi^2 = 4.82$; $p < .10$ for hospitals). The logics of federal involvement and market orientation tend to increase hospital exits. These results are consistent with the expectation that hospitals exhibit low-to-moderate fitness in these institutional environments. HHAs experience somewhat lower exit rates in state-oriented institutional contexts, as predicted, although this result did not reach statistical significance. Unexpectedly, HHAs were substantially more likely to suffer increased exit rates under market-oriented logics ($p < .01$), despite exhibiting greater entry rates under the same conditions (see table 9.5). Market-oriented environments appear to stimulate a "churning" of this population, encouraging both entries and exits.

The addition of material-resource factors, in model 2, corroborates some of the earlier evidence from organizational entries. As predicted, the relatively low-tech population of HHAs suffers increased exits in an environment that favors technological solutions while enjoying reduced

Table 9.7 Impact of Field-Level Forces on Exits from Bay Area Hospital and HHA Populations

| | Organizational Population | | | |
| | Hospitals | | Home Health Agencies | |
Variable	Model 1 (1948–91)	Model 2 (1948–91)	Model 1 (1966–91)	Model 2 (1966–91)
Intercept	−1.411 (0.527)**	−1.652 (0.529)**	−2.675 (0.236)**	−2.441 (0.273)**
Organizational				
Age (× 10)	0.039 (0.047)	0.030 (0.047)	−0.668 (0.191)**	−0.668 (0.195)**
Size	−0.622 (0.128)**	−0.624 (0.127)**	—	—
Integration	−0.839 (0.355)**	−0.952 (0.358)**	−0.625 (0.235)**	−0.641 (0.234)**
Material Environment				
Medical technology	—	1.154 (0.499)*	—	0.747 (0.301)**
Medical costs	—	0.021 (0.014)#	—	−0.023 (0.009)**
Institutional Environment				
Federal involvement	1.018 (0.542)*	0.830 (0.567)#	−0.862 (1.263)	−0.220 (1.001)
Market orientation	2.187 (1.267)*	−2.754 (2.341)	2.957 (0.965)**	3.048 (1.110)**
Number of cases	3878	3878	1756	1756
Number of events	64	64	117	117
−2 Log likelihood (d.f.)	618.04 (6)	608.62 (8)	826.98 (6)	816.52 (8)

# $p < .10$; * $p < .05$; ** $p < .01$ (one-tailed test)

mortality in environments that emphasize cost efficiency. Also consistent with expectations, hospitals tend to exhibit slightly higher exit rates under conditions of cost escalation. The only material-resource effect that does not necessarily match earlier hypotheses concerns the positive effect of marginal increases in medical innovation on hospital exits. This result runs counter to the characterization of hospitals as enjoying greater fitness in technologically complex environments. On the one hand, entries of hospital organizations are encouraged by their compatibility with a faith in technology; on the other hand, it appears that the "medical arms race" has become a double-edged sword for many of these venerable institutions. The central role attributed to sophisticated diagnostic and information-processing tools has increasingly served as a motivation for consolidating formerly separate hospital facilities.

SUMMARY AND CONCLUSION

In this chapter, we have stretched the data employed in previous analyses to attempt to probe broader, field-level forces. In some cases, our data have proved adequate to the challenge and, we believe, the results are both provocative and convincing. In other cases, our data exhibit their limitations, and we must be content to show tendencies and directions.

What we have been able to establish, based on a composite of indicators, is the trajectory of three different institutional logics, each promoting different claims and interests regarding healthcare delivery. We have documented the decline of professional hegemony, captured the sudden rise of federal responsibility, and recorded the recent rapid ascendance of corporate and market logics. We have been able to track these developments over a fifty-year period and have observed how their changing combinations have produced the varying institutional frameworks that support and constrain different actors and actions.

We have also provided evidence that the rise of market logics was not itself responsible for the decline of professional dominance. Rather, professional power was dislodged by the sudden escalation of federal involvement in the healthcare sector. Of greater interest, our data suggest that it was not the content of the new public logics that undermined professional dominance, but the fragmentation of governance structures that followed in the wake of the federal programs. Conflicting logics and contending institutional regimes weaken the legitimacy of entrenched interests and provide openings for new actors and interests. The corporate and managerial actors, both individual and collective, exploited this opportunity, bringing in their new procedures, ideologies, and structures. However, it may well prove difficult for even these new arrangements to establish themselves firmly amid the continuing cacophony of contending logics and divided regimes.

Finally, we explored the effects of these changing logics and other field-level forces on our organizational populations. We acknowledge that our organizational population data, based on a single geographic area, have no doubt been overextended for the analyses reported in this chapter. All too quickly, we have run out of events and other available observations to support our analyses. Still, we have sought to indicate directions and explore analytic procedures that studies such as our own need to pursue. We believe that organizations respond not only to local conditions—demographic and economic—but also to wider institutional parameters. National and state policies as well as broader cultural logics and the texture of governance structures affect the fate of specific organizations and, in aggregate, of organizational populations. Large data sets and long periods of time are required to detect such effects. Our own data set registers tremors and tendencies but cannot produce definitive proof.

We do provide general evidence that different kinds of organizations are advantaged and disadvantaged by their congruence with fieldwide forces. Those organizational populations that embrace dominant logics and exhibit appropriate attributes—whether an emphasis on cost effectiveness or the enshrinement of high technology—are more likely to flourish than organizations whose attributes are "out-of-joint" with their times. Specifically, the current field logics are more supportive of specialist players, such as home health agencies and kidney disease centers, than of more traditional generalist forms, such as hospitals.

Ten

INSTITUTIONAL CHANGE AND STRUCTURATION PROCESSES

IN THIS CONCLUDING CHAPTER, we draw together the threads connecting our arguments and highlight the main findings and conclusions from our inquiry. In addition, we consider the relationship between our framework and broader issues as we attempt to link our depiction of healthcare eras to a more abstract conception of field structuration. We begin by addressing the connection between our evidence of changing governance structures in healthcare and current debates regarding the contest of government- and market-centered controls in the evolution of the welfare state.

MODES OF GOVERNANCE AND THE WELFARE STATE

In our analysis of developments during the past half century in the healthcare sector, we have not ventured far above the level of our particular organizational field and its relevant institutional environment. We have taken note of some of the wider societal-level influences—for example, social movements targeting inequality or social rights—identifying their effects on the sector, but we have not attempted to locate our subject on the broader canvas of changing societal organization. We do so now but only briefly to sketch out possible connections. The subject of governance structures at the societal level is a large one and the scholarship vast; we treat here only the most obvious and direct connections to our own subject.

In chapter 6, we introduced a typology of governance structures devised by Streeck and Schmitter (1985) distinguishing between community, association, state, and market models. Obviously, these are ideal types, with existing governance structures consisting of varying combinations of these elements. Diverse governance structures may operate within a given society, each pertaining to a different sector. We suggested in our discussion that the evolution of governance structures in the U.S. healthcare field might be characterized as a movement from an associational- to a state- to a market-centered governance framework.

From early in this century up to 1965, professional medical associations exercised primary control in the sector, exemplifying an associational model. Backed by public agencies, they exercised legitimate control over the central bodies and activities within the sector. The primary advantages of this governance arrangement, according to Streeck and Schmitter, is that it affords closer congruence in a sector between decision making and implementation than under alternative governance systems:

> The same associations that negotiate the terms of regulation of their members' behavior, are charged as private governments with responsibility to enforce them. [In addition] the agents of implementation—the professional staff and the officials of the association—are closer to the target group (their members) than state bureaucracies, and they have more intimate knowledge of its situation and concerns (Streeck and Schmitter 1985: 22).

Such considerations, it is argued, render attempts at control more intelligent and increase the probability of conformity to them. Limitations of the associational model include the problem that the norms and incentives governing private associations may not necessarily be conducive to serving wider public interests.

Medicare/Medicaid legislation ushered in a vastly expanded role for the nation-state in sector governance in 1965—a more state-centered model, but, as we have noted, the state did not at first challenge the existing arrangements, merely providing additional resources to enable professionals to redirect their services to broader public goals. Ruggie has characterized this arrangement as a "segmented" regime:

> Segmentation in health care relations describes a situation in which the role of government is essentially to fund some portion of provision and the role of decentralized and/or professional actors is to decide how funds are to be expended and to implement those decisions. The mode of decision making thus reflects the separate domains of authority and competence (Ruggie 1996: 17).

This arrangement is characteristic of many other service sectors in U.S. society, where "funding decisions are more highly centralized than programmatic decisions" (Scott and Meyer 1991: 129).

Pressures to modify this arrangement in the direction of more centralized programmatic authority are particularly likely to occur when (1) there is a perceived funding crisis, as in healthcare; or (2) there is a perceived crisis in performance levels or quality, as is currently the case in education (see National Commission on Excellence in Education 1983; National Governors' Association 1986). As public expenditures for healthcare continued to climb rapidly from 1950 onward (see fig. 6.9), federal regulatory agencies also grew in numbers and size (see fig. 6.10), giving rise during the late 1960s to what Ruggie (1996) has termed an "interventionist" regime characterized by increased political activity and more contentious relations in the sector.

Students of the nation-state point to yet a third, more general, explanation for expansion in state structures and authority. They argue that for most of this century, modern nations have witnessed the growth of the "welfare state," as political authorities have expanded the definitions of entitlements to their citizens. In most European states, this development commenced earlier and has progressed faster and further than in the United States, which is generally regarded as late and relatively slow in embracing social welfare policies (Skocpol and Amenta 1986; Quadagno 1987).

Regardless of their stage of development, however, all contemporary welfare states experienced a "crisis" during the 1970s and 1980s, when tax revenues were unable to keep pace with expanding entitlements, in part because of a slowdown in economic growth. Theorists from the right argued that governments had promised more than they could deliver and that the expansion of state power and programs was stifling private enterprise and individual initiative (Anderson 1978; Murray 1984). Theorists from the left argued that the state's need to legitimate its authority by expanding benefits had undermined its ability to carry out the financial investment programs necessary to sustain capital accumulation (O'Connor 1973; Habermas 1976). Multiple voices called for reform if not retrenchment.

In a number of western democracies, including the United States, neo-conservatives came to power on a platform condemning the overexpanded nature of the welfare state. These critics insisted that governments were not only trying to do too much, they were ineffective in many of their efforts to remedy problems (Murray 1984). The solution was to rein in government programs and to unleash private initiative. Wherever possible, privatization of public programs was to take place. If this was not possible, then public agencies should attempt to separate policy making from implementation and utilize private firms to carry out programs under the guidance of the public sector. In all cases, organizational designers should employ marketlike incentives to motivate officials to pursue appropriate goals (Savas 1982; Osborne and Gaebler 1992). These ideas took command in Washington in the early 1970s and were quickly applied to healthcare, as reformers encouraged privatization, fostered the development of HMOs and other managed care systems, and attempted to rearrange the incentives directed toward consumers and, particularly, providers.

Nevertheless, while important changes have occurred in rhetoric and in the instruments of public policy, it is not apparent that the welfare state has been severely curtailed in size or scope, let alone dismantled. Numerous studies conducted during the late 1980s and into the 1990s suggest little if any change in the scope or advance of the welfare state (see Brown 1988).

More specifically, our own study has depicted a change in the institutional logics and in the "vocabulary" of organizational forms within the healthcare sector—for example, a decline in the proportion of public sector organizations, a rise of for-profit forms, and the emergence of types of organizations utilizing financial incentives to reduce medical care costs. There is, however, little evidence of healthcare costs being dramatically reduced or of government agencies withering away. While some healthcare plans and purchasing coalitions have been successful in negotiating lower costs (see Robinson 1995; Enthoven and Singer 1996), more recent developments suggest that such savings may have been short lived. In one recent year, medical premiums in the Bay Area jumped from 2 to 21 percent, "with giant insurer Kaiser Permanente at the high end" (Krieger 1998). Marmor, Mashaw, and Harvey (1990: 187) suggest that, at best, competitive negotiations effect savings for particular firms but not for the nation as a whole. Competition for patients, employees, and insurers reduces the amount of fiscal control that can be exercised, resulting in cost "shifting" rather than cost reduction. Moreover, as these authors point out, the most effective device for containing costs, the PPS program, is not a competitive program but an exercise in price controls (1990: 188).

Federal agencies in healthcare experienced a slight dip in their rate of increase between 1975 and 1980 but have resumed their path of growth since 1980 (fig. 6.10). Ruggie (1996) suggests that the policy regime now overseeing healthcare in the United States is not in the process of being dismantled but is shifting its mode of governance from an "interventionist" to an "integrative" regime. Her description of this mode depicts more rationality and cooperation among bureaucrats, professionals, and managers than we have observed. But we are in agreement with her general claim that the change we are currently observing does not involve "a swing along the axis from state to market because . . . the introduction of marketlike factors is occurring within a continuing strong framework of government regulation" (p. 234).

Thus, on balance, our first inclination to embrace the application of Streeck and Schmitter's typology, suggesting a simple transition in the U.S. healthcare sector from associational- to state- to market-centered governance structures, appears incorrect. All three modes of governance remain simultaneously active in this sector, although our indicators intimate that the associational mode of professional governance is in decline (see fig. 9.1).[1] Market mechanisms have joined, but not replaced, state controls. What we see is a change in rhetoric and in the policy mechanisms that governmental actors employ as they attempt to steer the development of this sector specifically and govern the welfare state more generally.

The current situation seems to us to represent substantial, even profound, change, but not revolution. Associational and state actors and mechanisms of governance have not been replaced but joined by new actors and logics. In a process referred to as *bricolage* (Douglas 1986), sector actors, both individual and collective, have constructed new combinations of governance structures out of preexisting forms and logics. The previous institutional regimes provide "a repertoire of already existing institutional principles (e.g., models, analogies, conventions, concepts) that actors use to create new solutions in ways that lead to evolutionary change" (Campbell 1997: 22). There are some novel elements but also innovative combinations of old elements. The governance structures, logics, and actors are altered but many of their components remain recognizable.

It is thus possible to emphasize the amount of continuity between earlier and current features of healthcare. Herzlinger adopts this stance:

> But the long-awaited transformation [of the U.S. healthcare system] has yet to occur. . . . Although its size grew enormously, from a staggering $70 billion of expenditures in 1970 to an incomprehensible $604 billion in 1989, the structure of the system changed very little: In 1970, hospitals consumed 37 percent of the total, physicians 19 percent, and other professional services 8 percent, and in 1990, they consumed 39 percent, 19 percent, and 6 percent of the total, respectively. No structural revolution is in sight (Herzlinger 1992: ix).

This conclusion is, in our view, overly conservative. It overstates the amount of continuity and persistence of traditional arrangements in this sector. Herzlinger's views, we believe, are a consequence of her focus on aggregate expenditure levels, causing her to overlook the quite extraordinary changes that have occurred in the nature of hospitals, the organization of physicians, and the linkages between them and other, newer delivery forms.

1. Note that these measures tap only medical associations, not those of managerial groups such as the AHA.

We argue, rather, that while elements of the old regime remain, much is new and that former elements now operate in a different context. We believe, in short, that this sector has undergone profound change. We turn now to revisit the criteria we proposed for identifying profound change and to juxtapose them to the evidence presented throughout this volume.

IDENTIFYING PROFOUND CHANGE IN SOCIAL SYSTEMS: REVIEWING CRITERIA AND EVIDENCE

Chapter 1 offered a set of nine criteria for assessing the presence and extent of profound change in a social system. Our empirical case focuses on a geographically bounded organizational field in the San Francisco Bay Area that includes, as a part of its environment, the wider material-resource and institutional structures at the local, state, and national levels that impinge on the focal field. As a way of summarizing our principal arguments and evidence, we review these criteria, examining their application to our case.

Multilevel Change

The data and diagrams distributed throughout this volume provide ample evidence that the changes observed are not just occurring at the level of individual participants or particular types of organizations but involve multiple kinds of actors and systems operating at various micro and macro levels. Individual physicians have become, on average, less active and engaged in the leading professional association, the AMA, and more likely to belong to specialist medical associations (fig. 6.1); undoubtedly, this is due, in part, to the increasing specialization of the profession itself (figs. 6.3, 6.5). In their workplace, physicians are more apt to be employees rather than independent operators or owners, and, even if they remain in "private" practice, are much more likely to belong to a group practice and to participate in one or more managed care service plans (fig. 3.14, chap. 6).

At the organizational level, traditional units such as hospitals are learning new ways of acting, for example, identifying "cost" and "profit" centers and engaging in strategic planning. New types of organizations, such as HMOs and PPOs, and employer purchasing groups have emerged, and older forms, such as hospitals, are more likely to be "hollowed out" and serve fewer patients, to fail altogether, or to become component units of wider healthcare systems (figs. 3.14, 3.15, 8.1). Organizations that deliver healthcare services under public auspices have been declining in numbers, while private organizations, both nonprofit and for-profit, have become more prevalent during the period of our study (fig. 3.5, chaps. 3, 4).

At broader, societal levels, ways of financing medical services undergo change. Indemnity insurance plans give way to prepaid healthcare plans, and public funding develops to rival private coverage in scale (figs. 5.2, 6.2). The numbers and types of professional associations proliferate, reflecting the increasing complexity and diversity of the health professions (fig. 6.5), and public regulatory agencies at various levels—federal, state, and local—multiply (fig. 6.10). Cultural beliefs affecting healthcare have also undergone change. More patients accept the legitimacy of and seek care from a widening range of alternative providers, and more patients are willing to view healthcare services as a customer-supplier relation not unlike those of other commercial transactions in which "the customer" knows best and is expected to look after his or her own interests (fig. 6.12, 6.13). Having long been regarded as a privileged professional sanctuary, healthcare services are rapidly undergoing bureaucratization and becoming subject to managerial logics stressing efficiency and cost consciousness.

There is no need to assume that all of these changes involving differing units and types of phenomena are highly integrated or tightly coupled. Indeed, much effort has been devoted to obtain sufficiently detailed information to exhibit the variegated nature of change and the loose coupling between various units and forces. The organizational case studies, in particular, illustrate the nuance and complexity of change (e.g., Case Illustrations 3.B, 4.B, 6.B, 8.C). Moreover, there remain important elements that exhibit continuity. For example, patients still seek healthcare services primarily from physicians, and hospitals are still the primary locus providing acute care for complex cases.

Nevertheless, there is much evidence that the changes occurring in healthcare are multileveled and multifaceted, involving both individual and collective actors and both local and more global social structures and cultural systems.

Discontinuous Change

Discontinuous, radical, or revolutionary change is, almost by definition, rare. All social processes exhibit change, but for the great majority of them and over the course of most of their history, the change involved is continuous or incremental in nature. A cursory review of the many figures in this volume depicting time trends reveals that virtually all of the instances of change described are incremental, not discontinuous. We have discussed some of the underlying change mechanisms, such as adaptation and hybridization, that are conducive to incremental change (chap. 4).

Two instances of discontinuous change appear in our history, the one strong and clear-cut, the other less dramatic, but sufficiently powerful and abrupt to be a viable candidate. The first involves the entry by the federal government in 1965 into the healthcare services arena, at the outset in the guise of a major purchaser of healthcare services. The government's increased involvement is dramatic. Signified by the passage of the Medicare/Medicaid Act, the graph lines charting these developments rise in almost a perpendicular fashion (figs. 5.3, 9.1). While preparation for this entry took place over several years, including earlier failed attempts to enlist public support for medical services (chap. 6), the legislative event unleashing vast new amounts of federal funding burst on the scene. Revolutionary committees and reform-oriented cabals may be years in formation, but when they succeed, their programs can engender large changes in short periods.

The second instance of discontinuous change is also precipitated by public legislation, federal acts in 1982 and 1983 to curtail hospital costs and encourage competitive processes in healthcare markets. These legislative acts are part of a broader initiative to reduce the exceptionalism that had long characterized healthcare transactions and organizational forms and bring them under the rubric of modern managerial and corporate controls (chap. 6). The discontinuous nature of these changes is reflected in the rapid rise of health service corporations, physician executives, and managerial-market logics (figs. 6.17, 9.1, chap. 6). The changes depicted are not quite so dramatic as those revealed by the onslaught of federal funding, but arise quickly and develop at a rapid rate. The difference in the speed with which the two events unfold is partly accounted for by the types of indicators employed: the former tracking the movement of funds, which are relatively fluid and maneuverable; the latter involving the generation of new behaviors (changes in individuals' memberships) and new organizations and activities that require more time to develop. And, as with the first event, the second also involved earlier ground-breaking and preparation extending over several years (chap. 6). Economists honed their theories in quiet corridors of universities and think tanks and only gradually crafted a new agenda for policy planners and politicians.

The two episodes of discontinuous change, which we highlight, involve forces that are not isolated or disconnected from other factors of interest but are ones that induce related change in many other variables. Both are precipitated by federal legislation but are set apart from routine law-making in that these acts instantiate new conceptions of healthcare delivery: who is to receive medical treatment, how it is to be financed, and how these decisions are to be made. They represent "breakthrough" policies rather than incrementalist efforts to "rationalize" existing policies (Brown 1983a). They are richly connected events that, if they do not quite "bring down the house," reconfigure its structure, rearrange the furniture, and change the lifestyle of its inhabitants. They are sufficiently important developments that we have treated them as markers and instigators of profound institutional change.

New Rules and Governance Mechanisms

The "rules" we have in mind are broadly defined, incorporating norms, formal and informal expectations and understandings, and formal and informal governance structures and mechanisms. At the most general level, it is possible to speak of the emergence, ascendance, and eventual weakening of three types of rule systems or regimes: the first involving professional medical authority and the exercise of formal and informal occupational controls; the second, the activation of public funding and growth of regulatory authority at both the federal and state levels; and the third, the increased employment of managerial and market control mechanisms. As we have emphasized, one regime does not displace another completely, although, over the course of our study, we observe a pattern in which first one and then another of the regimes appears to dominate (chaps. 6, 7, fig. 9.1).

Associated with the three regimes are differences in the types of control mechanisms utilized. Professional controls operate primarily via normative channels, professional associations and societies determining the distribution of discretionary authority, who has access to treatment facilities and which participants can legitimately perform what tasks (chap. 6). Although there is occasional resort to legal action, controls are exercised primarily through "voluntary" accreditation activities and the exercise of informal controls and sanctions (e.g., access to staff privileges in hospitals) operating at local levels (chap. 7).

When federal authorities enter, a bargain is struck with existing professional powers, such that their criteria and concerns continue to be honored in governmental decisions. The regimes constructed now, however, take on a more formal, regulatory character, with specific benefits and sanctions backing up the rules. Conformity to formalized professional standards becomes the basis of eligibility for federal funding and, hence, a key to survival (tables 7.3, 7.4). Healthcare planning is no longer voluntary but mandatory, and there are costs for noncompliance when organizational decisions involve the location or enlargement of facilities or the purchase of major equipment (table 6.A.1). Quality control in hospital utilization and treatment, while still carried out by physicians, takes place under the auspices of federally mandated professional review bodies (chap. 6).

Federal regulatory controls continue into the third era but are now supplemented by the "private government" controls of healthcare corporations, whose managers have suddenly become empowered by the new priority given to cost reduction and efficiency concerns. To the operation of the multitude of "visible hands" busily managing the internal operation of healthcare corporations is added the "invisible hand" of competition between provider forms. Professional and public controls still operate but are joined by managerial and market mechanisms (chaps. 6, 9, fig. 9.1).

New Logics

When institutional change is profound, participants not only do things differently, they do different things. There are shifts in the values that orient, guide, and motivate behavior. While a complete revolution has not occurred in the values served by healthcare systems—patients still look primarily to physicians for their healthcare services—we have proposed that important changes are apparent in the relative salience of central values over the course of our study. Accompanying the rise in the status and power of the medical profession was the importance placed on healthcare quality. Following a period of jurisdictional competition (early in this century), physicians claimed and were largely granted the privilege of being the arbiters of medical quality. The quest for quality fueled the growth of medical schools, increases in the relative numbers of physicians, and the rise in public expenditures for health-related research (figs. 5.4, 6.6); it also encouraged the great majority of physicians to seek additional training so as to qualify as specialists (fig. 6.3).

Physicians stressed the value of providing quality care for patients, but a new logic advocated by liberal reformers pointed out that many of the most needy individuals in our society, particularly the poor and elderly, lacked access to such care. While not contesting the importance of quality or the physicians' prerogatives in defining it and controlling its delivery, the new logic stressed the need to broaden coverage and increase equity (chap. 6).

This commitment was enacted into law in 1965 and resulted in the federal government becoming a major new presence in the healthcare sector. But the new partnership had unexpected effects. New entrants placed heavy demands on the system, and the reimbursement formulae employed encouraged practitioners to provide more rather than fewer services. The costs of medical care borne by the public sector rose rapidly. Congress sought ways to curb costs, attempting to rationalize the delivery system through mechanisms such as mandatory health planning. Regulatory programs and agencies grew.

Fueled largely by escalation in the costs of healthcare—as well as by the fact that healthcare expenditures were increasingly funded by public expenditures—a new logic emerged in the 1980s that stressed the value of efficiency. While some advocates still talk broadly to the effect that "health care is a right of every citizen," it is much less permissible now than formerly to argue that "health is to be assured at any cost." Economic arguments emphasizing limitations, constraints, and trade-offs increasingly dominate discourse in the healthcare arena. Such assertions can produce a backlash, and there is recent support for a patients' "bill of rights." But the fine print in these proposals suggests the extent to which the rights being defended are relatively restricted in character (e.g., to be told about options not covered by one's current insurance plan). While individuals who can afford it may continue to search for optimal quality, the system increasingly recognizes the value of cost savings and the need to provide a financial return to investors.

Medical costs have been relatively high and on the increase throughout the last half century—the period of our study (figs. 5.7, 5.8). But the interpretation of these costs has varied over time, being framed and filtered by dominant logics. In the first era, increasing costs were often interpreted as a sign of the increased salience and quality of healthcare (chap. 6); during the second era, increasing costs became a signal that the welfare state was reeling out of control, with expectations and entitlements outpacing revenues (chap. 10); and during the third era, cost-containment provided the legitimating rationale for corporate controls and market-oriented mechanisms (chaps. 6, 10).

The source of resources also reflects underlying institutional logics. Early healthcare systems were dependent on private philanthropy, charitable societies, and private elites expressing a "voluntary ethos" (fig. 6.4). Indemnity insurance and the "Blues" enabled the middle classes to cover their hospital bills while protecting physician prerogatives (fig. 5.2). During and following the war, employers increasingly extended health insurance coverage to their employees as a valued benefit. The passage of Medicare/Medicaid signals a major new public commitment to insuring access to care to the elderly and unprivileged. But, as the proportion of hospital bills covered by third-party payors—private and public—increased, so did the cost of medical care, surpassing and then rapidly outpacing the consumer price index from the early 1980s up to the present (fig. 5.8). More recently, healthcare organizations have become more dependent on investor financing and on their ability to compete for consumer dollars in the medical marketplace.

New Types of Actors

We have made much in previous chapters of the central role played in change processes by the creation of new types of actors, both individual and collective. Actors are socially constructed, through processes imperfectly understood, as comprising distinctive capacities and capabilities. They embody and serve as carriers of specific constellations of interests and logics of action (chaps. 2, 6).

Some of the actors described, for example, economists, are not "new" to the world, but are new to the sector. While not unknown in earlier eras, throughout the period of our study they grow in numbers and influence, bringing in their distinctive set of assumptions, perspectives, and analytic problem-solving capabilities (chap. 6). Their orientation, once regarded as foreign and inapplicable to healthcare issues, becomes more salient. By the third era of our study, they occupy some of the most important policy-setting and decision-making positions. Healthcare administrators become increasingly professionalized, developing their own powerful associations. Their training programs are increasingly linked to programs in business administration rather than to schools of public health (fig. 6.14). Other types of actors, for example, physician executives, represent new combinations of capabilities and interests: physician skills and capacities are supplemented with managerial training (chap. 6). The hope is that such hybrid roles can find a way of reconciling the multiple values and interests at large in the field.

Among the new collective entities that arise are a set of more specialized medical care forms, including home health agencies and kidney disease centers. These organizations are "new" types of actors only in the sense that they have carved out and contain a somewhat specific set of functions formerly performed in more generalist forms—as with the relation of ESRDCs to hospitals—or because they represent a revival and reconfiguration of an earlier, traditional form—as in the relation of HHAs to visiting nurses associations (chap. 3).

Of more interest are the new managed care forms and plans, including HMOs, PPOs, and POSs. These arrangements represent truly novel forms in that they combine functions—financial and risk-bearing together with medical service delivery—that earlier logics insisted should be insulated from one another (chaps. 2, 3). It is instructive to note that these functions were not separated in previous eras because of legal or regulatory requirements[2] but because of normative beliefs enforced by the medical profession. From the outset, organized medicine strongly opposed any financial or insurance arrangements that created an intermediary between patient and physician who might be in a position to influence physicians' patient care decisions because of the physician's financial dependence (Starr 1982).

Such new forms often grow out of unusual circumstances. The pioneer HMO, Kaiser Permanente, originated out of the need to provide medical services to workers in remote areas and was able to perfect its organizational template through a decade of development by servicing a closed clientele of company employees. The shortage of quality medical services in the immediate aftermath of World War II provided a large and ready pool of clients when KP opened its doors to the public in 1945 (chap. 2, Case Illustrations 3.A, 5.A, 6.B).

HMOs and related forms not only combine functions in innovative ways. They have also stimulated a reexamination of the traditional status ordering of physicians' specialties and alternative providers. Because of the new emphasis placed on cost-cutting approaches, medical organizations begin to place increased value on preventive care and measures to maintain wellness. Hence, primary care physicians, long regarded as residing on the lowest rung of the medical hierarchy, see their value reappraised and their functions upgraded. Group practices, which had formerly been restricted to a collection of multispecialty practitioners, are reconfigured to emphasize the central role played by primary care physicians (including physicians involved in internal medicine, family practice, and pediatrics). And there is increased acceptance of alternative providers, such as acupuncturists and chiropractors (table 6.13), as well as physician's assistants and nurse practitioners.

2. New organizational forms often arise as a result of deregulation or similar types of legal changes that permit the formation of previously proscribed forms. Such changes have recently occurred in the arena of financial services (see Gart 1994, Cohen 1996).

The new forms thus differ from those formerly occupying the field. They are built around different archetypes, and they represent new combinations of interests, personnel, and capabilities. And, of critical importance, it is the new forms of actors, both individual and organization, that are on the ascendance, growing in numbers, size, and distribution throughout the period of study. Traditional forms—private practice, commercial insurance vendors, independent hospitals—on the other hand, are stagnant or have declined in numbers and importance (fig. 3.15).

New Meanings

Meanings are necessarily elusive and difficult to measure. But if we are to insist that institutions supply "meaning and order" to social behavior (Scott 1995: 33), then we should attempt to provide evidence of such change. Much of the evidence adduced in relation to previous criteria can be recalled and reframed in this connection. New rule systems or governance mechanisms, new values and logics, and new types of actors and complexes of actions necessarily partake of and manifest new meanings. Physician roles that once connoted autonomy and independence are less likely to do so today. Corporate bodies and managerial logics that for so long were excluded from the medical care sector are increasingly recognized as legitimate types of actors and bases of decision making (fig. 6.17). Of course, such new logics are more rapidly embraced by the newer actors and structures and resisted by the more traditional players (figs. 6.16a–b).

Changed meanings can involve transvaluation of actors and actions. Formerly devalued actors, such as primary care physicians, see their value being reappraised, and historically central organizational players, such as hospitals, find that they are being forced to play a more circumscribed role in medical care provision, as managers and planners embed them in wider and more differentiated care networks.

Basic concepts can undergo changes in their connotations. Concepts such as "health planning" have been shown to change the company they keep, engaging first voluntary, community activities, then being championed and mandated by public agencies, and, more recently, enlisting corporate and purchaser interests (tables 6.A.1, 6.A.2). Clearly, what "planning" means—who participates and to what end—varies substantially under these different arrangements.

When the broader institutional context undergoes change, the "same" actors and activities can exhibit different meanings. The changing eras of the evolution of the American healthcare sector provide shifting symbolic frameworks for interpreting action. We observed, for example, a tendency for competitive intensity to have variable effects on the entries and exits of hospitals and HHAs depending on era (tables 5.4, 5.5). And, the normative assessments of the technical functions of hospitals were observed to have their strongest impact on hospital survival during the era of federal involvement, whereas the assessments of managerial functions had their strongest effects during the era of managerial logics (table 7.3). The relative salience of similar functions appears to vary depending on the value configurations within the wider institutional context.

New Relations among Actors

Changes in the extent and the ways in which actors are connected are as important in their effects on social behavior as changes in the characteristics of the actors themselves. Indeed, many social network theorists would assert that relational properties are more important because they provide the supportive or constraining contexts within which activities are carried out.

Our discussion has provided evidence of change in both intra- and inter-organizational relations. Within healthcare settings, for example, physicians are more likely to find themselves in the position of employee rather than owner, and, even if still in independent practice, to be subject to the managerial authority of those who administer managed care plans (chaps. 5, 6). Current newspapers are full of accounts describing the protests of unhappy physicians unaccustomed to taking orders from "glorified clerks" and "bean-counters." In addition, various categories of technicians, paraprofessionals, and other professionals increasingly share power with physicians.[3]

Most of our research attention, however, has been devoted to examining changes in the relations among organizations within the healthcare sector. In particular, we have described and analyzed the increasing numbers and types of linkages between hospitals and other types of healthcare organizations, first involving primarily horizontal ties and later more vertical connections (chap. 8, Case Illustrations 8.A, 8.C). We have also chronicled the development of new kinds of connections, more loosely coupled virtual ties, as organizations enter into various types of networks and alliances (figs.

---

3. Fundamental changes have also occurred in the relation between physicians and the wide range of other professional and paraprofessional healthcare providers, as complex technologies generate new forms of technical expertise giving rise to increased decentralization of authority, as well as encouraging the employment of more elaborate interprofessional teams of caregivers (see Barley 1986, Begun and Lippincott 1993).

8.4–8.7). In addition, connections that formerly were largely limited to the local area have been greatly extended so that a great many healthcare organizations are linked not only into local service networks but into national and even international systems (fig. 8.7).

At a more general level, we have also described changes occurring over time in the connections between principal types of organizational actors: governance units, purchasers, intermediaries, and providers (fig. 2.2). We have emphasized throughout our discussion the changes occurring between and among organizational forms making up the governing units of the sector (professional associations, public agencies, corporate entities), and have also emphasized the importance of developments that have induced two formerly quiescent sets of participants—purchasers and financial intermediaries—to become increasingly active in attempting to influence providers' behavior (chap. 6).

Much of the interest and complexity of today's healthcare arena, compared with its condition at midcentury, is due not simply to the numbers of new types of social actors now active but also to the multiple ways in which these actors have become interpenetrated and richly connected.

Changes in Organizational Boundaries

Organizational boundaries are notoriously difficult to define, in part because they are multiplex. Participants and observers variously emphasize normative, relational, and activity criteria (Scott 1998: 183–84)—criteria that never exactly coincide for social phenomena that are always experiencing change. In dealing with institutional transformation, our attention is directed above the level of the individual organization to consider the boundaries defining an organizational form, a discrete type of organization that serves as the basis for an organizational population. At this level too, there exists little consensus on how organizational forms are to be defined and their boundaries delimited (chaps. 1, 2).

Hannan and Freeman (1989) have advanced the debate by helpfully shifting the focus from organizational forms to boundary-setting processes. Stable institutional frameworks are characterized by the dominance of "segregating" processes that specify and delimit the boundaries of collective units in the field. By contrast, changing institutional arrangements give rise to "blending" processes, as lines between existing forms become obscured and displaced. In this formulation, then, changed and confusing organizational and organizational population boundaries can be considered a hallmark of profound institutional change.

As we have noted, any shifting or blending of organizational boundaries poses problems for analysts pursuing a conventional population ecology study (chap. 1). Our own attempt to define and pursue the historical evolution of five organizational populations across a span of five decades has been somewhat compromised by this problem (chap. 3, Case Illustration 3.A). But because our principal focus has been at the wider field rather than the population level of analysis, we have been in a position to document not only the rise and fall of specific forms but also the erosion over time in the boundaries of these forms (chap. 3, table 3.3).

We have provided substantial evidence of boundary confusion. Among our specialized populations, HHAs exhibit such diversity—with some emphasizing medical, some nonmedical functions—that we were forced to use certification criteria in an attempt to isolate the subset of the form most relevant to the healthcare sector, narrowly defined (chap. 2). And HMOs display such internal diversity of features that analysts routinely refer to them as reflecting a continuum of forms, varying along several dimensions (table 2.1). The hospitals in our sample variously include or exclude within their portfolio home health and renal disease services (figs. 3.11, 3.13). And, the largest and most prominent single provider in the Bay Area, Kaiser-Permanente is engaged in healthcare services that span the full spectrum of all our organizational populations combined (Case Illustration 3.A).

The fifth population studied, integrated healthcare systems, is virtually impossible to define at this moment in time: some of the "systems" are linked horizontally, some vertically, and still others, by virtual ties. They are made up of different component units, connected in diverse ways. Some are regionally restricted while others operate nationally. Some are nonprofit, some are for-profit and others exhibit exotic combinations of both (chap. 8).

In short, all of the organizational populations surveyed are, to a substantial degree, in flux. There exists little current consensus on which organizational archetypes or templates are best suited to the tasks at hand. And this will continue to be the case as long as there remains conflict among contending parties regarding the appropriate mode of governance and nature of institutional logics to be employed.

Change in Field Boundaries

At the time when our study commenced, the healthcare sector was arguably the most distinctive and most insulated of all major U.S. societal sectors from conventional business practices and institutions. Industrialization and its accompanying twin, bureaucratization, had long been prevented from invading and transforming the ways in which healthcare was delivered. Most physicians operated as independent practitioners; most hospitals were independent, community-based, nonprofit entities. There were few other organizational forms available for dispensing healthcare services.

By the end of the century, many of these distinctive features have disappeared or are under siege. The organizational forms and managerial agents that have long characterized most of American society have invaded and are currently in the process of transforming healthcare. Physicians are increasingly involved in and employed by healthcare organizations (chap. 6). A multitude of specialist healthcare organizations has arisen (chap. 3), and independent hospitals are rapidly being incorporated into broader integrated healthcare systems (chap. 8). Most healthcare services are now dispensed under managed care arrangements in which fiscal and administrative controls constrain medical decision-making.

How did this profound transformation occur? The process, as we have observed it, appears to be one in which the ideological barriers erected to insulate the healthcare field have been delegitimated and discredited. The data support the argument that the new and somewhat alien logics acting to limit professional prerogatives entered the field as a result of the fragmentation of existing governance structures, both professional and public. The unity that once characterized and upheld the privileged position claimed by the medical establishment became unraveled and fractured around specialists' diverse interests. Added to this rupture was the growing number and diversity of public regulatory systems at all levels. Institutionalists such as Meyer and Scott (1983) have argued that organizational arrangements that are subjected to numerous and conflicting authorities become delegitimated. Fragmentation of institutional governance structures paves the way for profound institutional change (fig. 9.4, table 9.3).

The weakening of professional unity together with the continuing escalation of healthcare costs rendered the sector vulnerable to the introduction of a new set of logics and governance mechanisms. Why was it that corporate interests and managerial logics that had long and unsuccessfully attempted to gain a foothold in the healthcare field, were finally able to do so in the early 1980s? The "barbarians" had long been at the gates; how did they finally succeed in entering? In part, the way was paved by the emergence in the 1970s of alternative logics broadening the conception of health and healers (table 9.4). But the major impetus for the victory of managerial logics was that they were packaged as a new and effective set of tools of public policy consistent with an ascendant political ideology (chap. 9). Throughout the 1970s, the courts were increasingly disinclined to view professionals as exempt from antitrust legislation; and legislative acts passed in the early 1980s legitimated managerial controls and competitive practices (chap. 6). The introduction of market logics ultimately rested on a series of legal/political decisions and acts.

The Structuration and Destructuration of Organizational Fields

In their seminal paper on the forces shaping organizational fields, DiMaggio and Powell propose the concept of structuration as an indicator of the extent of institutionalization of a field:

> Fields only exist to the extent that they are institutionally defined. The process of institutional definition, or "structuration," consists of four parts: an increase in the extent of interaction among organizations in the field; the emergence of sharply defined interorganizational structures of domination and patterns of coalition; an increase in the information load with which organizations in a field must contend; and the development of a mutual awareness among participants in a set of organizations that they are involved in a common enterprise (DiMaggio and Powell 1983: 65).

As indicated in chapter 1, we embrace this general definition of structuration, but believe that it is important to identify somewhat more specific dimensions to guide empirical research. Moreover, we are as interested in examining destructuration processes—processes that undermine coherence and unity—as in those processes that increase stability and order.

Throughout this volume, we have employed a number of distinctions and categories. Some, like the concepts of logics, governance structures, and actors, are quite general; others, like the concept of professional dominance, federal involvement, and market orientation, are more particular to the subject of this study. In order to place our study in a wider context that will allow comparisons with the specific sector we have studied—in a particular society, at a given time—we propose a set of dimensions along which the structuration of fields can vary (see also, Scott 1994). These dimensions are implicit in our preceding analysis but here we make them explicit. Eight dimensions are identified:

• *Funding centralization*—the extent to which financial resources employed by field actors are concentrated. At one end of this continuum, the field would be occupied by many, small buyers. At the other end, a single entity, perhaps a nation-state or a single corporation would be the only source of demand and of revenues.

• *Unity of governance*—the extent to which governance structures are congruent in jurisdiction and consistent in the rule systems enunciated and enforced. At one end of this continuum, there would exist multiple competing governance structures, fragmented and inconsistent in jurisdiction and rule enforcement. At the other end would exist a single, integrated, governance unit.

• *Public/private mode of governance*—the extent to which different types of governance structures exercise uncontested power and authority over an organizational field. At one extreme, only public authorities control activities within the field. At the other, private systems of control (i.e. "private governments") exercise exclusive authority. Most existing fields are characterized by mixtures of public and private governance structures.

• *Structural isomorphism*—the extent to which organizational actors in the field conform to a single archetype or structural model. At one extreme, all actors performing a similar function would reflect the same basic structural features in their organizational design. At the other extreme, organizational actors would embrace many, diverse structural templates.

• *Coherence of organizational boundaries*—the extent to which organizational forms in the sector exhibit clear, well-demarcated boundaries. A field with high coherence might include many different types of organizational forms (populations), but these forms would be clearly differentiated and readily distinguished from one another. By contrast, a field with low coherence would exhibit a kind of organizational "soup" in which distinctive forms are difficult to discern and there is much overlap and blending of forms.

• *Consensus on institutional logics*—the extent to which actors in the sector embrace and adhere to the same general beliefs and recipes of action in carrying out sector activities. Low consensus would be indicated by disagreements and disputations over the priorities and goals of the sector and lack of agreement on the appropriate means to be employed in reaching them. High consensus would be indicated by a unity of purpose and approach.

• *Organizational linkages*—the extent to which there is a relatively high number of formal connections between organizational actors in the sector. At one pole would exist a field in which the actors are relatively disconnected, unfettered by formal ties of relations to one another. At the other, actors would be associated with one another in dense, reciprocal networks of relations.

• *Clarity of field boundaries*—the extent to which there exists relatively high insulation and separation of field actors and structures from neighboring fields. Participants in fields with porous or weak boundaries cannot agree on who is a legitimate player in the field and experience high penetration of the sector by "foreign" actors and ideas. By contrast, actors in fields with clear boundaries agree on who is in the field and encounter relatively few unknown actors or alien ideas.

While we have not been completely successful in developing operational indicators of each of these dimensions, we have provided examples of measures in table 10.1—some of which we employed, others which could have been used in our analyses. We recognize that some of the indicators are relatively crude and may tap more than one dimension, for example, measures of funding, which reflect the resource environment as well as governance structures and logics.

Another way to portray the utility of the dimensions identified is to show the ways in which they relate to the three institutional eras we have defined in our study. These associations are summarized in table 10.2. The story depicted in this table suggests a number of dimensions along which the degree of structuration of the healthcare field has decreased. The unity of governance has been disrupted: governance structures have become much more fragmented. Structural isomorphism has been reduced: a much higher diversity of organizational forms now operates in the field. The coherence of organizational boundaries has been greatly reduced, with forms undergoing transformation with increasing frequency and many more hybrid forms existing. Practitioners and patients alike are confused by the array of alternative plans and providers and unclear about the differences among them. Consensus about institutional logics has been reduced; field participants do not agree on the routines for carrying out the work of the field nor the aims toward which those routines are directed. And, field boundaries have become less clearly defined. The healthcare sector is no longer seen as a distinctive and protected sector but is more subject to external influences and invaded by alien actors and ideas. In all of these ways, destructuration of the field has proceeded during the past fifty years.

On the other hand, structuration processes are complex and do not all proceed in the same direction at the same pace. Centralization of funding—an important stimulant to further structuration (DiMaggio, 1983)—increased between the first and second eras. But increased centralization in funding authority in the healthcare sector has not had the effect of unifying programmatic authority. Instead, governance structures became less unified and coherent.

Table 10.1 Field Dimensions and Indicators

Dimensions	Indicators
Funding centralization	federal, state, local government funding enrollment in health insurance plans
Unity of governance	regulatory and planning bodies professional associations accreditation regimes policy maps field fragmentation
Public/private mode of governance	proportion of public to private governance structures proportion of public to private funding
Structural isomorphism	numbers of differentiated organizational populations
Coherence of organizational boundaries	blending of organizational populations
Consensus on logics	discourse (professional journals, medical school curricula) professional training programs
Organizational linkages	multihospital associations integrated healthcare systems relational contracting purchasing coalitions
Clarity of field boundaries	appearance of new field-level actors appearance of organizational actors operating in more than one field acceptance of logics originating outside the sector

Linkages among organizational actors in the field have also increased considerably. A field once made up of independent and isolated actors has become much more richly connected, in local as well as geographically dispersed systems. It appeared for a time that these large corporate structures would produce greater field coherence. But these trends seem to have peaked during the 1990s and have engendered a backlash in which consumers are turning to politicians with demands that they be protected from "normal" business practices, regarded as inappropriate in this context.

It is difficult to identify precisely the causal structure at work in determining the direction and nature of change of field structuration processes. Our analysis in chapter 9 suggests that the high level of structuration that characterized the era of professional dominance was undermined by the increasing fragmentation of governance structures. This fragmentation had two components: a breakup of the unity of the governance structures associated with the medical profession and the rise of public authorities to

Table 10.2   Field Dimensions and Institutional Eras

	Professional dominance	Federal involvement	Market orientation
Funding centralization	low	high	intermediate
Unity of governance	high	intermediate	low
Public/private mode of governance[a]	low	intermediate	intermediate
Structural isomorphism	high	intermediate	low
Coherence of organizational boundaries	high	intermediate	low
Consensus on logics	high	intermediate	low
Organizational linkages	low	intermediate	high
Clarity of field boundaries	high	intermediate	low

NOTE: a. Scale reflects public in relation to private mode of governance.

oversee the expenditure of increased levels of public funding. Fragmentation of governance structures led to a delegitimation of existing professional authorities. Reduced consensus on field logics and increased diversity of organizational forms followed in the wake of these changes. The ascendance of market logics was stimulated by the rise in alternative health and healers, associated with the decline in medical authority. They were also supported by increasing medical costs and bolstered by their congruence with a broader program of neo-conservative reform.

Structuration is the master process operating at the level of the organizational field as it relates to its wider environments—both material-resource and institutional. Each individual organization is variably related to this field in a more or less tightly or loosely coupled manner. Many organizations are relatively tightly connected to the field, both in relational and cognitive terms (e.g., in that they closely embrace field logics). These organizations reflect and are strongly affected by forces operating at the field level. Other organizations are more loosely connected, being less embedded in relational attachments and/or being relatively distinctive in their characteristics and behavior. They can often evade or ignore field influences.

The more highly structured the field, the less impetus or room there is for disconnected and distinctive actors. The less structured the field, the more latitude and stimulation there is for autonomy and innovation at the organizational level. It is a bellwether of the state of the wider healthcare field that we currently observe such vigorous organizational experimentation and exploration.

A CONCLUDING COMMENT

This research has been guided by many objectives. We have attempted to demonstrate the value of integrating multiple theoretical perspectives and diverse research methods. We have hoped to illustrate the utility of employing a field-level perspective as a means of comprehending changes occurring among many different types of organizations providing related services. We have embraced an open systems perspective to emphasize the effects of environmental factors—at local, state, and national levels—on organizational forms and functions. But, we have also attended, through case studies, to the ways in which organizations act to shape, challenge, and construct the environments in which they operate. And, most important, we have stressed the value of taking into account the impact of institutional features on social structures and processes.

The effects of institutional environments on social structures and processes are all too frequently ignored. This oversight occurs because, in many studies, such forces are ubiquitous but invariant. Much social science research is content to examine structures and behavior in one relatively homogeneous area of social life and is restricted to one point in time, employing a cross-sectional approach. In order to detect institutional effects, analysts must design studies that compare and contrast different institutional conditions, for example, differing sectors within a society or similar sectors in differing societies, or compare and contrast conditions in a given sector experiencing substantial change over time. The present study has opted for the latter design, selecting the arena of healthcare services because, in the United States at least, this sector has experienced great, even profound, change.

When comparisons across diverse sectors or across time for the same sector are possible, broader institutional forces often become evident. All social structures and processes operate within a context whose values and assumptions are framed by taken-for-granted or broadly enforced cognitive, normative, and regulative beliefs and rules. While social actors create and carry these beliefs (and construct and conform to these rules), institutional arrangements provide the cultural milieu that determines what kinds of actors can exist, what they can do, and what meanings their actions have. We believe that an important component of the agenda of contemporary social science is to generate designs that will enable researchers to uncover these larger frameworks and detect their important and pervasive, but often overlooked, effects on social life. Our study provides one example of such a design.

DATA SOURCES FOR ORGANIZATIONAL POPULATIONS

Table A.1   Summary of Principal Data Sources

Organizational Population	Data Sources	Years Available	Total Records	Total Organizations
Event History Data				
Hospitals	American Hospital Directory Hospitals AHA Guide to the Healthcare Field OSHPD reports	1945–48 1949–/1 1972–92 1976–92	4596	163
Home health agencies	OSHPD reports Health Care Directory SSA listings[a]	1978–92 1977 1969–76	1789	255
HMOs	Interstudy national HMO census	1945–92[b]	397	36
ESRDCs	HCFA provider directory Health Care Directory SSA listings[a,c]	1978–92 1977 1973–76	670	58
Multihospital systems	Annual reports, web sites, histories AHA Guide to Multihospital Systems AHA Guide to the Healthcare Field	1945–79 1979–85 1986–92	717[d]	45[d]
Event Count Data				
Medical groups	PHS Medical Groups in the U.S. MGMA Directory Kaiser Permanente Annual Reports	1946, 1959 1961–93[e] 1960–93[e]	—[f]	—[f]
Preferred provider organizations	PPOs: The California Experiment AMCRA Directory of PPOs AMCRA Managed Healthcare Directory	1983 1985–91[e] 1994	—[f]	—[f]

NOTES: a. Limited variable subsets only.

b. Although the census did not begin until 1976, it also includes information on HMO foundings prior to that year.

c. Prior to 1973, all Bay Area ESRDCs were hospital-based. Data for these facilities were collected from the AHA Guide and *Hospitals*.

d. Total only includes system-level data.

e. Selected years only.

f. Count data do not distinguish the total number of distinct organizations or records.

Table A.2   Summary of Measures Collected for the Focal Populations

	Hospitals	**HHAs**	**HMOs**	**ESRDs**	**MHSs**
Accreditation and quali- fication	AHA, Blue Cross, CHA, interns, JCAHO, medical school, Medicare, nursing, resi- dents, surgeons, teaching	Medicare, MediCal	Federal, NCQA	—	—
Events	Entry, exit, founding date, location change, name change	Entry, exit, founding date, location change, name change	Entry, exit, founding date, name change	Entry, exit, founding date, name change, location change	Entry, exit, founding date, name change
Linkages	HMO contracts, system affiliation	System affili- ation, vertical integration	National affilia- tion	System affili- ation, vertical integration	
Market niche	Hospital type, length of stay	HHA type, reimbursement sources	HMO type	ESRD type	System type
Services	General services, outpatient services	General services, AIDS services	—	General services, outpatient services	—
Size	Admissions, bassinets, beds, payroll, plant valuation, staff, total expenses	Home visits, patients (total), patients (seniors)	Enrollments	Dialysis stations	Member hospitals
Utilization	Census bassinets, census beds	—	Hospital days, physician en- counters	—	—
Ownership	✔	✔	✔	✔	✔

STATISTICAL COMPARISON OF ECOLOGICAL AND ADAPTIVE CHANGE

As noted in chapter 4, changes observed at the level of an organizational population can be parsed into two basic components—"ecological" change, due to entries into and exits from the population, and "adaptive" change, due to transformations on the part of population members. The ecological and adaptive components of change can be isolated by: (1) computing the distribution statistics for an organizational characteristic at some time period t; (2) considering rates of change in those distribution statistics by time period $t + 1$, allowing only ecological dynamics to operate (i.e., holding attributes for *existing* organizations at the same level as period t); and (3) determining the residual difference between the "ecological" distribution obtained in $t + 1$ and the empirical distribution for that period (with the difference being accounted for by adaptive changes). While this methodology can, in principal, be applied to any statistic that describes a characteristic's distribution (e.g., variance, skewness, kurtosis), we restrict our analytic attention to shifts in population means.

The decomposition procedure yields one observation per annum for each characteristic that is considered, indicating the proportion of change in that characteristic due to ecological and adaptive factors. Pooling these observations across the organizational characteristics allows us to consider whether statistically significant differences exist in terms of their susceptibility to adaptive transformation. The structural inertia theory of Hannan and Freeman (1984) intimates the following rank-ordering among organizational characteristics:

Inertia (goal orientation) > *Inertia* (formal structure)
> *Inertia* (technology, linkages)

where adaptability is inversely related to structural inertia. A statistical test of the ordering can be performed using an analysis of variance procedure, with a Scheffé test of pairwise comparisons between each class of organizational attributes.

As an empirical example, we can consider annual observations of ecological change proportions for various hospital characteristics (see table 4.1). For the 1946–91 timeframe, there are $46 \times 7 = 322$ potential cases; 36 cases are missing, representing years in which there was no adaptive or ecological change in some class of attributes.[1] Reviewing the comparisons (table B.1), we find that population-level changes in linkages (e.g., accreditations/AHA membership) and technology (service portfolios) are significantly less likely ($p < .05$) to be generated by ecological dynamics than are changes in formal structure and goals. The distinction between goals and formal structure is not as pronounced. Nevertheless, on the whole there appears to be remarkable support for the inertial hierarchy as a heuristic device, if not necessarily as an empirical generalization.

EVIDENCE OF DISCONTINUOUS CHANGE

Our characterization of institutional eras relies on discontinuous period effects bounded by major changes in governance structures, specifically, legislative and regulative events (chap. 6). Thus, the era of federal involvement

Table B.1 One-Way ANOVA with Scheffé Multiple Comparison Test of Structural Inertia (N = 286)

	Mean[a]	**(1)**	**(2)**	**(3)**	**(4)**
(1) Linkages	0.276				
(2) Technology	0.301				
(3) Formal Structure	0.477	*	*		
(4) Goals	0.602	*	*		
	F-Ratio = 14.753**				

NOTES: * $p < .05$; ** $p < .01$ (two-tailed test)

a. Because of missing values, means need not correspond to the average of overall proportions in table 4.1.

1. The time series nature of this data may lead to concerns about serial autocorrelation. Durbin-Watson tests conducted in conjunction with the ANOVA analysis suggest that a null hypothesis of no positive autocorrelation cannot be rejected at the $p < .01$ level (in other words, there is no clear evidence of positive autocorrelation).

was ushered in with the passage of the Medicare and Medicaid programs in 1965 and their implementation the following year. The beginning of the era of managerial and market orientation was marked by the establishment of the prospective payment system (PPS) at the federal level and selective contracting with healthcare providers at the state level in California during the early 1980s.

However, an alternative perspective may view these changes in institutional arrangements as having been incremental rather than discontinuous. The associated null hypothesis would be that the regulatory events we have treated as definitive do not significantly explain change in organizational populations when the incremental, linear time trend underlying these processes is taken into account.

In addition, a second alternative perspective would acknowledge that the healthcare field has been shaken by discontinuous changes but that regulatory events other than the ones we have selected better reflect the timing of these episodic shifts. The 1973 HMO Act is a particularly obvious alternative event to consider. Numerous observers have pointed to its significance in according regulative legitimacy to HMOs—the leading new model of managed care organizations.

In this section, we evaluate both these propositions with a set of trend analyses of one of the most important transformations in healthcare organizations, privatization, among our three largest organizational populations—hospitals, home health agencies, and end-stage renal disease centers.

Impact on Facility Privatization

Recall that privatization is operationalized as the changing proportion of nongovernmental (either for-profit or nonprofit) to publicly owned organizations (see chap. 3). As is the case throughout our study, federal providers are excluded because of their highly specific niches.[2]

Empirical studies of the healthcare field, including our own research, have reported a gradual decline in the proportion of public facilities in the U.S. from World War II to the present (see chaps. 3 and 4). This general trend is reconfirmed by model 1 in table B.2, which shows a positive and significant association between the linear time trend and the privatization

2. Thus, public providers are limited to those operated by state, county, municipal, or special district jurisdictions.

Table B.2   Fixed-Effect Models of Regulatory Impact on Bay Area Hospital Privatization, 1945–92

Event	Model 1	Model 2	Model 3
Linear trend	0.003 (0.000)**	−0.001 (0.001)	−0.002 (0.001)
Medicare/Medicaid	—	0.105 (0.023)**	0.104 (0.023)**
PPS/DRG implementation	—	0.037 (0.020)*	0.036 (0.020)*
HMO Act	—	—	0.023 (0.020)
Number of cases	432	432	432
Log likelihood (model df)	344.92 (9)	355.83 (11)	356.50 (12)

* $p < .05$; ** $p < .01$ (one-tailed test)

Table B.3   Fixed-Effect Models of Regulatory Impact on Bay Area HHA and ESRDC Privatization

	Home Health Agencies		End-Stage Renal Disease Centers	
	1966–92		1979–92	
Event	Model 1	Model 2	Model 1	Model 2
Linear trend	0.008 (0.001)**	0.012 (0.003)**	0.008 (0.002)**	0.006 (0.003)**
PPS/DRG	—	−0.103 (0.041)**	—	0.013 (0.022)
HMO Act	—	0.053 (0.038)	—	—
Number of cases	243	243	117	117
Log likelihood (df)	123.06 (9)	131.36 (11)	159.21 (9)	159.40 (10)

* $p < .05$; ** $p < .01$ (one-tailed test)

of Bay Area hospitals during the period 1945–92.[3] Table B.3 reports similar results for both HHAs and ESRDCs.

We have argued throughout, however, that major regulatory events, such as the implementation of Medicare/Medicaid and PPS, have generated "punctuated equilibria" with respect to this population dynamic, providing occasions for discontinuous change. At the end of the first proposed era, the Medicare/Medicaid legislation abruptly blurred a boundary that had long separated governmental from private facilities by initiating direct funding of health services to both public and private providers. Private and public facilities now vied for the same public funds. Governmental facilities had lost their distinctive, protective niche, while at the same time

3. These models use fixed effects in order to control for county-level heterogeneity, in lieu of material-resource indicators employed in previous analyses (e.g., in chap. 5).

continuing to be subject to a set of environmental pressures and public expectations that made it difficult for them to compete (Rainey, Backoff, and Levine 1976). This possibility is confirmed in model 2 of table B.2, in which Medicare/Medicaid legislation is shown to have a positive, significant impact on privatization of hospitals.

Model 2 of table B.2 also indicates that the PPS legislation, which led to implementation of substantial cost-containment incentives for healthcare organizations, was significantly and positively related to hospital privatization. Since the intent of this act was to favor those organizations best able to respond to market-based criteria of performance (i.e., private providers), this effect is not unexpected.

Most important for our present concern, when the two legislative events demarcating eras were included (model 2 of table B.2), the linear time trend no longer had a significant effect on privatization processes. These models provide statistical support for our assumption that the organizational processes of interest, such as privatization in healthcare, have reflected a discontinuous, rather than incremental, pattern of institutional change.

On the other hand, similar analyses conducted on two other organizational populations in the Bay Area, HHAs and ESRDCs provided less clear evidence. Sufficient data were not available for these populations to test the effects of the first event, the Medicare/Medicaid programs, but the PPS legislation shows significant effects only for HHAs, and not ESRDCs. Moreover, the time trend for these populations maintained its significant relation to privatization, even when the PPS initiative was entered into the equation (table B.3, model 2).

The argument that the HMO Act passed in 1973 had a significant effect on these population processes receives little support from any of our analyses. Despite only weak effects nationally of the legislation on HMO growth (Brown 1983),[4] the Bay Area HMO population did show a rise beginning in the mid-1970s (see fig. 3.7).[5] But model 3 of table B.2 and model 2 of table B.3 reveal no significant effects of this regulatory event on the privatization of either hospitals or HHAs in the Bay Area.[6] Thus, the possibility that we have overlooked a significant regulatory event equal or greater in strength to that of the selected markers seems remote.

4. The numbers of HMOs for the United States as a whole did not begin its rapid increase until the early 1980s (Brown 1983).

5. Unfortunately, not enough cases for Bay Area HMOs exist to conduct similar statistical tests.

6. We could not test the effects of the HMO Act on ESRDCs, because we do not have the necessary data for this population before 1979.

Conclusion

In sum, we find considerable support for our two assumptions regarding eras. For the populations considered, the markers we identified to delineate eras were observed to have stronger effects on the organizational population process of interest than an alternative legislative event. And, for two populations, the selected markers had a significant effect even after taking into account a linear time trend. Yet the results also suggest that institutional changes are nuanced and multifaceted. As noted in chapter 1, environmental effects may vary substantially in salience to differing field participants and populations. In the current analyses, for example, hospitals appear to have been the primary targets of both Medicare/Medicaid and PPS legislation. Although events may generate "punctuated equilibria" in institutional environments, it is important to chart the differing impact of these shifts across varying sectors and dimensions of a field.

Quantitative
Methodology

This appendix provides a technical overview of the quantitative methods employed in chapters 4, 5, 7, 8, and 9. Four classes of analytic methods are reviewed: (1) methods for modeling organizational entries; (2) methods for modeling organizational exits; (3) methods for analyzing organizational adaptation; and (4) factor analysis methods for measuring latent variables.

Organizational Entries

Entries into the organizational populations are modeled as continuous-time stochastic processes that generate annual event counts. Estimation proceeds via maximum likelihood techniques, which are applied to the following Poisson regression model (Greene 1997):

$$\Pr\{Y_t = y_t\} = e^{-\lambda(t)}\lambda(t)^{y_t}/y_t!$$

where Y_t is the estimated entry count in year t, y_t is the corresponding observed entry count, and $\lambda(t)$ is a linear function of the specified covariates and their coefficients. This model is employed using the nine Bay Area counties as its units of analysis—i.e., counts include any entries into an organizational population within each county and covariates are likewise measured at this level of analysis.

Because the Poisson regression model relies on a statistical assumption of equal means and variances for event count distributions, special steps need to be taken to handle *overdispersion,* a violation of this assumption when a distribution's variance exceeds its mean (Greene 1997; Barron 1992). The assumption is met for the entry process governing our hospital and ESRDC populations but does not hold for HHAs. In the latter case, a negative binomial regression model was used, introducing an overdispersion error term (ϕ) into the Poisson equation. This specification corresponds to the NegBin II model introduced by Cameron and Trivedi (1986). Greene's (1995) LIMDEP software was used to estimate both the Poisson and negative binomial models.

ORGANIZATIONAL EXITS

Event history analyses are used to model exits from the organizational populations. Left-truncation of some of the data sets (e.g., a lack of complete hospital event histories before 1945) led us to observe some precautions in specifying the time-parametric form of the hospital survivor models (Tuma and Hannan 1984). Nonparametric exploratory analyses were conducted to obtain Nelson-Aalen estimates of the hazard rates over time. Broad variations in these hazard rates generally matched the substantively interesting institutional eras of professional dominance, federal involvement, and market reform. Since piecewise exponential survivor models can readily capture these variations and produce unbiased results even when left-truncation is present (Guo 1993), we opted for the following functional form for transition rates (r):

$$r(t) = \exp\{\gamma_n + A\alpha_n + B\beta\} \quad \text{if } t \in n$$

where γ_n is a constant coefficient associated with the nth time period, $\mathbf{A}$ is a vector of covariates (also associated with the nth period), α_n is the corresponding vector of coefficients, $\mathbf{B}$ is a vector of covariates with time-stationary effects, and β is the coefficient vector corresponding to $\mathbf{B}$. The vector of covariates with time-varying effects ($\mathbf{A}$) allows us to explore changes in the institutional salience of different organizational and environmental characteristics—e.g., legitimacy, competition, and performance—in promoting or impeding exit rates (see chaps. 5 and 7). The survivor models were estimated using maximum likelihood techniques and Rohwer's (1994) Transition Data Analysis program.

Many of the survivor models presented in the text involve multiple levels of analysis. For instance, the models of resource environment effects presented in chapter 5 include both organization-level and county-level covariates. In conjunction with the previous piecewise exponential specification, the higher-level (i.e., county) effects can most easily be accommodated by disaggregating them to the lower level organizational units, which are nested within them. This approach raises two potential statistical problems: (1) random errors between organizational units may no longer be independent since they contain components attributable to common higher-level county units; and (2) statistical tests of the impact of county-level variables tend to be based on an inflated number of (organization-level) cases. Unfortunately, the standard hierarchical linear modeling approach (Bryk and Raudenbush 1992) typically used to deal with these problems cannot be applied very reliably because of the small number of Bay Area counties considered ($N = 9$). Future analyses, based on a broader selection of counties, will be required to formally separate out the hierarchical layers affecting organizational exits.

ORGANIZATIONAL ADAPTATION

Exploratory analyses of organizational adaptation require the calculation of transition rates from one state (e.g., for-profit ownership) to another (nonprofit ownership). When these states are discrete in character, the *hazard rate* (r) for state transitions can simply be computed as:

$$r(t) = \lim_{\Delta t \to 0} \frac{\Pr(t \leq T < t + \Delta t | T \geq t)}{\Delta t}$$

where the numerator expresses a conditional probability that an organization will have a state transition in the time interval between t and $t + \Delta t$, provided that the event has not occurred before time t (Rohwer 1994). Descriptive statistics in chapter 4 offer estimates of mean hazard rates for various discrete organizational adaptations.

Confirmatory analysis of organizational adaptation (with respect to discrete characteristics) builds on this basic specification (see chap. 8). Insofar as the temporal heterogeneity of adaptive changes is not of theoretical interest, in and of itself, we can employ a semiparametric approach that treats such heterogeneity as an underlying "nuisance" function. The following Cox (1972) specification can then be applied:

$$r(t) = h(t) \exp(\boldsymbol{B}(t)\beta)$$

where $r(t)$ is the transition rate, $h(t)$ is an unspecified baseline rate (which controls for temporal variation), $\boldsymbol{B}$ is a vector of covariates, and β is the corresponding vector of coefficients. Partial likelihood estimation is used to obtain the parameter estimates.

In the case of organizational attributes measured on an interval scale (e.g., number of hospital beds), basic rates of transition can be obtained as first-order derivatives of the continuous variable (Y):

$$r(t) = \frac{dY}{dt}$$

When annual time intervals are involved, this rate is simply computed by differencing sequential values of the continuous variable: $r(t) = Y_t - Y_{t-1}$. It can be divided by Y_t in order to obtain the percentage change in a continuous variate by unit of time.

FACTOR ANALYSIS

In the institutional analysis of organizational fields, there are typically a large number of organizational and environmental processes that lack directly observable referents. Chapters 7 and 9 have provided such examples as normative legitimation of hospitals; institutional logics linked to professional dominance, federal responsibility, or market orientation; and fragmentation of governance and funding structures. These concepts themselves are represented by *latent,* or unobserved, variables. In order to measure these latent variables, a model must be specified that ties the latent variable to a series of observed indicators. The general measurement model employed in factor analytic approaches to latency can be written as:

$$X_{ij} = \sum_k f_{ik}\lambda_{jk} + e_{ij}$$

where X_{ij} is the observation for the jth indicator variable and ith individual, f_{ik} is the kth latent factor for the same individual, λ_{jk} is the coefficient describing the estimated effect of the kth latent factor on the jth indicator variable, and e_{ij} is the error term (sometimes called the unique factor).

Indicator variables (X_j's) proposed in the text have included accreditation measures for normative legitimacy (table 7.1) and AMA membership for the logic of professional dominance (table 9.1). Given such indicators, a final step involves estimating the measurement model. We have employed two basic techniques for performing this step: *exploratory* factor analysis (chap. 7) and *confirmatory* factor analysis (chap. 9) (Bollen 1989).

Exploratory factor analysis (EFA) is typically applied when there is limited a priori certainty regarding the measurement model associated with a set of latent variables. We encountered this scenario with normative legitimacy, where the complexity of interrelationships among different sources of legitimacy rendered our preliminary empirical intuitions somewhat suspect. Accordingly, we conducted an exploratory factor analysis.

Three sets of procedures were employed in this process: (1) missing values for legitimacy indicators, which were unavailable for some sets of years (i.e., JCAHO, 1945–53 and CHA, 1964–90), were replaced with the means of the respective indicators; (2) latent factors were extracted using a principal components method; factors were retained based on the conventional criteria that their eigenvalues were greater than one (Kim and Mueller 1978); (3) a varimax rotation technique was applied to generate statistically independent factors. Because of the ordinal character of the accreditation indicators, a separate estimation technique was also applied to provide special treatment for the categorical measures (Lee, Poon, and Bentler 1994). We found, however, virtually no difference between the resulting factor scores and those computed using standard exploratory factor analysis.

When stronger theoretical intuitions guide the measurement model of a latent variable, then confirmatory factor analysis (CFA) can appropriately be applied. Unlike the EFA approach, the CFA requires that the analyst identify the number of latent variables underlying a series of indicators in advance, as well as the connections between latent and observed constructs. The CFA approach has the advantage that it allows correlation among the measurement errors of latent variables.

All confirmatory factor models in chapter 9 were estimated with the AMOS 3.61 structural equation modeling program (Arbuckle 1997). For these analyses, we did not include covariation among the latent factors since our purpose was to generate factor scores for use in time series regression models. But in order to understand the relationship between the primary logics factors in particular, we did estimate a joint model with covariation among these three latent variables (see chap. 9, n. 4).

Factor scores provide an estimated metric of the latent factor for each data case (corresponding, in our design, to each annual time point). Factor scores were calculated using a regression weighted method, computed as $\mathbf{W} = \mathbf{S}^{-1}\mathbf{B}$, where $\mathbf{W}$ is the matrix of regression weights, $\mathbf{S}$ is the matrix of covariances among the observed variables, and $\mathbf{B}$ is the matrix of covariances between the observed and unobserved variables. Factor score trends were standardized for comparability (with mean of 0 and standard deviation of 1) before graphing or inclusion in time series analyses.

Glossary of Abbreviations and Acronyms

AAFRC	American Association of Fundraising Councils
AAAHC	Accreditation Association for Ambulatory Health Care
AACSB	American Assembly of Collegiate Schools of Business
AAMD	American Academy of Medical Directors
ABMS	American Board of Medical Specialties
ACEHSA	Accrediting Commission on Education for Health Services Administration
ACGME	Accreditation Council for Graduate Medical Education
ACPE	American College of Physician Executives
ACS	American College of Surgeons
AHA	American Hospital Association
AMA	American Medical Association
AMCRA	American Managed Care and Review Association
AUPHA	Association of University Programs in Hospital Administration
BACHPC	Bay Area Comprehensive Health Planning Council
BCA	Blue Cross Association
BC/BS	Blue Cross/Blue Shield
CalPERS	California Public Employees' Retirement System
CHA	California Hospital Association
CHW	Catholic Healthcare West
CMA	California Medical Association
CON	certificate of need
DRG	diagnostic-related group
ESRD	end-stage renal disease
ESRDC	end-stage renal disease center
FFS	fee-for-service
FTC	Federal Trade Commission
HCA	Hospital Corporation of America

HCFA	U.S. Health Care Financing Administration
HEDIS	Health Plan Employer Data and Information Set
HFPC	Health Facility Planning Council (Bay Area)
HHA	home health agency
HHI	Herfindahl-Hirschman Index
HIAA	Health Insurance Association of America
HIPA	Health Information and Promotion Act
HIPC	Health Insurance Plan of California
HMO	health maintenance organization
HPEA	Health Professions Educational Act
HSA	Health Systems Agency
IPA	independent practice association
JAMA	*Journal of the American Medical Association*
JCAHO	Joint Commission on Accreditation of Healthcare Organizations
KP	Kaiser Permanente Medical Care Program
LCME	Liaison Committee for Medical Education
MBA	master of business administration
MD	doctor of medicine
MHA	master of health administration
MGMA	Medical Group Management Association
MHS	multihospital system
MPH	master of public health
MSO	management service organization
NCHS	National Center for Health Statistics
NCQA	National Committee for Quality Assurance
NIH	National Institutes of Health
OBRA	Omnibus Budget Reconciliation Act
OMB	U.S. Office of Management and Budget
OSHPD	California Office of Statewide Health Planning and Development
OTA	Office of Technical Assessment
PAMC	Palo Alto Medical Clinic
PBGH	Pacific Business Group on Health
PHO	physician-hospital organization
PHS	U.S. Public Health Service
POS	point-of-service
PPO	preferred provider organization
PPS	prospective payment system

PRO	peer review organization
PSRO	professional standards review organization
SJH	San Jose Hospital
SSA	U.S. Social Security Administration
SUH	Stanford University Hospital
TEFRA	Tax Equity and Fiscal Responsibility Act
UCSF	University of California at San Francisco
URAC	Utilization Review Accreditation Commission
USHC	University of California-Stanford Health Care
VNA	visiting nurse association

AACSB (American Assembly of Collegiate Schools of Business). 1995. "The Need for Greater Efficiency and Lower Costs in Health Care Creates New Opportunities for Business Schools." *Newsline* Summer: 14–16.

AAFRC (American Association of Fundraising Councils). 1997. *Giving USA: The Annual Report on Philanthropy for the Year 1996.* New York: AAFRC Trust for Philanthropy.

AAHP (American Association of Health Plans). 1997. *National Directory of Health Plans and Utilization Review Organizations.* Washington, DC: AAHP.

Abbott, Andrew. 1988. *The System of Professions: An Essay on the Division of Expert Labor.* Chicago: University of Chicago Press.

Abbott, Carl. 1981. *The New Urban America: Growth and Politics in Sunbelt Cities.* Chapel Hill: University of North Carolina Press.

———. 1994. "The Federal Presence." In *The Oxford History of the American West,* edited by Clyde A. Milner II, Carol A. O'Connor, and Martha A. Sandweiss, 469–99. New York: Oxford University Press.

ABMS (American Board of Medical Specialties). 1996. *1996 Annual Report & Reference Handbook.* Evanston, IL: ABMS.

ACEHSA (Accrediting Commission on Education for Health Services Administration). 1995. "The Official List of Accredited Programs in Health Services Administration in Canada and the United States." July 1. Arlington, VA: ACEHSA.

ACPE (American College of Physician Executives). 1996. *Year-end Membership Figures* [Phone Interview]. Membership Office.

ACS (American College of Surgeons). 1966. *Manual for Cancer Programs.* Chicago: ACS.

Aday, Lu Ann, Charles E. Begley, David R. Lairson, and Carl H. Slater. 1993. *Evaluating the Medical Care System: Effectiveness, Efficiency and Equity.* Ann Arbor, MI: Health Administration Press.

Adventist Healthcare West. 1998. Internet site. URL: <www.AdventistHealth.org>.

AHA (American Hospital Association). 1945–49. *American Hospital Directory.* Chicago: AHA.

———. 1949–71. *Hospitals.* Chicago: AHA.

———. 1972–97. *Guide to the Health Care Field.* Chicago: AHA.

———. 1974–87. *Policies, Policy Statements, Policy Strategies, Guidelines, Technical Advisory Bulletins.* Chicago: AHA.

———. 1980–85b. *AHA Directory of Multihospital Systems.* Chicago: AHA.

————. 1986, 1992. *Directory of Health Care Coalitions in the United States.* Chicago, IL: Published on behalf of the Dunlop Group of Six.

Aldrich, Howard. 1979. *Organizations and Environments.* Englewood Cliffs, NJ: Prentice-Hall.

Aldrich, Howard E., and C. Marlene Fiol. 1994. "Fools Rush In? The Institutional Context of Industry Construction." *Academy of Management Review* 19: 645–70.

Aldrich, Howard, and Jeffrey Pfeffer. 1976. "Environments of Organizations." *Annual Review of Sociology* 2: 79–105.

Alexander, Jeffrey A., and Terry L. Amburgey. 1987. "The Dynamics of Change in the American Hospital Industry: Transformation or Selection?" *Medical Care Review* 44: 279–322.

Alexander, Jeffrey A., James G. Anderson, and Bonnie L. Lewis. 1985. "Toward an Empirical Classification of Hospitals in Multihospital Systems." *Medical Care* 23: 913–32.

Alexander, Jeffrey A., and Thomas A. D'Aunno. 1990. "Transformation of Institutional Environments: Perspectives on the Corporatization of U.S. Health Care." In *Innovations in Health Care Delivery: Insights for Organization Theory,* edited by Stephen S. Mick, 53–85. San Francisco: Jossey-Bass.

Alexander, Jeffrey A., Thomas A. D'Aunno, and Melissa J. Succi. 1996. "Determinants of Profound Organizational Change: Choice of Conversion or Closure among Rural Hospitals." *Journal of Health and Social Behavior* 37: 238–51.

Alexander, Jeffrey A., and Mary L. Fennell. 1986. "Patterns of Decision Making in Multihospital Systems." *Journal of Health and Social Behavior* 27: 14–27.

Alexander, Jeffrey A., Arnold D. Kaluzny, and Suann Middleton. 1986. "Organizational Growth, Survival and Death in the U.S. Hospital Industry." *Social Science and Medicine* 22: 303–8.

Alexander, Jeffrey A., and Michael A. Morrisey. 1988. "Hospital Selection into Multihospital Systems: The Effects of Market, Management, and Mission." *Medical Care* 26: 159–76.

Alexander, Jeffrey A., and W. Richard Scott. 1984. "The Impact of Regulation on the Administrative Structure of Hospitals." *Hospitals and Health Services Administration* 29 (May/June): 71–85.

Alexander, Jeffrey A., Thomas Vaughn, Lawton R. Burns, Howard S. Zuckerman, Ronald M. Anderson, Paul Torrens, and Diana W. Hilberman. 1996. "Organizational Approaches to Integrated Health Care Delivery: A Taxonomic Analysis of Physician-Organizational Arrangements." *Medical Care Research and Review* 53: 71–93.

Alexian Brothers Healthcare System. 1998. Internet site. URL: <www.AlexianBros.org>.

Alford, Robert R. 1972. "The Political Economy of Health Care: Dynamics Without Change." *Politics and Society* 2(Winter): 127–64.

————. 1975. *Health Care Politics: Ideological and Interest Group Barriers to Reform.* Chicago: University of Chicago Press.

Alvarado, Donna. 1994a. "Hospitals Readying Major Cuts; Staff Reductions Possible at SJ Medical Center." *San Jose Mercury News.* February 8, p. 1B, 8B.

————. 1994b. "Downsize or Die, Hospitals Told Cutbacks Can Avert Closings, Report Says." *San Jose Mercury News.* May 11, p. 1B, 8B.

————. 1995a. "$45 million Cut for Good Sam? Health System Chief Apparently Confirms Doctors' Warning." *San Jose Mercury News.* March 31, pp.1B, 4B.

———. 1995b. "3 Area Hospitals to Join Huge Chain." *San Jose Mercury News.* September 19, pp. 1A, 9A.

———. 1995c. "Good Sam Price Called Too Low Health System Sale: Consumer Group Wants State to Block $165 Million Deal." *San Jose Mercury News.* December 23, pp. 1B, 5B.

———. 1995d. "Huge Hospital Chain Called 'Pac-Man' of the Industry." *San Jose Mercury News.* December 29, pp. 1A, 26A.

———. 1996. "Dispute over Sale Profits: State Wants Good Sam to Provide Care to Needy." *San Jose Mercury News.* January 1, pp. 1B, 4B.

AMA (American Medical Association). 1942, 1950. *American Medical Directory.* Chicago: AMA.

———. 1959–73. *Physician Distribution in the U.S.* Chicago: Department of Economic Research, AMA.

———. 1968. *Reclassification of Physicians: A New Base for Health Manpower Studies.* Chicago: Center for Health Services Research and Development, AMA.

———. 1974–79. *Physician Characteristics and Medical Licensure.* Chicago: Department of Statistical Analysis, AMA.

———. 1981–98. *Physician Characteristics and Distribution in the US.* Chicago: Division of Survey and Data Resources, AMA.

———. 1982. *Multihospital Systems Data Book 1980–1981.* Chicago: AMA.

———. 1995. *Graduate Medical Education Directory.* Chicago: AMA.

———. 1997. *AMA Membership 1847–96.* [Internal reports]. Chicago: Division of Library and Information Services, AMA.

Amburgey, Terry L., Tina Dacin, and Dawn Kelly. 1994. "Disruptive Selection and Population Segmentation: Interpopulation Competition as a Segregating Process." In *Evolutionary Dynamics of Organizations,* edited by Joel A. C. Baum and Jitendra V. Singh, 240–56. New York: Oxford University Press.

Amburgey, Terry L., Dawn Kelly, and William P. Barnett. 1993. "Resetting the Clock: The Dynamics of Organizational Change and Failure." *Administrative Science Quarterly* 38: 51–73.

AMCRA (American Managed Care and Review Association). 1985–91. *Directory of Preferred Providers Organizations and the Industry Report on PPO Development.* Washington, DC: AMCRA.

———. 1994–95. *Managed Health Care Directory.* Washington, DC: AMCRA.

American Medical International (AMI). 1972–75. Annual Reports.

American Medicorp, Inc. 1968–70. Annual Reports.

Anders, George. 1996. *Health Against Wealth: HMOs and the Breakdown of Medical Trust.* Boston: Houghton Mifflin.

Andersen, Ronald M., and Pamela L. Davidson. 1996. "Measuring Access and Trends." In *Changing the U.S. Health Care System: Key Issues in Health Services, Policy and Management,* edited by Ronald M. Andersen, Thomas H. Rice, and Gerald F. Kominski, 13–40. San Francisco: Jossey-Bass.

Anderson, Martin. 1978. *Welfare: The Political Economy of Welfare Reform.* Stanford, CA: Hoover Institution.

Anderson, Odin. 1975. *Blue Cross Since 1929: Accountability and the Public Trust.* Cambridge, MA: Ballinger.

Andreopoulos, Spyros. 1993. "Medical Center has a History of Changing to Fit the Times." *Medical Center Report* (special issue of *Campus Report*). June 22. Stanford, CA.
———. 1994. Memo to Harry Press. April 23.
Ansley, David. 1991. "SJ Clinic Severs 35-year Partnership with Medical Center." *San Jose Mercury News.* November 21, p. 1B.
Appleby, Julie. 1997. "Operating on Kaiser." *The Sunday Times.* Sunday August 3, pp. D1, D6.
Arbuckle, James L. 1997. *AMOS Version 3.61.* Chicago: SmallWaters Corporation.
Archer, Margaret S. 1988. *Culture and Agency: The Place of Culture in Social Theory.* Cambridge: Cambridge University Press.
Arndt, Margarete, and Barbara Bigelow. 1992. "Vertical Integration in Hospitals." *Medical Care Review* 49: 93–116.
Arrow, Kenneth J. 1963. "Uncertainty and the Welfare Economics of Medical Care." *American Economic Review* 53: 941–73.
Astin, John A. 1998. "Why Patients Use Alternative Medicine: Results of a National Study." *Journal of the American Medical Association* 279(19): 1548–53.
Astley, W. Graham. 1985. "The Two Ecologies: Population and Community Perspectives on Organizational Evolution." *Administrative Science Quarterly* 30: 224–41.
BACHPC (Bay Area Comprehensive Health Planning Council). 1971. *Health Planning CHPC 1971.* (newsletter), November.
———. 1972. *Health Planning CHPC 1972.* (newsletter), May.
Baer, Hans A. 1987. "Divergence and Convergence in Two Systems of Manual Medicine: Osteopathy and Chiropractic in the United States." *Medical Anthropology Quarterly* 1: 176–93.
Bain, Joe Staten. 1951. "Relation of Profit Rate to Industry Concentration: American Manufacturing, 1936–40." *Quarterly Journal of Economics* 65: 293–324.
———. 1956. *Barriers to New Competition.* Cambridge: Harvard University Press.
Barger, S. Brian, David G. Hillman, and H. Randall Garland. 1985. *The PPO Handbook.* Rockville, MD: Aspen.
Barley, Stephen R. 1986. "Technology as an Occasion for Structuring: Evidence from Observations of CT Scanners and the Social Order of Radiology Departments." *Administrative Science Quarterly* 31: 78–108.
Barnett, William P. 1994. "The Liability of Collective Action: Growth and Change among Early Telephone Companies." In *Evolutionary Dynamics of Organizations,* edited by Joel A. C. Baum and Jitendra V. Singh, 337–54. New York: Oxford University Press.
Barnett, William P., and Glenn R. Carroll. 1987. "Competition and Mutualism among Early Telephone Companies." *Administrative Science Quarterly* 32: 400–421.
Baroody, William J. 1981. "Foreword." In *A New Approach to the Economics of Health Care,* edited by Mancur Olson, xv-xvi. Washington, DC: American Enterprise Institute.
Barron, David. 1992. "The Analysis of Count Data: Overdispersion and Autocorrelation." *Sociological Methodology 1992,* edited by Peter Marsden, 179–220. Washington, DC: American Sociological Association.
Barron, David, Elizabeth West, and Michael T. Hannan. 1994. "A Time to Grow and a Time to Die: Growth and Mortality of Credit Unions in New York City, 1914–1990." *American Journal of Sociology* 100: 381–421.
Baum, Joel A. C. 1996. "Organizational Ecology." In *Handbook of Organizational Studies,*

edited by Stewart R. Clegg, Cynthia Hardy, and Walter Nord, 77–114. Thousand Oaks, CA: Sage.

Baum, Joel A. C., and Christine Oliver. 1991. "Institutional Linkages and Organizational Mortality." *Administrative Science Quarterly* 36: 187–218.

———. 1992. "Institutional Embeddedness and the Dynamics of Organizational Populations." *American Sociological Review* 57: 430–59.

Baum, Joel A. C., and Walter W. Powell. 1995. "Cultivating an Institutional Ecology of Organizations: Comment on Hannan, Carroll, Dundon, and Torres." *American Sociological Review* 60: 529–38.

Baum, Joel A. C., and Jitendra V. Singh, eds. 1994. *Evolutionary Dynamics of Organizations.* New York: Oxford University Press.

Begun, James W., and Ronald C. Lippincott. 1993. *Strategic Adaptation in the Health Professions: Meeting the Challenges of Change.* San Francisco: Jossey-Bass.

Belknap, Ivan, and John G. Steinle. 1963. *The Community and its Hospitals: A Comparative Analysis.* Syracuse, NY: Syracuse University Press.

Bell, Daniel. 1973. *The Coming of Post-Industrial Society: A Venture in Social Forecasting.* New York: Basic Books.

Bennett, Ivan L., Jr. 1977. "Technology as a Shaping Force." In *Doing Better and Feeling Worse: Health in the United States,* edited by John H. Knowles, 125–33. New York: W. W. Norton.

Bentler, Peter. 1990. "Comparative Fit Indexes in Structural Models." *Psychological Bulletin* 107: 238–46.

Berger, Peter L., and Thomas Luckmann. 1967. *The Social Construction of Reality.* New York: Doubleday.

Bergman, Rhonda. 1994. "No Accreditation, No Contract, Say Most Managed Care Plans." *Hospital and Health Networks* 68(21): 64.

Bergthold, Linda. 1984. "Crabs in a Bucket: The Politics of Health Care Reform in California." *Journal of Health Politics, Policy and Law* 9(2): 203–22.

———. 1990. *Purchasing Power in Health: Business, the State, and Health Care Politics.* New Brunswick, NJ: Rutgers University Press.

Berk, Richard. 1983. "An Introduction to Sample Selection Bias in Sociological Data." *American Sociological Review* 58: 386–98.

Beyers, Bob. 1997. "Command and Control of Merger." *Palo Alto Weekly.* June 11, p. 25.

Blau, Peter M. 1970. "A Formal Theory of Differentiation in Organizations." *American Sociological Review* 35: 201–18.

Blau, Peter M., and Richard A. Schoenherr. 1971. *The Structure of Organizations.* New York: Basic Books.

Blau, Peter M., and W. Richard Scott. 1962. *Formal Organizations: A Comparative Approach.* San Francisco: Chandler.

Bloom, Floyd E., and Mark A. Randolph, eds. 1990. *Funding Health Sciences Research: A Strategy to Restore Balance.* Washington DC: National Academy Press.

Blum, Henrik L. 1976. "From a Concept of Health to a National Health Policy." *American Journal of Health Planning* 1(1): 3–22.

Bollen, Kenneth A. 1989. *Structural Equations with Latent Variables.* New York: John Wiley & Sons.

Bourdieu, Pierre. 1977. *Outline of a Theory of Practice.* New York: Columbia University Press.

Boychuk, Terry. 1994. *Bordering on Universality: The Transformation of Hospital Politics and Policy in the United States and Canada.* Unpublished Ph.D. dissertation, Department of Sociology, Princeton University.

Bresnahan, Timothy F. 1989. "Empirical Studies of Industries with Market Power." In *Handbook of Industrial Organization,* vol. 2, edited by Richard Schmalensee and Robert D. Willig, 1001–57. New York: North-Holland.

Brittain, Jack W. 1994. "Density-Independent Selection and Community Evolution." In *Evolutionary Dynamics of Organizations,* edited by Joel A. C. Baum and Jitendra V. Singh, 355–78. New York: Oxford University Press.

Brodie, Mollyann, Lee Ann Brady, and Drew A. Altman. 1998. "Media Coverage of Managed Care: Is There A Negative Bias?." *Health Affairs,* 17(1): 9–25.

Brown, E. Richard, and Michael R. Cousineau. 1984. "Effectiveness of State Mandates to Maintain Local Government Health Services for the Poor." *Journal of Health Politics, Policy and Law* 9(2): 223–36.

Brown, Lawrence D. 1983a. *New Policies, New Politics.* Washington, DC: Brookings.

———. 1983b. *Politics and Health Care Organization: HMOs as Federal Policy.* Washington, DC: Brookings.

———. 1986. "Introduction to a Decade of Transition." *Journal of Health Politics, Policy and Law* 11: 569–83.

Brown, Michael K., ed. 1988. *Remaking the Welfare State: Retrenchment and Social Policy in America and Europe.* Philadelphia: Temple University Press.

Brown, Montague. 1996. "Mergers, Networking, and Vertical Integration." In *The Economic Era of Health Care: A Revolution in Organized Delivery Systems,* edited by Everett A. Johnson, Montague Brown, and Richard L. Johnson, 21–39. San Francisco: Jossey-Bass.

Brown, Montague, and Howard L. Lewis. 1976. *Hospital Management Systems: Multi-unit Organization and Delivery of Health Care.* Germantown, MD: Aspen Systems Corporation.

Brown, Raymond E., ed. 1972. *Economies of Scale in the Health Services Industry: Proceedings of an Invitational Seminar.* HRA-74-3100. Washington, DC: National Center for Health Services Research.

Bryant, Keith L., Jr. 1994. "Entering the Global Economy." In *The Oxford History of the American West,* edited by Clyde A. Milner II, Carol A. O'Connor, and Martha A. Sandweiss, 195–235. New York: Oxford University Press.

Bryk, Anthony, and Stephen Raudenbush. 1992. *Hierarchical Linear Models.* Newbury Park, CA: Sage.

Buhler-Wilkerson, Karen. 1989. *False Dawn: The Rise and Decline of Public Health Nursing, 1900–1930.* New York: Garland.

———. 1991. "Home Care the American Way: An Historical Analysis." *Home Health Care Services Quarterly* 12: 5–18.

Burda, David, Elizabeth Gardner, and Jay Greene. 1992. "Waves of Mergers, Affiliations Starts Year for Hospitals." *Modern Healthcare* 22(2): 2–3.

Burns, Lawton. 1990. "The Transformation of the American Hospital: From Community Institution toward Business Enterprise." In *Comparative Social Research,* vol. 12, edited by Craig Calhoun, 77–112. Greenwich, CT: JAI Press.

California Board of Chiropractic Examiners. 1925–84. *Directory of Doctors of Chiropractic.* Sacramento, CA.

California Department of Consumer Affairs. 1971–95. *Annual Report.* Sacramento, CA.

———. 1998. Active Chiropractic and Acupuncture Licenses. [requested reports]. Sacramento, CA: Department of Consumer Affairs, Consumer Information- Public Sales Division.

California Department of Finance. 1967–69. *Population Estimates for California Counties.* Sacramento, CA: Financial and Population Research Section.

———. 1997. *California Statistical Abstract.* Sacramento, CA: Demographic Research Unit.

California Department of General Services. 1970–95. *State of California Telephone Directory.* Sacramento, CA.

California Department of Health Services. 1968–69. *Annual Statistical Report, Medical Assistance Program.* Sacramento, CA: Medical Care Statistics Section.

———. 1970–97. *California's Medical Assistance Program Annual Statistical Report.* Sacramento, CA: Health and Welfare Agency, Medical Care Statistics Section.

———. 1997. Personal communication with Phyllis Barnhouse, Medical Care Statistics Section, June 18, 1997.

California Hospitals and Related Health Facilities and Services Planning Committee. 1968. "Voluntary Regional Planning: Hospitals and Related Health Facilities and Services." Report to the California Legislature and to the State Advisory Hospital Council.

California Office of the Governor. 1975–91. *Central Appointments Registry.* Sacramento, CA.

———. 1992–96. *State Appointments List.* Sacramento, CA.

California Secretary of State. 1940–75. *California Blue Book and State Roster.* Sacramento, CA.

California Task Force for the Development of the State Plan for Health. 1971. *California State Plan for Health.* Sacramento, CA: California Department of Public Health, State Office of Comprehensive Health Planning.

Callahan, Daniel. 1977. "Health and Society: Some Ethical Imperatives." In *Doing Better and Feeling Worse: Health in the United States,* edited by John H. Knowles, 23–33. New York: W. W. Norton.

CalPERS (California Public Employees' Retirement System). 1994. *Comprehensive Annual Financial Report 1993/1994.* Sacramento, CA: CalPERS.

———. 1997. Personal communication with Mark Desio, CalPERS Public Affairs Office, July 3, 1997.

Cameron, A. C., and P. K. Trivedi. 1986. "Econometric Models Based on Count Data: Comparisons and Applications of Some Estimators and Tests." *Journal of Applied Econometrics* 1: 29–53.

Campbell, John L. 1997. "Mechanisms of Evolutionary Change in Economic Governance: Interaction, Interpretation and Bricolage." In *Evolutionary Economics and Path Dependence,* edited by Lars Magnusson and Jan Ottosson, 10–31. Cheltenham, UK: Edward Elgar.

Campbell, John L., Rogers Hollingsworth, and Leon N. Lindberg, eds. 1991. *Governance of the American Economy.* New York: Cambridge University Press.

Campbell, John L., and Leon N. Lindberg. 1990. "Property Rights and the Organization of Economic Activity by the State." *American Sociological Review* 55: 634–47.

Campion, Frank D. 1984. *The AMA and U.S. Health Policy Since 1940.* Chicago: Chicago Review Press.

Caronna, Carol A., Seth S. Pollack and W. Richard Scott. 1997. "Cases and Contexts: Investigating Micro-Macro Linkages through an Embedded Case Design." Paper presented to the Annual meetings of the American Sociological Association, Toronto, Canada.

Carroll, Glenn R. 1984. "Organizational Ecology." *Annual Review of Sociology* 10: 71–93.

————. 1985. "Concentration and Specialization: Dynamics of Niche Width in Populations of Organizations." *American Journal of Sociology* 90: 1262–83.

Carroll, Glenn R., and Michael T. Hannan. 1989. "Density Dependence in the Evolution of Populations of Newspaper Organizations." *American Sociological Review* 54: 524–48.

Carroll, Marjorie Smith, and Ross H. Arnett, III. 1979. "Private Health Insurance Plans in 1977: Coverage, Enrollment, and Financial Experience." *Health Care Financing Review* 1(2): 3–22.

————. 1981. "Private Health Insurance Plans in 1978 and 1979: A Review of Coverage, Enrollment, and Financial Experience." *Health Care Financing Review,* 3(1): 55–87.

Carter, Phillip. 1996. "UCSF, Stanford Merger Continues to See Resistance." *Daily Bruin.* November 13. Berkeley, CA.

Casalino, Lawrence. 1997. *Medical Groups and the Transition to Managed Care in California.* Unpublished Ph.D. dissertation, School of Public Health, University of California, Berkeley.

Casalino, Lawrence, and James Robinson. 1997. "The Evolution of Medical Groups and Capitation in California." Report of the Henry J. Kaiser Family Foundation, Menlo Park, CA, September.

Chanco Medical and Electronics Industries. 1968–71. Annual Report.

Chandler, Alfred D., Jr. 1977. *The Visible Hand: The Managerial Revolution in American Business.* Cambridge, MA: Belknap Press of Harvard University Press.

————. 1990. *Scale and Scope: The Dynamics of Industrial Capitalism.* Cambridge, MA: Belknap Press of Harvard University Press.

Child, John. 1972. "Organizational Structure, Environment, and Performance: The Role of Strategic Choice." *Sociology* 6: 2–22.

Chirot, Daniel. 1977. *Social Change in the Twentieth Century.* New York: Harcourt Brace Jovanovich.

Christianson, Jon B., Ira S. Moscovice, and Anthony Wellever. 1995. "The Structure of Strategic Alliances: Evidence from Rural Hospital Networks." In *Partners for the Dance: Forming Strategic Alliances in Health Care,* edited by Arnold D. Kaluzny, Howard S. Zuckerman and Thomas C. Ricketts III, 99–117. Ann Arbor, MI: Health Administration Press.

Christianson, Jon B., Susan M. Sanchez, Douglas R. Wholey, and Maureen Shadle. 1991. "The HMO Industry: Evolution in Population Demographics and Market Structures." *Medical Care Review* 48: 3–46.

Christy, Jack E. 1993. "The PROs 4th Scope of Work: The Maturing of Federal Peer Review." Presented on behalf of the California Medical Review to the National Health Lawyers' Association, Conference on the The Law of Utilization Management and Quality Assurance. April 20.

Chui, Glennda. 1999. "UCSF Stanford to Cut Jobs." *San Jose Mercury News,* March 30, pp. 1B, 4B.

Cisneros, Linda. 1997. "UCSF Academic Senate Hosts Second, Less Volatile Forum on Merger." *Stanford Report,* July 16. 29(36): 9.

Clark, Peter M., and James Q. Wilson. 1961. "Incentive Systems: A Theory of Organizations." *Administrative Science Quarterly* 6: 129–66.

Clement, Jan P. 1988. "Vertical Integration and Diversification of Acute Care Hospitals: Conceptual Definitions." *Hospital and Health Services Administration* 33(1): 99–110.

CMA (California Medical Association). 1941–96. *Membership Recap by Component Society* [Internal Reports]. San Francisco: CMA Scientific and Educational Division.

Cohen, Michael, and Sean L. King. 1996. *California Health Care Fact Book.* Sacramento, CA: Office of Statewide Health Planning and Development.

Cohen, Randi-Charlene. 1996. *Who's Planning for your Future? Jurisdictional Competition among Organizations and Occupations in the Personal Financial Planning Industry.* Unpublished doctoral dissertation, Department of Sociology, Stanford University.

Coleman, James C. 1974. *Power and the Structure of Society.* New York: W. W. Norton.

Connors, Edward J. 1979. "Generic Problems in the Development and Operation of Multi-Hospital Systems." In *Multi-Institutional Hospital Systems,* edited by Howard S. Zuckerman and Lewis E. Weeks, 199–206. Chicago: Hospital Research and Educational Trust.

Conrad, Douglas, Stephen Mick, Carolyn Madden, and Geoffrey Hoare. 1988. "Vertical Structures and Control in Health Care Markets: A Conceptual Framework and Empirical Review." *Medical Care Review* 45: 49–100.

Cox, David. 1972. "Regression Models and Life-Tables." *Journal of the Royal Statistical Society* 34: 187–220.

Crozier, Michel. 1964. *The Bureaucratic Phenomenon.* Chicago: University of Chicago Press.

Cutting, Windsor. 1955. "The First Hundred Years." Stanford University Hospital.

D'Aunno, Thomas A., and Howard S. Zuckerman. 1987 "The Emergence of Hospital Federations: An Integration of Perspectives from Organizational Theory." *Medical Care Review* 44: 323–44.

Daughters of Charity Healthcare System. 1998. Internet site. URL: <www.dcnhs.org>.

Davis, Gerald F. 1991. "Agents without Principles? The Spread of the Poison Pill through the Intercorporate Network." *Administrative Science Quarterly* 36: 583–613.

Davis, Gerald F., Kristina A. Diekmann, and Catherine H. Tinsley. 1994. "The Decline and Fall of the Conglomerate Firm in the 1980s: The Deinstitutionalization of an Organizational Form." *American Sociological Review* 59: 547–70.

Davis, Karen. 1975. *National Health Insurance: Benefits, Costs, and Consequences.* Washington, DC: Brookings Institution.

Denison, D. R., and Robert I. Sutton. 1990. "Operating Room Nurses." In *Groups That Work (And Those That Don't): Creating Conditions for Effective Teamwork,* edited by J. Richard Hackman, 293–308. San Francisco: Jossey-Bass.

Department of Economics, University of Michigan, and Bureau of Public Health Economics. 1964. *The Economics of Health and Medical Care.* Ann Arbor, MI: University of Michigan Press.

Dezalay, Yves, and Bryant G. Garth. 1996. *Dealing in Virtue: International Commercial Arbitration and the Construction of a Transnational Legal Order.* Chicago: University of Chicago Press.

DHHS (Department of Health and Human Services). 1976–92. *National HMO Census.*

Rockville, MD: DHHS, U.S. Public Health Service, Office of Health Maintenance Organizations.

Dietz, Thomas, and Tom R. Burns. 1992. "Human Agency and the Evolutionary Dynamics of Culture." *Acta Sociologica* 35(3): 187–200.

DiMaggio, Paul J. 1983. "State Expansion and Organizational Fields." In *Organization Theory and Public Policy,* edited by Richard H. Hall and Robert E. Quinn, 147–61. Beverly Hills, CA: Sage.

———. 1986. "Structural Analysis of Organizational Fields: A Block Model Approach." In *Research in Organizational Behavior,* vol. 8, edited by Barry M. Staw and L. L. Cummings, 335–70. Greenwich, CT: JAI Press.

———. 1988. "Interest and Agency in Institutional Theory." In *Institutional Patterns and Organizations,* edited by Lynne G. Zucker, 3–22. Cambridge, MA: Ballinger.

———. 1991. "Constructing an Organizational Field as a Professional Project: U.S. Art Museums, 1920–1940." In *The New Institutionalism in Organizational Analysis,* edited by Walter W. Powell and Paul J. DiMaggio, 267–92. Chicago: University of Chicago Press.

———. 1994. "The Challenge of Community Evolution." In *Evolutionary Dynamics of Organizations,* edited by Joel A. C. Baum and Jitendra V. Singh, 444–50. New York: Oxford University Press.

DiMaggio, Paul J., and Helmut K. Anheier. 1990. "The Sociology of Nonprofit Organizations and Sectors." *Annual Review of Sociology* 16: 137–59.

DiMaggio, Paul J., and Walter W. Powell. 1983. "The Iron Cage Revisited: Institutional Isomorphism and Collective Rationality in Organizational Fields." *American Sociological Review* 48: 147–60.

———. 1991. "Introduction." In *The New Institutionalism in Organizational Analysis,* edited by Walter W. Powell and Paul J. DiMaggio, 1–38. Chicago: University of Chicago Press.

Donabedian, Avedis. 1980–85. *Explorations in Quality Assessment and Monitoring.* 3 vols. Ann Arbor, MI: Health Administration Press.

Donahue, John D. 1989. *The Privatization Decision: Public Ends, Private Means.* New York: Basic Books.

Donaldson, Lex. 1996. *For Positivist Organization Theory: Proving the Hard Core.* London: Sage.

Dornbusch, Sanford M., and W. Richard Scott, with the assistance of Bruce C. Busching and James D. Laing. 1975. *Evaluation and the Exercise of Authority.* San Francisco: Jossey-Bass.

Douglas, Mary. 1986. *How Institutions Think.* Syracuse, NY: Syracuse University Press.

Dowling, William L. 1995. "Strategic Alliances as a Structure for Integrated Delivery Systems." In *Partners for the Dance: Forming Strategic Alliances in Health Care,* edited by Arnold D. Kaluzny, Howard S. Zuckerman, and Thomas C. Ricketts III, 139–75. Ann Arbor, MI: Health Administration Press.

Dranove, David, and Mark Shanley. 1995. "Cost Reductions or Reputation Enhancement as Motives for Mergers: The Logic of Multihospital Systems." *Strategic Management Journal* 16: 55–74.

Duffy, Sarah. 1992. "Do Competitive Hospitals Really Adopt Technology Faster? An Analysis of the Influence of Alternative Relevant Market Definitions." *Eastern Economic Journal* 18: 187–208.

Duncan, Otis Dudley, W. Richard Scott, Stanley Lieberson, Beverly Davis Duncan, and Hal H. Winsborough. 1960. *Metropolis and Region.* Baltimore, MD: Johns Hopkins Press.

Edelman, Lauren. 1992. "Legal Ambiguity and Symbolic Structures: Organizational Mediation of Civil Rights Law." *American Journal of Sociology* 97: 1531–76.

Edmunds, Margaret, Richard Frank, Michael Hogan, Dennis McCarty, Rhonda Robinson-Beale, and Constance Weisner, eds. 1997. *Managing Managed Care: Quality Improvement in Behavioral Health.* Washington, DC: National Academy Press.

Eisenberg, David M., Ronald C. Kessler, Cindy Foster, Frances E. Norlock, David R. Calkins, and Thomas L. Delbanco. 1993. "Unconventional Medicine in the United States: Prevalence, Costs, and Patterns of Use." *New England Journal of Medicine* 328(4): 246–52.

Eldrege, Niles, and Stephen Jay Gould. 1972. "Punctuated Equilibria: An Alternative to Phyletic Gradualism." In *Models of Paleobiology,* edited by Thomas J. M. Schopf, 82–115. San Francisco: Freeman Cooper.

Ellwood, Paul M., Jr. 1971. "Testimony Presented to the Subcommittee on Health of the Senate Committee on Labor and Public Welfare." Oct. 6. Minneapolis, MN: InterStudy.

———. 1972. "Models for Organizing Health Services and Implications of Legislative Proposals." *Milbank Memorial Fund Quarterly/Health and Society* 50: 73–101.

Enthoven, Alain C. 1980. *Health Plan: The Only Practical Solution to the Soaring Cost of Medical Care.* Reading, MA: Addison-Wesley.

Enthoven, Alain C., and Sara J. Singer. 1996. "Managed Competition and California's Health Care Economy." *Health Affairs* 15(1): 39–55.

Ermann, Daniel, and Jon Gabel. 1984. "Multihospital Systems: Issues and Empirical Evidence." *Health Affairs* 3: 50–64.

———. 1986. "Investor-Owned Multihospital Systems: A Synthesis of Research Findings." In *For-Profit Enterprise in Health Care,* edited by Bradford H. Gray, 474–91. Washington, DC: National Academy Press.

Estes, Carroll L., Charlene Harrington, and A. E. Benjamin. 1994. *Uncertified Homecare: Structure and Performance.* San Francisco: Institute for Health and Aging.

Estes, Carroll L., James H. Swan, Linda A. Bergthold, and Pamela H. Spohn. 1992. "Running as Fast as They Can: Organizational Changes in Home Health Care." *Home Health Care Services Quarterly* 13(1–2): 35–69.

Evan, William M. 1966. "The Organization Set: Toward a Theory of Interorganizational Relations." In *Approaches to Organizational Design,* edited by James D. Thompson, 173–88. Pittsburgh: University of Pittsburgh Press.

Evans, R. W., C. R. Blagg, and F. A. Bryan, Jr. 1981. "Implications for Health Care Policy: A Social and Demographic Profile of Hemodialysis Patients in the United States." *Journal of the American Medical Association* 245: 487–91.

Falk, I. S. 1970. "National Health Insurance: A Review of Policies and Proposals." *Law and Contemporary Problems* 35: 669–96.

Faxon, Nathaniel W., ed. 1949. *The Hospital in Contemporary Society.* Cambridge, MA: Harvard University Press.

Federation of Chiropractic Licensing Boards. 1963–98. *Official Directory.* Greeley, Colorado: Federation of Chiropractic Licensing Boards.

Feldstein, Martin. 1971. *The Rising Cost of Hospital Care.* Washington, DC: Information Resources Press for the National Center for Health Services Research and Development.

———. 1983. *Hospital Costs and Health Insurance.* Cambridge, MA: Harvard University Press.

Feldstein, Paul J. 1966. "Research on the Demand for Health Services." *Milbank Memorial Fund Quarterly* 44(3),Part 2: 126–62.

———. 1986. "The Emergence of Market Competition in the U.S. Health Care System: Its Causes, Likely Structure, and Implications." *Health Policy* 6: 1–20.

———. 1988. *Health Care Economics.* New York: Wiley.

Fennell, Mary L. 1980. "The Effect of Environmental Characteristics on Structure of Hospital Clusters." *Administrative Science Quarterly* 25: 485–510.

Fennell, Mary L., and Jeffrey A. Alexander. 1987. "Organizational Boundary Spanning and Institutionalized Environments." *Academy of Management Journal* 30: 456–76.

———. 1993. "Perspectives on Organizational Change in the US Medical Care Sector." *Annual Review of Sociology* 19: 89–112.

Fennell, Mary L., and Kevin T. Leicht. 1998. "The Changing Nature of Professional Work and Professional Organizations: Diversification of Interests and Career Paths in Medicine." Paper presented to the Annual Meetings of the Academy of Management, August, San Diego, California.

Fennell, Mary L., and Richard B. Warnecke. 1988. *Diffusion of Medical Innovations: An Applied Network Analysis.* New York: Plenum.

Field, John W. 1976. *Group Practice Development.* Germantown, MD: Aspen.

Fink, Donald L. 1976. "Holistic Health: Implications for Health Planning." *American Journal of Health Planning* 1(1): 23–31.

Fligstein, Neil. 1985. "The Spread of the Multidivisional Form among Large Firms, 1919–1979." *American Sociological Review* 50: 377–91.

———. 1990. *The Transformation of Corporate Control.* Cambridge, MA: Harvard University Press.

Flood, Ann Barry, and W. Richard Scott. 1987. *Hospital Structure and Performance.* Baltimore, MD: Johns Hopkins Press.

Flood, Ann Barry, Stephen M. Shortell, and W. Richard Scott. 1997. "Organizational Performance: Managing for Efficiency and Effectiveness." In *Essentials of Health Care Management,* edited by Stephen M. Shortell and Arnold D. Kaluzny, 381–429. Albany, NY: Delmar Publishers.

Foley, Henry A., and Stephen S. Sharfstein. 1983. *Madness and Government: Who Cares for the Mentally Ill?* Washington, DC: American Psychiatric Press.

Folland, Sherman. 1983. "Predicting Hospital Market Shares." *Inquiry* 20: 34–44.

Fortney, Mary T. 1980. *Palo Alto Medical Clinic: The First Fifty Years.* Unpublished manuscript.

Foster, Mark S. 1989. *Henry J. Kaiser: Builder in the Modern American West.* Austin, TX: University of Texas Press.

Fox, Renee C. 1977. "The Medicalization and Demedicalization of American Society." In *Doing Better and Feeling Worse: Health in the United States,* edited by John H. Knowles, 9–22. New York: W. W. Norton.

Fox, Wende L. 1989. "Vertical Integration Strategies: More Promising than Diversification." *Health Care Management Review* 14: 19–56.

Frabotta, Judy. 1996. "Proposed UCSF Collaboration Detailed in Town Hall Meetings." *Stanford Report.* April 24, p. 11.

Fredrickson, Donald S. 1977. "Health and the Search for Knowledge." In *Doing Better and Feeling Worse: Health in the United States,* edited by John H. Knowles. 159–70. New York: W. W. Norton.

Freeman, John, and Alessandro Lomi. 1994. "Resource Partitioning and Foundings of Banking Cooperatives in Italy." In *Evolutionary Dynamics of Organizations,* edited by Joel A. C. Baum and Jitendra V. Singh, 255–68. New York: Oxford University Press.

Freidson, Eliot. 1970a. *Profession of Medicine: A Study in the Sociology of Applied Knowledge.* New York: Dodd, Mead.

———. 1970b. *Professional Dominance: The Social Structure of Medical Care.* Chicago: Aldine.

———. 1975. *Doctoring Together: A Study of Professional Social Control.* New York: Elsevier.

———. 1984. "The Changing Nature of Professional Control." *Annual Review of Sociology* 10: 1–20.

———. 1985. "The Reorganization of the Medical Profession." *Medical Care Review* 42: 11–35.

———. 1986. *Professional Powers: A Study of the Institutionalization of Formal Knowledge.* Chicago: University of Chicago Press.

Freidson, Eliot, and Buford Rhea. 1963. "Processes of Control in a Company of Equals." *Social Problems* 11: 119–31.

Friedland, Roger, and Robert R. Alford. 1991. "Bringing Society Back In: Symbols, Practices, and Institutional Contradictions." In *The New Institutionalism in Organizational Analysis,* edited by Walter W. Powell and Paul J. DiMaggio, 232–63. Chicago: University of Chicago Press.

Friedman, Emily. 1996. "A Matter of Value: Profits and Losses in Healthcare." *Health Progress* 77(3): 28–34, 48.

Fuchs, Victor. 1968. "The Growing Demand for Medical Care." *New England Journal of Medicine* 279(4): 190–95.

———. 1974. *Who Shall Live? Health, Economics, and Social Choice.* New York: Basic Books.

———. 1996. "Economics, Values, and Health Care Reform." *American Economic Review,* 86: 1–24.

Furrow, Barry R., Thomas L. Greany, Sandra H. Johnson, Timothy Stolzfus Jost, and Robert L. Schwartz. 1995. *Health Law.* St. Paul, MN: West.

Galbraith, Jay. 1973. *Designing Complex Organizations.* Reading, MA: Addison-Wesley.

Gamm, Larry D. 1992. "Health Care Markets as Interorganizational Fields: A Conceptual Perspective." *Health Services Management Research* 5: 44–53.

Gamm, Larry D., Cathy D. Kassab, S. Diane Brannon, and Mary L. Fennell. 1996. "Linkage Strategies of Rural Hospitals—Independent Hospital, Local Health System, and/or Externally Linked Facility." *Hospital and Health Services Administration* 41: 236–54.

Garceau, Oliver. 1941. *The Political Life of the American Medical Association.* Cambridge, MA: Harvard University Press.

Garnick, Deborah W., Harold S. Luft, James C. Robinson, and Janice Tetreault. 1987. "Appropriate Measures of Hospital Market Areas." *Health Services Research* 22: 69–89.

Gart, A. 1994. *Regulation, Deregulation, Reregulation: The Future of the Banking, Insurance and Securities Industries.* New York: John Wiley & Sons.

Geertz, Clifford. 1973. *The Interpretation of Cultures.* New York: Basic Books.

Georgopoulos, Basil S. 1972. "The Hospital as an Organization and Problem-Solving System." In *Organization Research on Health Institutions,* edited by Basil S. Georgorpoulos, 9–48. Ann Arbor: Institute for Social Research, University of Michigan.

Giddens, Anthony. 1979. *Central Problems in Social Theory: Action, Structure and Contradiction in Social Analysis.* Berkeley: University of California Press.

———. 1984. *The Constitution of Society.* Cambridge: Cambridge University Press.

Gillies, Robin R., Stephen M. Shortell, David A. Anderson, John B. Mitchell, and Karen L. Morgan. 1996. "Conceptualizing and Measuring Integration: Findings from the Health Systems Integration Study." *Hospital and Health Services Administration* 38: 467–89.

Glaser, William A. 1963. "American and Foreign Hospitals: Some Sociological Comparisons." In *The Hospital in Modern Society,* edited by Eliot Freidson, 37–72. New York: Free Press of Glencoe.

Godfrey, Brian John. 1984. *Inner-City Neighborhoods in Transition: The Morphogenesis of San Francisco's Ethnic and Nonconformity Communities.* Unpublished Ph.D. dissertation, University of California, Berkeley.

Goldberg, Carey. 1999. "Teaching Hospitals Battling Cutbacks in Medicare Money." *New York Times,* May 6, pp. A1, A22.

Goodrick, Elizabeth, and Gerald R. Salancik. 1996. "Organizational Discretion in Responding to Institutional Practices: Hospitals and Cesarean Births." *Administrative Science Quarterly* 41: 1–29.

Goodstein, Jerry, Johann Peter Murmann, and Warren Boeker. 1993. "Determinants of Entry into Multihospital Systems: the Important Role of Hospital Boards." Paper Presented at the Annual Meetings of the Academy of Management, Atlanta, Georgia.

Goss, Mary E. W. 1961. "Influence and Authority among Physicians in an Outpatient Clinic." *American Sociological Review* 26: 39–50.

———. 1963. "Patterns of Bureaucracy among Hospital Staff Physicians." In *The Hospital in Contemporary Society,* edited by Eliot Freidson, 170–94. New York: Free Press of Glencoe.

Grant, Peter N. 1988. *The Struggle for Control of California's Health Care Marketplace.* Unpublished Ph.D. dissertation, Harvard University.

Gray, Bradford H., ed. 1986. *For-Profit Enterprise in Health Care.* Washington, DC: National Academy Press.

Greene, William. 1992. *LIMDEP Version 6.0.* Bellport, NY: Econometric Software, Inc.

———. 1997. *Econometric Analysis.* Upper Saddle River, NJ: Prentice-Hall.

Greenhouse, Steven. 1999. "AMA's Delegates Decide to Create Union of Doctors." *New York Times,* June 24, pp. A1, A17.

Greenwood, Royston, and C. R. Hinings. 1988. "Organizational Design Types, Tracks, and the Dynamics of Strategic Change." *Organization Studies* 9: 293–316.

———. 1993. "Understanding Strategic Change: The Contribution of Archetypes." *Academy of Management Journal* 36: 1052–81.

————. 1996. "Understanding Radical Organizational Change: Bringing Together the Old and New Institutionalism." *Academy of Management Review* 21: 1022–54.

Gruber, Lynn R., Maureen Shadle, and Cynthia L. Polich. 1988. "From Movement to Industry: The Growth of HMO's." *Health Affairs* 7(3): 197–208.

Guo, Guang. 1993. "Event-History Analysis for Left-Truncated Data." In *Sociological Methodology 1993*, edited by Peter Marsden, 217–43. Cambridge, MA: Basil Blackwell.

Habermas, Jürgen. 1976. *Legitimation Crisis*. London: Heinemann.

Hafferty, Frederic W., and Donald W. Light. 1995. "Professional Dynamics and the Changing Nature of Medical Work." *Journal of Health and Social Behavior* (Extra Issue): 132–53.

Hafferty, Frederic W., and John B. McKinlay, eds. 1993. *The Changing Medical Profession*. New York: Oxford University Press.

Hall, Oswald. 1946. "The Informal Organization of the Medical Profession." *Canadian Journal of Economics and Political Science* 12(1): 30–41.

Hannan, Michael T., M. Diane Burton and James N. Baron. 1996. "Inertia and Change in the Early Years: Employment Relations in Young, High-Technology Firms." *Industrial and Corporate Change* 5(2): 503–36.

Hannan, Michael T., and Glenn R. Carroll. 1992. *Dynamics of Organizational Populations: Density, Legitimation, and Competition*. New York: Oxford University Press.

————. 1995. "An Introduction to Organizational Ecology." In *Organizations in Industry: Strategy, Structure and Selection*, edited by Glenn R. Carroll and Michael T. Hannan, 17–31. New York: Oxford University Press.

Hannan, Michael T., and John Freeman. 1977. "The Population Ecology of Organizations." *American Journal of Sociology* 82: 929–64.

————. 1984. "Structural Inertia and Organizational Change." *American Sociological Review* 49: 149–64.

————. 1989. *Organizational Ecology*. Cambridge, MA: Harvard University Press.

Hansmann, Henry. 1987. "Economic Theories of Nonprofit Organization." In *The Nonprofit Sector: A Research Handbook*, edited by Walter W. Powell, 27–42. New Haven: Yale University Press.

Harrison, Bennett. 1994. *Lean and Mean: The Changing Landscape of Corporate Power in the Age of Flexibility*. New York: Basic Books.

Haug, Marie R. 1973. "Deprofessionalization: An Alternative Hypothesis for the Future." *Sociological Review Monographs* 20: 195–211.

Haveman, Heather, and Hayagreeva Rao. 1998. "Hybrid Forms and Institutional Change in the Early California Thrift Industry." Paper Presented at the Annual Meetings of the American Sociological Association, San Francisco.

Havighurst, Clark C. 1980. "Antitrust Enforcement in the Medical Services Industry." *Milbank Memorial Fund Quarterly/Health and Society* 58: 89–124.

————. 1986. "The Changing Locus of Decision Making in the Health Care Sector." *Journal of Health Politics, Policy and Law* 11: 697–735.

Havlicek, Penny L., Mary Ann Eiler, and Ondria T. Neblett. 1993. *Medical Groups in the U.S.: A Survey of Practice Characteristics*. Chicago: American Medical Association.

Hawes, Catherine, and Charles D. Phillips. 1986. "The Changing Structure of the Nursing Home Industry and the Impact of Ownership on Quality, Cost, and Access." In

For-Profit Enterprise in Health Care, edited by Bradford H. Gray, 492–541. Washington, DC: National Academy Press.

Hawley, Amos. 1950. *Human Ecology.* New York: Ronald Press.

HCFA (Health Care Financing Administration). 1978–80. *Renal Provider List.* Baltimore, MD: HCFA.

———. 1981–92. *Annual MediCare [Medicare] Program Statistics.* Baltimore, MD: Department of Health and Human Services, Bureau of Data Management and Strategy.

———. 1981–97. *National Listing of Providers Furnishing Kidney Dialysis and Transplant Services.* Baltimore, MD: HCFA.

———. 1987. "National Health Expenditures, 1986–2000." *Health Care Financing Review,* Summer 8(4): 1–36.

———. 1995. *Health Care Financing Review, Medicare and Medicaid Statistical Supplement.* Washington, DC: Office of Research and Demonstrations.

———. 1997. Personal communication with Jan Drexler, Bureau of Data Management and Strategy, July 1.

Heiner, Albert P. 1989. *Henry J. Kaiser, American Empire Builder: An Insider's View.* New York: Peter Lang.

Hendricks, Rickey. 1991. "Medical Practice Embattled: Kaiser Permanente, the American Medical Association, and Henry J. Kaiser on the West Coast, 1945–1955." *Pacific Historical Review* 60: 439–73.

———. 1993. *A Model for National Health Care: the History of Kaiser Permanente.* New Brunswick, NJ: Rutgers University Press.

Herzlinger, Regina E. 1992. *Creating New Health Care Ventures: The Role of Management.* Gaithersburg, MD: Aspen Publications.

———. 1997. *Market-Driven Health Care: Who Wins, Who Loses in the Transformation of America's Largest Service Industry.* Reading, MA: Addison-Wesley.

Heydebrand, Wolf V. 1973. *Hospital Bureaucracy: A Comparative Study of Organizations.* New York: Dunellen Press.

HIAA (Health Insurance Association of America). 1959–98. *Source Book of Health Insurance Data.* Washington, DC: HIAA.

———. 1993. "Historical Insurance Facts." *Source Book of Health Insurance Data.* Washington, DC: HIAA.

Hickson, David J., C. R. Hinings, C. A. Lee, R. E. Schneck, and J. M. Pennings. 1971. "A Strategic Contingencies' Theory of Intraorganizational Power." *Administrative Science Quarterly* 14: 378–97.

HIPC (Health Insurance Plan of California). 1997. Personal communication with Carl Martin, Director of Marketing, June 3, 1997.

Hirsch, Paul M., and Michael Lounsbury. 1997. "Ending the Family Quarrel: Toward a Reconciliation of 'Old' and 'New' Institutionalisms." *American Behavioral Scientist* 40: 406–18.

Hodgson, Geoffrey. 1991. "Institutional Economic Theory: The Old versus the New." In *After Marx and Sraffa: Essays in Political Economy,* edited by Geoffrey Hodgson, 194–213. New York: St. Martin's.

Hoechst Marion Roussel. 1995. *HMO-PPO Digest.* Kansas City, MO: HMR.

Hospital Affiliates International. 1973–78. Annual Reports.

Hospital Corporation of America. 1970–75. Annual Reports.

HRHFSPC (Hospitals and Related Health Facilities and Services Planning Committee).

1968. "Voluntary Regional Planning: Hospitals and Related Health Facilities and Services." Report to the California Legislature and to the State Advisory Hospital Council.

Hulka, Barbara S., and J. R. Wheat. 1985. "Patterns of Utilization." *Medical Care* 23: 438–60.

Hult, Karen M., and Charles Walcott. 1990. *Governing Public Organizations: Politics, Structures, and Institutional Design.* Pacific Grove, CA: Brooks/Cole.

Humana. 1975–78. Annual Reports.

Hunt, Courtney Shelton, and Howard E. Aldrich. 1998. "The Second Ecology: Creation and Evolution of Organizational Communities." In *Research in Organizational Behavior,* vol. 20, edited by Barry Staw, 267–301. Greenwich, CT: JAI Press.

Hunt, G. Halsey. 1947. *Medical Groups in the United States, 1946.* Washington, DC: Federal Security Agency, U.S. Public Health Service.

Hurley, Robert E., and Mary L. Fennell. 1990. "Managed-Care Systems as Governance Structures: A Transaction-cost Approach." In *Innovations in Health Care Delivery: Insights for Organization Theory,* edited by Stephen S. Mick, 241–68. San Francisco: Jossey-Bass.

Iglehart, John K. 1992. "The American Health Care System: Managed Care." *New England Journal of Medicine* 327(10): 742–47.

Interstudy. 1976–94. *National HMO Census.* Washington, DC: Interstudy.

Jaspen, Bruce. 1997. "Empire of the Air?" *Modern Healthcare* 27(46): 14.

Jepperson, Ronald L. 1991. "Institutions, Institutional Effects, and Institutionalism." In *The New Institutionalism in Organizational Analysis,* edited by Walter W. Powell and Paul J. DiMaggio, 143–63. Chicago: University of Chicago Press.

Joskow, Paul J. 1981. *Controlling Hospital Costs: The Role of Government Regulation.* Cambridge, MA: MIT Press.

Kaluzny, Arnold D., and Richard B. Warnecke. 1996. *Managing a Health Care Alliance.* San Francisco: Jossey-Bass.

Kaluzny, Arnold D., Howard S. Zuckerman, and Thomas C. Ricketts III, eds. 1995. *Partners for the Dance: Forming Strategic Alliances in Health Care.* Ann Arbor, MI: Health Administration Press.

Katz, Alfred H., and Donald M. Proctor. 1969. *Social-Psychological Characteristics of Patients Receiving Hemodialysis Treatment for Chronic Renal Failure: Report of a Questionnaire Survey of Dialysis Centers and Patients during 1967.* Rockville, MD: Public Health Service, Kidney Disease Control Program.

Katz, Daniel, and Robert L. Kahn. 1978. *The Social Psychology of Organizations.* New York: Wiley, 2d ed.

Keene, Clifford H. 1971. "Kaiser Industries and the Kaiser-Permanente Health Care Partnership." In *The Kaiser-Permanente Medical Care Program: One Valid Solution to the Problem of Health Care Delivery in the United States,* edited by Anne R. Somers, 13–16. New York: The Commonwealth Fund.

Kertesz, Louise. 1995. "Catholic System Merger Approved." *Modern Healthcare* 27(13): 6.

Kessel, Reuben A. 1970. "The AMA and the Supply of Physicians." *Law and Contemporary Problems* 35: 167–83.

Kim, Jae-On, and Charles Mueller. 1978. *Factor Analysis: Statistical Methods and Practical Issues.* Beverly Hills, CA: Sage.

Kimberly, John R. 1976. "Organizational Size and the Structuralist Perspective: A Review, Critique and Proposal." *Administrative Science Quarterly* 21: 571–97.

———. 1980. "Initiation, Innovation, and Institutionalization in the Creation Process." In *The Organizational Life Cycle*, edited by John R. Kimberly and Robert H. Miles, 18–43. San Francisco: Jossey-Bass.

Kimberly, John R., and Robert H. Miles, eds. 1980. *The Organizational Life Cycle*. San Francisco: Jossey-Bass.

Klarman, Herbert. 1965. *The Economics of Health*. New York: Columbia University Press.

Kletke, Phillip R., David W. Emmons, and Kurt D. Gillis. 1996. "Current Trends in Physicians' Practice Arrangements." *Journal of the American Medical Association* 276(7): 555–60.

Knoke, David. 1986. "Associations and Interest Groups." *Annual Review of Sociology* 12: 1–21.

Knowles, John H. 1977. "The Responsibility of the Individual." In *Doing Better and Feeling Worse: Health in the United States*, edited by John H. Knowles, 57–80. New York: W. W. Norton.

Knox, Richard A. 1979. "Stanford Medical School Suffers Fiscal Ideological Crisis." *Science* 23: 148–52.

Kongstvedt, Peter, ed. 1996. *The Managed Health Care Handbook*. Gaithersburg, MD: Aspen.

Koury, Renee. 1997a. "Hospital Merger gets Key Support." *San Jose Mercury News*. September 18, pp. 1A, 18A.

———. 1997b. "Hospital Merger Approved by UC." *San Jose Mercury News*. September 20, pp. 1B, 6B.

KP (Kaiser Permanente Medical Care Program). 1960–94. *Annual Report*. Oakland, CA: Kaiser Permanente Medical Care Program.

———. 1994b. *How We Measure Up: A Report on our Performance*.

Kramon, Glenn. 1989. "Why Kaiser is Still the King." *New York Times*, July 2, section 3, pp. 1, 9.

Krasner, Stephen D. 1988. "Sovereignty: An Institutional Perspective." *Comparative Political Studies* 21: 66–94.

Krause, Elliot. 1997. *Death of the Guilds: Professions, States, and the Advance of Capitalism, 1930 to the Present*. New Haven, CT: Yale University Press.

Krieger, Lisa M. 1998. "Health Insurance Costs Rising Again." *San Jose Mercury News*, July 5.

———. 1999. "Health Merger Defended." *San Jose Mercury News*, May 21, pp. 1B, 2B.

Kutner, Nancy. 1982. "Cost-Benefit Issues in U.S. National Health Legislation: The Case of the End-Stage Renal Disease Program." *Social Problems* 30: 51–64.

Kuttner, R. 1996. "Columbia/HCA and the Resurgence of the For-Profit Hospital Business." *New England Journal of Medicine* 5: 445–51.

LaMont, B., D. Marlin, and J. Hoffman. 1993. "Porter's Generic Strategies, Discontinuous Environments, and Performance: A Longitudinal Study of Changing Strategies in the Hospital Industry." *Health Services Research* 28: 623–40.

Lapin, Lisa. 1991. "Hospital Goes on Sick List Prescription for Staff Cuts." *San Jose Mercury News*. March 21, pp. 1B, 2B.

Larmac. 1945–94. *Consolidated Index to the Constitution and Laws of California*. San Francisco: Recorder Printing and Publishing Company.

Larson, Magali Sarfatti. 1977. *The Rise of Professionalism: A Sociological Analysis.* Berkeley: University of California Press.

Laumann, Edward O., and David Knoke. 1987. *The Organizational State: Social Choice in National Policy Domains.* Madison, WI: University of Wisconsin Press.

Lawrence, Paul R., and Jay W. Lorsch. 1967. *Organization and Environment: Managing Differentiation and Integration.* Boston: Graduate School of Business Administration, Harvard University.

Leblebici, Husayin, and Gerald R. Salancik. 1982. "Stability in Interorganizational Exchanges: Rulemaking Processes of the Chicago Board of Trade." *Administrative Science Quarterly* 27: 227–42.

Leblebici, Husayin, Gerald R. Salancik, Anne Copay, and Tom King. 1991. "Institutional Change and the Transformation of Interorganizational Fields: An Organizational History of the U.S. Radio Broadcasting Industry." *Administrative Science Quarterly* 36: 333–63.

Lee, Philip R. 1976. "The Frontiers of Health Planning." *American Journal of Health Planning* 1(2): 1–6.

Lee, Sik-Yum, Wai-Yin Poon, and P. M. Bentler. 1994. "Covariance and Correlation Structure Analysis with Continuous and Polytomous Variables." In *Multivariate Analysis and Its Applications,* edited by Theodore W. Anderson, Kai-Tai Fang, and Ingram Olkin, 13: 347–58. Hayward, CA: Institute of Mathematical Statistics.

Levander, Michelle. 1996. "Panel Backs UCSF, Stanford Merger." *San Jose Mercury News.* November 14, pp. 1A, 19A.

———. 1997. "Accountability Sought in Hospitals' Merger." *San Jose Mercury News.* May 21, pp. 1B, 4B.

Levine, Sol, and Paul E. White. 1961. "Exchange as a Conceptual Framework for the Study of Interorganizational Relationships." *Administrative Science Quarterly* 5: 583–601.

Lewis, Bonnie L., and Jeffrey Alexander. 1986. "A Taxonomic Analysis of Multihospital Systems." *Health Services Research* 21: 29–56.

Light, Donald W. 1991. "The Restructuring of American Health Care." In *Health Politics and Policy,* edited by T. J. Litman and L. S. Robins, 53–65. New York: Wiley, 2d ed.

Limbacher, Patricia B. 1997. "Frist: It's Time for a Culture Shock." *Modern Healthcare* 27(31): 2, 12.

Lindblom, Charles E. 1977. *Politics and Markets: The World's Political-Economic Systems.* New York: Basic Books.

Lohr, Kathleen N., ed. 1990. *Medicare: A Strategy for Quality Assurance.* Washington, DC: National Academy Press.

Long, Millard F., and Paul J. Feldstein. 1967. "The Economics of Hospitals Systems: Peak Loads and Regional Coordination." *American Economic Review: Papers and Proceedings of the 79th Annual Meetings of the American Economic Association* 57(2): 119–29.

Longest, Buford B. 1990. "Interorganizational Linkages in the Health Sector." *Health Care Management Review* 15: 17–28.

Lowi, Theodore J. 1969. *The End of Liberalism: Ideology, Policy, and the Crisis of Public Authority.* New York: W. W. Norton.

Luft, Harold S. 1981. *Health Maintenance Organizations: Dimensions of Performance.* New York: Wiley.

Luft, Harold S., D. W. Garnick, D. H. Mark, D. J. Peltzman, C. S. Phibbs, E. Lichtenberg, and S. J. McPhee. 1990. "Does Quality Influence Choice of Hospital?" *Journal of the American Medical Association* 263(21): 2899–906.

Luke, Roice D., and James W. Begun. 1994. "Strategy Making in Health Care Organizations." In *Health Care Management: Organization Design and Behavior,* edited by Stephen M. Shortell and Arnold Kaluzny, 355–91. Albany: Delmar, 3d ed.

Luke, Roice D., James W. Begun, and Dennis D. Pointer. 1989. "Quasi Firms: Strategic Interorganizational Forms in the Health Care Industry." *Academy of Management Review* 14: 9–19.

Luke, Roice D., Yasar A. Ozcan, and James W. Begun. 1990. "Birth Order in Small Multihospital Systems." *Health Services Research* 25: 305–25.

Luke, Roice D., Yasar A. Ozcan, and Peter C. Olden. 1995. "Local Markets and Systems: Hospital Consolidations in Metropolitan Areas." *Health Services Research* 30: 555–75.

Lumsdon, K., and M. Hagland. 1994. "For-Profits: The Right Medicine for Some Markets?" *Hospitals and Health Networks* 12: 34.

Lutz, Sandy. 1995. "NME's New Day Dawns." *Modern Healthcare* 25(10): 68, 70, 72, 74.

———. 1996. "Let's Make a Deal: Health Care Mergers, Acquisitions Take Place at Dizzying Pace." *Modern Healthcare* 24(51): 27.

MacColl, William A. 1966. *Group Practice and Prepayment of Medical Care.* Washington, DC: Public Affairs Press.

Martin, Joseph B., Haile T. Debas, and Bruce Schroffel. 1997. "UCSF Letter Addresses Merger Concerns." *Stanford Report* April 9, 29(24): 12.

March, James G. 1990. "Exploration and Exploitation in Organizational Learning." *Organization Science* 2: 71–87.

March, James G., and Herbert A. Simon. 1958. *Organizations.* New York: John Wiley & Sons.

Marion Merrell Dow. 1993. *Managed Care Digest, PPO Edition 1993.* Kansas City, MO: Marion Merrell Dow.

Marmor, Theodore R. 1970. *The Politics of Medicare.* Chicago: Aldine.

Marmor, Theodore R., Jerry L. Mashaw, and Philip L. Harvey. 1990. *America's Misunderstood Welfare State: Persistent Myths, Enduring Realities.* New York: Basic Books.

Marmor, Theodore R., Mark Schlesinger, and Richard W. Smithey. 1987. "Nonprofit Organizations and Health Care." In *The Nonprofit Sector: A Research Handbook,* edited by Walter W. Powell, 221–39. New Haven, CT: Yale University Press.

Marsteller, Jill A., Randall R. Bovbjerg, Len M. Nichols, and Diana K. Verrilli. 1997. "The Resurgence of Selective Contracting Restrictions." *Journal of Health Politics, Policy and Law* 22(5): 1133–89.

May, Joel J. 1967. *Health Planning: Its Past and Potential.* Center for Health Administration Studies, Health Administration Perspectives, no. A5.

McCready, Linda A., and Billy Harris. 1995. *From Quackery to Quality Assurance: The First Twelve Decades of the Medical Board of California.* Sacramento, CA: Medical Board of California.

McFall, Violet, ed. 1989. *Fairmont Hospital, 125 Years.* Unpublished document.

McKelvey, William. 1982. *Organizational Systematics.* Berkeley: University of California Press.

———. 1994. "Evolution and Organizational Science." In *Evolutionary Dynamics of*

Organizations, edited by Joel A. C. Baum and Jitendra V. Singh, 314–26. Oxford: Oxford University Press.

McKinlay, John B. 1982. "Toward the Proletarianization of Physicians." In *Professionals as Workers: Mental Labor in Advanced Capitalism,* edited by Charles Derber, 37–62. Boston, MA: G. K. Hall.

McMillan, J. 1992. *Games, Strategies and Managers.* New York: Oxford University Press.

Mechanic, David. 1994. "Managed Care: Rhetoric and Realities." *Inquiry,* 31(Summer): 124–28.

Melhado, Evan M. 1988. "Competition versus Regulation in American Health Policy." In *Money, Power and Health Care,* edited by Evan M. Malhado, Walter Feinberg, and Harold M. Swartz, 15–102. Ann Arbor, MI: Health Administration Press.

Meyer, Alan D., Geoffrey R. Brooks, and James B. Goes. 1990 "Environmental Jolts and Industry Revolutions: Organizational Responses to Discontinuous Change." *Strategic Management Journal* 11: 93–110.

Meyer, Alan D., James B. Goes, and Geoffrey R. Brooks. 1993. "Organizations Reacting to Hyperturbulence." In *Organizational Change and Redesign: Ideas and Insights for Improving Performance,* edited by George P. Huber and William H. Glick, 66–111. New York: Oxford University Press.

Meyer, John W. 1977. "The Effects of Education as an Institution." *American Journal of Sociology* 83: 55–77.

———. 1983. "Centralization of Funding and Control in Educational Governance." In *Organizational Environments: Ritual and Rationality,* edited by John W. Meyer and W. Richard Scott, 179–98. Beverly Hills, CA: Sage.

Meyer, John W., John Boli, and George W. Thomas. 1987. "Ontology and Rationalization in the Western Cultural Account." In *Institutional Structure: Constituting State, Society, and the Individual,* edited by George M. Thomas, John W. Meyer, Francisco O. Ramirez, and John Boli, 1–40. Newbury Park: Sage.

Meyer, John W., and Brian Rowan. 1977. "Institutionalized Organizations: Formal Structure as Myth and Ceremony." *American Journal of Sociology* 83: 340–63.

Meyer, John W., and W. Richard Scott. 1983. "Centralization and the Legitimacy Problems of Local Government." In *Organizational Environments: Ritual and Rationality,* edited by John W. Meyer and W. Richard Scott, 199–215. Beverly Hills, CA: Sage.

Meyer, John W., W. Richard Scott, and David Strang. 1987. "Centralization, Fragmentation, and School District Complexity." *Administrative Science Quarterly* 32: 186–201.

MGMA (Medical Group Management Association). 1961–93. *Medical Group Management Association Directory.* Denver, CO: MGMA.

Michaels, Hal. 1981. *Alameda Hospital, 1894–1981.* Alameda, CA: Alameda Hospital.

Mick, Stephen S. 1990a. "Explaining Vertical Integration in Health Care: An Analysis and Synthesis of Transaction-Cost Economics and Strategic-Management Theory." In *Innovations in Health Care Delivery: Insights for Organization Theory,* edited by Stephen S. Mick, 207–40. San Francisco, CA: Jossey-Bass.

———. 1990b. "Themes, Issues and Research Avenues." In *Innovations in Health Care Delivery: Insights for Organization Theory,* edited by Stephen S. Mick, 1–19. San Francisco, CA: Jossey-Bass.

Miles, Robert H. 1982. *Coffin Nails and Corporate Strategies*. Englewood Cliffs, NJ: Prentice-Hall.

Miller, Danny, and P. Friesen. 1980. "Momentum and Revolution in Organization Adaptation." *Academy of Management Journal* 23: 591–614.

Miller, John L., and John D. Cochrane. 1994. "The Palo Alto Medical Foundation." *Integrated Healthcare Report,* October.

Miller, Robert H. 1996. "Health System Integration: A Means to an End." *Health Affairs* 15(2): 92–106.

Miller, Robert H., and Harold S. Luft. 1994. "Managed Care Plans: Characteristics, Growth, and Premium Performance." *Annual Review of Public Health* 15: 437–59.

Millman, Michael, ed. 1993. *Access to Health Care in America*. Washington, DC: National Academy Press.

Milner, Murray, Jr. 1980. *Unequal Care: A Case Study of Interorganizational Relations in Health Care*. New York: Columbia University Press.

Mintzberg, Henry. 1983. *Power In and Around Organizations*. Englewood Cliffs, NJ: Prentice-Hall.

Mitchell, John B. 1996. *Remaking Health Care in America: Building Organized Delivery Systems*. San Francisco: Jossey-Bass.

Moller, Gudrun, Ian Goldie, and Egon Jonsson. 1992. "Hospital Care versus Home Care for Rehabilitation after Hip Replacement." *International Journal of Technology Assessment in Health Care* 8(1): 93–101.

Money, William H., David P. Gilfillan, and Robert Duncan. 1976. "A Comparative Study of Multi-Unit Health Care Organizations." In *Organizational Research in Hospitals,* edited by Stephen M. Shortell and Montague Brown, 29–61. Chicago: Blue Cross Association Inquiry Book.

Monte, Thomas. 1993. *World Medicine: The East-West Guide to Healing Your Body.* New York: Jeremy P. Tarcher/Perigee.

Montgomery, Kathleen. 1990. "A Prospective Look at the Specialty of Medical Management." *Work and Occupations* 17: 178–97.

———. 1992. "Professional Dominance and the Threat of Corporatization." In *Current Research on Occupations and Professions,* edited by Helena Z. Lopata, 7: 221–40. Greenwich, CT: JAI Press.

Montgomery, Sister Alice. 1990. "The Sisters of Mercy: Caring for San Francisco since 1854." *Senior Life News* 22(5).

Moore, J. Stuart. 1993. *Chiropractic in America: The History of a Medical Alternative.* Baltimore: Johns Hopkins University Press.

Moran, Donald W. 1997. "Federal Regulation of Managed Care: An Impulse in Search of a Theory?" *Health Affairs,* 16(6): 7–21.

Morlock, Laura L., and Jeffrey A. Alexander. 1986. "Models of Governance in Multihospital Systems: Implications for Hospital and System-Level Decision-Making." *Medical Care* 24: 1118–35.

Morrisey, Michael A., and Jeffrey A. Alexander. 1987. "Hospital Participation in Multihospital Systems." In *Advances in Health Economics and Health Services Research,* edited by Richard M. Scheffler and Louis F. Rossiter, 7: 59–82. Greenwich, CT: JAI Press.

Morrisey, Michael A., Jeffrey A. Alexander, Lawton R. Burns, and Victoria Johnson. 1996. "Managed Care and Physician/hospital Integration." *Health Affairs* 15(4): 62–73.

Morrison, Ellen M., and Harold S. Luft. 1990. "Health Maintenance Organization Environments in the 1980s and Beyond." *Health Care Financing Review* 12(1): 81–90.

Murray, Charles. 1984. *Losing Ground: American Social Policy, 1950–1980*. New York: Basic Books.

Murray, J., J. Merrill, and J. Harrison. 1955. "Renal Homotransplantation in Identical Twins." *Surgical Forum* 6: 432–35.

Nadler, David A., and Michael L. Tushman. 1995. "Types of Organizational Change: From Incremental Improvement to Discontinuous Transformation" In *Discontinuous Change: Leading Organizational Transformation*, edited by David A. Nadler, Robert B. Shaw, and A. Elise Walton, 15–44. San Francisco: Jossey-Bass.

Nash, Gerald D. 1973. *The American West in the Twentieth Century: A Short History of an Urban Oasis*. Englewood Cliffs, NJ: Prentice-Hall.

———. 1985. *The American West Transformed: The Impact of the Second World War*. Bloomington, IN: Indiana University Press.

National Chiropractic Association. 1952. Data furnished to the President's Commission on the Health Needs of the Nation. In *Building America's Health*. Washington, DC: Government Printing Office, 1953, Vol. 3, p. 207.

National Commission on Excellence in Education. 1983. *A Nation at Risk: The Imperative for Educational Reform*. Washington, DC.

National Governors' Association. 1986. *Time for Results*. Washington, DC: National Governors' Association, Center for Policy Research and Analysis.

National Library of Medicine. 1998. *MEDLINE* [computer periodicals data base]. Bethesda, MD: Department of Health and Human Services.

National Medical Enterprises. 1968–80. Annual Reports.

NCHS (National Center for Health Statistics). 1995. *Health United States, 1994*. Hyattsville, MD: U.S. Public Health Service.

Neuhauser, Duncan. 1971 *The Relationship between Administrative Activities and Hospital Performance*. Chicago: Center for Health Administration Studies.

Newman, Andrew E. 1991. *Institutional, Political and Economic Factors Affecting Rates of Organization Change in California State Government, 1850–1975*. Unpublished Ph.D. dissertation, Department of Sociology, Stanford University.

NIH (National Institutes of Health). 1994. *Alternative Medicine: Expanding Medical Horizons*. NIH Publication No. 94–066. Prepared under the auspices of the Workshop on Alternative Medicine, Chantilly, VA, September 14–16, 1992. Washington, DC: U.S. Office of Alternative Health, Government Printing Office.

Norback, Craig, and Peter Norback, eds. 1977. *The Health Care Directory, 1977–78*. Orndell, NJ: Medical Economics Company.

Norman, George, and Manfredi La Manna. 1992. "Introduction." In *The New Industrial Economics: Recent Developments in Industrial Organization, Oligopoly, and Game Theory*, edited by George Norman and Manfredi La Manna, 1–11. Worcester, UK: Edward Elgar.

North, Douglass C. 1990. *Institutions, Institutional Change, and Economic Performance*. Cambridge: Cambridge University Press.

O'Connor, Carol A. 1994. "A Region of Cities." In *The Oxford History of the American West*, edited by Clyde A. Milner II, Carol A. O'Connor, and Martha A. Sandweiss, 535–63. New York: Oxford University Press.

O'Connor, James. 1973. *The Fiscal Crisis of the State*. New York: St. Martin's.

Offe, Claus. 1984. *Contradictions of the Welfare State*. Cambridge, MA: MIT Press.

Oliver, Christine. 1991. "Strategic Responses to Institutional Processes." *Academy of Management Review,* 16: 145–79.

Orru, Marco, Nicole Woolsey Biggart, and Gary G. Hamilton. 1991. "Organizational Isomorphism in East Asia." In *The New Institutionalism in Organizational Analysis,* edited by Walter W. Powell and Paul J. DiMaggio, 361–89. Chicago: University of Chicago Press.

Orton, J. Douglas, and Karl E. Weick. 1990. "Loosely Coupled Systems: A Reconceptualization." *Academy of Management Review* 15: 203–23.

Osborne, David, and Ted Gaebler. 1992. *Reinventing Government: How the Entrepreneurial Spirit is Transforming the Public Sector.* Reading, MA: Addison-Wesley.

OSHPD (California Office of Statewide Health Planning and Development). 1976–92. *Annual Hospital Disclosure Report.* Sacramento, CA: OSHPD.

———. 1978–92. *Home Health Agency Annual Report.* Sacramento, CA: OSHPD.

———. 1994. *Annual Utilization Report of Home Health Agencies: Licensed Services and Utilization Profiles.* Sacramento, CA: OSHPD.

OTA (Office of Technology Assessment). 1990. *Health Care in Rural America.* Washington, DC: Government Printing Office.

Palo Alto–Stanford Hospital Center. 1967. Annual Report.

Parsons, Talcott. 1960. "A Sociological Approach to the Theory of Organizations." In *Structure and Process in Modern Societies,* 16–58. Glencoe, IL: Free Press.

———. 1966. *Societies: Evolutionary and Comparative Perspectives.* Englewood Cliffs, NJ: Prentice-Hall.

———. 1990. "Prolegomena to a Theory of Social Institutions." *American Sociological Review* 55: 319–39. (Original essay written in 1934).

Pauly, Mark. 1974. "The Behavior of Non-Profit Hospital Monopolies: Alternative Models of the Hospital." In *Regulating Health Facilities Construction,* edited by Clark Havighurst, 143–61. Washington, DC: American Enterprise Institute.

Payton, Sallyanne, and Rhoda M. Powsner. 1980. "Regulation through the Looking Glass: Hospitals, Blue Cross, and Certificate-of-Need." *Michigan Law Review* 79: 201–77.

PBGH (Pacific Business Group on Health). 1995. *Pacific Currents* 1(1 2).

———. 1997. Personal Communication with Emma Hoo, June 17.

Perrow, Charles. 1963. "Goals and Power Structures—A Historical Case Study." In *The Hospital in Modern Society,* edited by Eliot Freidson, 112–46. New York: Free Press of Glencoe.

———. 1986. *Complex Organizations: A Critical Essay.* New York: Random House.

———. 1991. "A Society of Organizations." *Theory and Society* 20: 725–62.

Pfeffer, Jeffrey. 1973. "Size, Composition and Function of Hospital Boards of Directors: A Study of Organization-Environment Linkage." *Administrative Science Quarterly* 18: 349–64.

———. 1982. *Organizations and Organization Theory.* Boston: Pitman.

———. 1997. *New Directions for Organization Theory: Problems and Prospects.* New York: Oxford University Press.

Pfeffer, Jeffrey, and Gerald R. Salancik. 1978. *The External Control of Organizations.* New York: Harper & Row.

PHS (U.S. Public Health Service). 1954. *Health Manpower Source Book: County Data from 1950 Census and Area Analysis.* Prepared by Maryland Y. Pennell and Marion E.

Altenderfer. PHS Publication No. 263, Section 4. Washington, DC: Department of Health, Education, and Welfare, Division of Public Health Methods.

————. 1960. *Health Manpower Source Book: Physicians' Age, Type of Practice, and Location.* Prepared by William H. Stewart and Maryland Y. Pennell. PHS Publication No. 263, Section 10. Washington, DC: Department of Health, Education, and Welfare, Division of Public Health Methods.

————. 1962. *Health Manpower Source Book: Medical Specialists.* Prepared by Paul Q. Peterson and Maryland Y. Pennell. PHS Publication No. 263, Section 14. Washington, DC: Department of Health, Education, and Welfare, Division of Public Health Methods.

————. 1963a. *Medical Groups in the United States, 1959: Results of Questionnaire Survey, Including Comparison with Findings of 1946 Study.* Washington, DC: Department of Health, Education, and Welfare.

————. 1963b. *Health Manpower Source Book: Industry and Occupation Data from the 1960 Census, by State.* Prepared by Richard A. Prindle and Maryland Y. Pennell. PHS Publication No. 263, Section 17. Washington, DC: Department of Health, Education, and Welfare, Division of Public Health Methods.

————. 1968. *Health Resources Statistics, 1968.* Office of Health Research, Statistics, and Technology, with the National Center for Health statistics. Hyattsville, MD: Government Printing Office.

————. 1981. *Directory of Community Health Care Coalitions.* Hyattsville, MD: Department of Health and Human Services.

Piore, Michael J., and Charles F. Sabel. 1984. *The Second Industrial Divide: Possibilities for Prosperity.* New York: Basic Books.

Podolny, Joel. 1993. "A Status-Based Model of Market Competition." *American Journal of Sociology* 98: 829–72.

Pomrinse, S. David, and Marcus S. Goldstein. 1960. *A Preliminary Directory of Medical Groups in the United States, 1959.* Washington, DC: U.S. Department of Health, Education, and Welfare, Public Health Service.

Porter, Michael. 1980. *Competitive Strategy: Techniques for Analyzing Industries and Competitors.* New York: Free Press.

Powell, Walter W. 1990. "Neither Market nor Hierarchy: Network Forms of Organizations." In *Research in Organizational Behavior,* edited by Barry M. Staw and Larry L. Cummings, 12: 295–336. Greenwich, CT: JAI Press.

————. 1991. "Expanding the Scope of Institutional Analysis." In *The New Institutionalism in Organizational Analysis,* edited by Walter W. Powell and Paul J. DiMaggio, 183–203. Chicago: University of Chicago Press.

Powell, Walter W., and Jason Owen-Smith. 1998. "Commercialism in Universities: Life Sciences Research and Its Linkage with Industry." *Journal of Policy Analysis and Management* 17: 253–77.

Pryor, David B., Robert M Califf, Frank E. Harrell, Jr., Mark A. Hlatky, Kerry L. Lee, Daniel B. Mark, and Robert A Rosati. 1985. "Clinical Data Bases: Accomplishments and Unrealized Potential." *Medical Care* 23: 623–47.

Puzzanghera, Jim. 1995a. "Hospital Swinging Budget Ax." *San Jose Mercury News* (Peninsula edition). May 2, pp. 1B, 2B.

————. 1995b. "Hospitals Changing to Survive." *San Jose Mercury News.* October 10, p. 1B.

————. 1997a. "Columbia Sets Sail for Lofty Profit Goals." *San Jose Mercury News.* June 22, pp. 1A, 24A.

————. 1997b. "Columbia/HCA Chief Executive is Forced Out." *San Jose Mercury News.* July 26, pp. 1C, 2C.

————. 1997c. "Cuts Crimp Care at Columbia Hospitals." *San Jose Mercury News.* September 22, pp. 1A, 12A.

Quadagno, Jill. 1987. "Theories of the Welfare State." *Annual Review of Sociology* 13: 109–28.

Rainey, Hal G., Robert W. Backoff, and Charles H. Levine. 1976. "Comparing Public and Private Organizations." *Public Administration Review* 36: 233–44.

Ramada Inns, Inc. 1965–70. Annual Reports.

Readers' Guide to Periodical Literature. 1945–94. New York: H. W. Wilson.

Rettig, Richard, and Norman Levinsky, eds. 1991. *Kidney Failure and the Federal Government.* Washington, DC: National Academy Press.

Ricketts, Thomas C., Thomas R. Konrad, Jane S. Stein, and Gordon H. DeFriese. 1987. "Population Ecology and Health Policy Analysis: The Case of Rural Primary Care Centers." *Medical Care Review* 44: 345–73.

Robert Wood Johnson Foundation. 1994. *Trends in National Health Expenditures* [Pamphlet]. Princeton, New Jersey.

Robinson, James C. 1995. "Health Care Purchasing and Market Changes in California." *Health Affairs* 14(4): 117–30.

————. 1998. "Consolidation of Medical Groups into Physician Practice Management Organizations." *Journal of the American Medical Association.* 279(2): 144–49.

Robinson, James C., and Lawrence P. Casalino. 1995. "The Growth of Medical Groups Paid through Capitation in California." *The New England Journal of Medicine* 333: 1684–87.

————. 1996. "Vertical Integration and Organizational Networks in Health Care." *Health Affairs* 15(1): 7–22.

Roemer, Milton I. 1961. "Bed Supply and Hospital Utilization: A Natural Experiment." *Hospitals* 35 (November): 36–42.

Roemer, Milton I., and J. W. Friedman. 1971. *Doctors in Hospitals: Medical Staff Organization and Hospital Performance.* Baltimore: Johns Hopkins University Press.

Rogers, Barbara, and Stephen Dobbs. 1987. *The First Century: Mount Zion Hospital and Medical Center, 1887–1987.* San Francisco: Mt. Zion Hospital.

Rohwer, Götz. 1994. *Transition Data Analysis* (TDA) *5.7.* Working Papers. Institut für Empirische und Angewandte Soziologie, University of Bremen, Germany.

Romanelli, Elaine. 1991. "The Evolution of New Organizational Forms." *Annual Review of Sociology* 17: 79–103.

Rosen, George. 1963. "The Hospital: Historical Sociology of a Community Institution." In *The Hospital in Modern Society,* edited by Eliot Freidson, 1–36. New York: Free Press of Glencoe.

Ross Medical Corporation of San Rafael. 1969–70. Annual Report.

Rossiter, Louis F., and Gail R. Wilensky. 1983. "A Reexamination of the Use of Physician Services: The Role of Physician-Initiated Demand." *Inquiry* 20(2): 162–72.

Ruef, Martin. 1997. "Assessing Organizational Fitness on a Dynamic Landscape: An

Empirical Test of the Relative Inertia Thesis." *Strategic Management Journal* 18(11): 837–53.

Ruef, Martin, Peter Mendel, and W. Richard Scott. 1998. "An Organizational Field Approach to Resource Environments in Health Care: Comparing Entries of Hospitals and Home Health Agencies in the San Francisco Bay Region." *Health Services Research* 32: 775–803.

Ruef, Martin, and W. Richard Scott. 1998. "A Multidimensional Model of Organizational Legitimacy: Hospital Survival in Changing Institutional Environments." *Administrative Science Quarterly* 43: 877–904.

Ruggie, Mary. 1996. *Realignments in the Welfare State: Health Policy in the United States, Britain, and Canada.* New York: Columbia University Press.

Ruggles, Steven and Matthew Sobek. 1997. Integrated Public Use Microdata Series: Version 2.0 [on-line data base]. Minneapolis, MN: Historical Census Projects, University of Minnesota. URL: <http://www.ipums.umn.edu>.

Russell, Sabin. 1995. "Alternative Medicine Thrives in Bay Area." *San Francisco Chronicle,* May 17: A1, A12.

Ruzek, Sheryl Burt. 1978. *The Women's Health Movement: Feminist Alternatives to Medical Control.* New York: Praeger.

Ryder, Claire, Pauline Stitt, and William Elkin. 1969. "Home Health Services—Past, Present, and Future." *American Journal of Public Health* 59: 1720–29.

Ryle, Gilbert. 1971. *Collected Papers,* vol. 2. New York: Barnes and Noble.

Salkever, Davis S., and Thomas W. Bice. 1976. "The Impact of Certificate-of-Need Controls on Hospital Investment." *Milbank Memorial Fund Quarterly* 54: 185–214.

Salvatore, Tony. 1985. "Organizational Adaptation in the VNA: Paradigm Change in the Voluntary Sector." *Home Health Care Services Quarterly* 6: 19–31.

San Francisco Chamber of Commerce. 1952. *San Francisco and the Bay Area.* San Francisco: Chamber of Commerce Research Department.

Santa Rosa Memorial Hospital. 1990. *The Press Democrat,* April 8.

Savas, E. S. 1982. *Privatizing the Public Sector: How to Shrink Government.* Chatham, NJ: Chatham House.

Saward, Ernest W. 1977. "Institutional Organization, Incentives, and Change." In *Doing Better and Feeling Worse: Health in the United States,* edited by John H. Knowles, 193–202. New York: W. W. Norton.

Scalzi, Cynthia, Jacqueline S. Zinn, Michael J. Guilfoyle, and Sondra T. Perdue. 1994a. "Medicare-Certified Home Health Services: National and Regional Supply in the 1980's" *American Journal of Public Health* 84: 1646–48.

———. 1994b. "Growth and Decline in the Supply of Medicare-Covered Home Health Services in the 80's: National and Regional Experience." *Home Health Care Services Quarterly* 15(1): 3–17.

Schlesinger, Mark. 1998. "Mismeasuring the Consequences of Ownership: External Influences and the Comparative Performance of Public, For-Profit, and Private Nonprofit Organizations." In *Private Action and the Public Good,* edited by Walter W. Powell and Elisabeth S. Clemens, 85–113. New Haven, CT: Yale University Press.

Schmalensee, Richard. 1989. "Inter-Industry Studies of Structure and Performance." In *Handbook of Industrial Organizations,* v. 2, edited by Richard Schmalensee and Robert D. Willig, 951–1009. New York: North-Holland.

Schmidt, Laura. 1998. "How 'Things Fall Apart': An Institutional Approach to the

U.S. Health Care Crisis." Paper Presented at the Annual Meetings of the American Sociological Association, San Francisco.

Schmidt, R., M. Blumenkrantz, and T. Wiegmann. 1983. "The Dilemmas of Patient Treatment for End-Stage Renal Disease." *American Journal of Kidney Diseases* 3: 37–57.

Schmitter, Philippe. 1990. "Sectors in Modern Capitalism: Models of Governance and Variations in Performance." In *Labour Relations and Economic Performance,* edited by Renato Brunetta and Carol Dell-Aringa, 3–39. Houndmills, UK: Macmillan.

Schultze, Charles L. 1969. "The Role of Incentives, Penalties, and Rewards in Attaining Effective Policy." In *The Analysis and Evaluation of Public Expenditures: The PBB System, A Compendium of Papers."* U. S. Congress, I, 201–25, Joint Economic Committee, Subcommittee on Economy in Government, 91st Congress.

———. 1977. *The Public Use of Private Interest.* Washington, DC: Brookings Institution.

Schumpeter, Joseph. 1947. *Capitalism, Socialism, and Democracy.* New York: Harper & Row, 2d ed.

Scott, Lisa. 1997. "A Study in Regional Delivery: Big Catholic Player CHW tries to Balance System, Local Needs." *Modern Healthcare* 27(17): 30.

Scott, W. Richard. 1981. *Organizations: Rational, Natural and Open Systems.* Englewood Cliffs, NJ: Prentice-Hall, 1st ed.

———. 1982a. "Health Care Organizations in the 1980s: The Convergence of Public and Professional Control Systems." In *Contemporary Health Services: A Social Science Perspective,* edited by Allen W. Johnson, Oscar Grusky, and Bertram H. Raven, 177–95. Boston: Auburn House.

———. 1982b. "Managing Professional Work: Three Models of Control for Health Organizations." *Health Services Research* 17 (Fall): 213–40.

———. 1985. "Conflicting Levels of Rationality: Regulators, Managers and Professionals in the Medical Care Sector." *Journal of Health Administration Education* 3 (part 2): 113–31.

———. 1993. "The Organization of Medical Care Services: Toward an Integrated Theoretical Model." *Medical Care Review* 50: 271–303.

———. 1994. "Conceptualizing Organizational Fields: Linking Organizations and Societal Systems." In *Systemrationalitat und Partialinteresse,* edited by Hans-Ulrich Derlien, Uta Gerhardt, and Fritz W. Scharpf, 203–21. Baden Baden, Germany: Nomos Verlagsgesellschaft.

———. 1995. *Institutions and Organizations.* Thousand Oaks, CA: Sage.

———. 1998. *Organizations: Rational, Natural and Open Systems.* Upper Saddle River, NJ: Prentice-Hall, 4th ed.

Scott, W. Richard, and Søren Christensen. 1995. "Crafting a Wider Lens." In *The Institutional Construction of Organizations: International and Longitudinal Studies,* edited by W. Richard Scott and Søren Christensen, 302–13. Thousand Oaks, CA: Sage.

Scott, W. Richard, and John C. Lammers. 1985. "Trends in Occupations and Organizations in the Medical Care and Mental Health Sectors." *Medical Care Review* 42: 37–76.

Scott, W. Richard, Peter Mendel, and Seth Pollack. 2000. "Environments and Fields: Studying the Evolution of a Field of Medical Care Organizations." In *Bending the Bars of the Iron Cage: Institutional Dynamics and Processes,* edited by Walter W. Powell and Daniel L. Jones. Chicago: University of Chicago Press.

Scott, W. Richard, and John W. Meyer. 1983. "The Organization of Societal Sectors." In *Organizational Environments: Ritual and Rationality*, edited by John W. Meyer and W. Richard Scott, 129–53. Beverly Hills, CA: Sage.

———. 1991. "The Organization of Societal Sectors: Propositions and Early Evidence." In *The New Institutionalism in Organizational Analysis*, edited by Walter W. Powell and Paul J. DiMaggio, 108–40. Chicago: University of Chicago Press.

Searle, John R. 1969. *Speech Acts: An Essay in the Philosophy of Language*. New York: Cambridge University Press.

———. 1995. *The Construction of Social Reality*. New York: Free Press.

Selznick, Philip. 1949. *TVA and the Grass Roots*. Berkeley: University of California Press.

———. 1957. *Leadership in Administration: A Sociological Interpretation*. New York: Harper & Row.

Sewell, William. 1992. "A Theory of Structure: Duality, Agency, and Transformation." *American Journal of Sociology* 98: 1–29.

Shannon, Claude, and Warren Weaver. 1963. *The Mathematical Theory of Communication*. Urbana: University of Illinois Press (originally published in 1949).

Schiller, Zachary. 1995. "Balance Sheets That Get Well Soon." *Business Week,* September 4, pp. 80–81, 84.

Shortell, Stephen M. 1988. "The Evolution of Hospital Systems: Unfulfilled Promises and Self-fulfilling Prophecies." *Medical Care Review* 45: 177–214.

Shortell, Stephen M., Robin R. Gillies, and David A. Anderson. 1994. "The New World of Managed Care: Creating Organized Delivery Systems." *Health Affairs* 13: 46–64.

Shortell, Stephen M., Robin R. Gillies, David A. Anderson, Karen Morgan Erickson, and John B. Mitchell. 1996. *Remaking Health Care in America: Building Organized Delivery Systems*. San Francisco: Jossey-Bass.

Shortell, Stephen M., Ellen M. Morrison, and Bernard S. Friedman. 1990. *Strategic Choices for America's Hospitals*. San Francisco: Jossey-Bass.

Shortell, Stephen M., Ellen M. Morrison, Susan L. Hughes, Bernard S. Freidman, and Joan L. Vitek. 1987. "Diversification of Health Care Services: The Effects of Ownership, Environment, and Strategy." In *Advances in Health Economics and Health Services Research,* edited by Richard M. Scheffler and Louis F. Rossiter, 7: 3–40. Greenwich, CT: JAI Press.

Shortell, Stephen M., Ellen M. Morrison, and S. Robbins. 1985. "Strategy Making in Health Care Organizations: A Framework and Agenda for Research." *Medical Care Review* 42: 219–66.

Shortell, Stephen M., and Edward Zajac. 1990. "Health Care Organizations and the Development of the Strategic Management Perspective." In *Innovations in Health Care Delivery: Insights for Organization Theory,* edited by Stephen S. Mick, 144–80. San Francisco: Jossey-Bass.

Shriners. 1998. Internet site. URL: <www.shrinershq.org>.

Singh, Jitendra V., and Charles J. Lumsden. 1990. "Theory and Research in Organizational Ecology." *Annual Review of Sociology* 16: 161–95.

Singh, Jitendra V., David J. Tucker, and Robert J. House. 1986. "Organizational Legitimacy and the Liability of Newness." *Administrative Science Quarterly* 31: 171–93.

Skocpol, Theda. 1996. *Boomerang: Clinton's Health Security Effort and the Turn against Government in U.S. Politics*. New York: W. W. Norton.

Skocpol, Theda, and Edwin Amenta. 1986. "States and Social Policies." *Annual Review of Sociology* 12: 131–57.

Sloan, Frank A. 1988. "Property Rights in the Hospital Industry." In *Health Care in America,* edited by H. E. Frech, 103–41. San Francisco: Pacific Research Institute for Public Policy.

Sloan, Frank A., and A. B. Steinwald. 1980. *Insurance, Regulation, and Hospital Costs.* Lexington, MA: D. C. Heath, Lexington Books.

Smillie, John G. 1991. *Can Physicians Manage the Quality and Costs of Health Care?: The Story of the Permanente Medical Group.* New York: McGraw-Hill.

Smith, Harvey. 1955. "Two Lines of Authority: The Hospital's Dilemma." *Modern Hospital* 84: 59–64.

Smoller, Marvin. 1996. Interview conducted by Carol A. Caronna, Oakland, California, April 10.

Snow, Charlotte. 1997. "Renal-Care Biggies Plan Merger." *Modern Healthcare* 27(47): 20.

Somers, Anne R. 1969. *Hospital Regulation: The Dilemma of Public Policy.* Princeton, NJ: Industrial Relations Section, Princeton University.

————. 1971a. *Health Care in Transition: Directions for the Future.* Chicago: Health Research and Educational Trust.

————, ed. 1971b. *The Kaiser-Permanente Medical Care Program: One Valid Solution to the Problem of Health Care Delivery in the United States.* New York: The Commonwealth Fund.

Somers, Herman M., and Anne R. Somers. 1961. *Doctors, Patients, and Health Insurance.* Washington, DC: Brookings Institution.

————. 1967. *Medicare and the Hospitals: Issues and Prospects.* Washington, DC: Brookings Institution.

Spohn, Pamela H., Linda Bergthold, and Carroll L. Estes. 1988. "From Cottages to Condos: The Expansion of the Home Health Care Industry Under Medicare." *Home Health Care Services Quarterly* 8: 25–55.

SSA (U.S. Social Security Administration). 1966–72. *MediCare [Medicare]: Health Insurance for the Aged, Reimbursement by State and County.* Washington, DC: Department of Health, Education and Welfare, Office of Research and Statistics.

————. 1967–68. *Directory of Medicare Providers of Services: Home Health Agencies.* Washington, DC: SSA.

————. 1969–76. *Directory, Medicare Providers and Suppliers of Services; Hospitals, Extended Care Facilities, Home Health Agencies, Outpatient Physical Therapy, Independent Laboratories.* Washington, DC: SSA.

St. Helena Hospital History. 1998. Unpublished document.

Standard and Poor. 1996. *Compustat Industrial Commercial File* [Computer File]. Englewood, CO: Standard and Poor's Compustat Services.

Stanford University School of Medicine. 1940–95. *Stanford University Bulletin, School of Medicine Announcements.* Stanford, CA: Stanford University.

Starkweather, David B. 1981. *Hospital Mergers in the Making.* Ann Arbor, MI: Health Administration Press.

————. 1990. "Competition, Integration, and Diversification: Seven Hospitals of Growthville, U.S.A." *Journal of Health Administration Education* 8(4): 519–70.

Starkweather, David B., and James M. Carman. 1987. "Horizontal and Vertical

Concentrations in the Evolution of Hospital Competition." In *Advances in Health Economics and Health Services Research,* 7: 179–94. Greenwich, CT: JAI.

Starr, Paul. 1982. *The Social Transformation of American Medicine.* New York: Basic Books.

Stern, Robert N. 1979. "The Development of an Interorganizational Control Network: The Case of Intercollegiate Athletics." *Administrative Science Quarterly* 24: 242–66.

Stevens, Edward B. 1976. *The History of the Medical Group Management Association 1926–1976.* Denver, Colorado: Medical Group Management Association.

Stevens, Robert, and Rosemary Stevens. 1974. *Welfare Medicine in America: A Case Study of Medicaid.* New York: Free Press.

Stevens, Rosemary. 1971. *American Medicine and the Public Interest.* New Haven, CT: Yale University Press.

———. 1989. *In Sickness and in Wealth: American Hospitals in the Twentieth Century.* New York: Basic Books.

Stigler, George. 1958. "The Economies of Scale." *Journal of Law and Economics* 1: 54–71.

Stinchcombe, Arthur L. 1965. "Social Structure and Organizations." In *Handbook of Organizations,* edited by James G. March, 142–93. Chicago: Rand McNally.

———. 1968. *Constructing Social Theories.* Chicago: University of Chicago Press.

———. 1997. "On the Virtues of the Old Institutionalism." *Annual Review of Sociology* 23: 1–18.

Strang, David. 1990. "From Dependency to Sovereignty: An Event-History Analysis of Decolonization 1870–1987." *American Sociological Review* 55: 846–60.

———. 1995. "Health Maintenance Organization." In *Organizations in Industry: Strategy, Structure and Selection,* edited by Glenn R. Carroll and Michael T. Hannan, 163–82. New York: Oxford University Press.

Streeck, Wolfgang, and Philippe C. Schmitter. 1985. "Community, Market, State—and Associations? The Prospective Contribution of Interest Governance to Social Order." In *Private Interest Government: Beyond Market and State,* edited by Wolfgang Streeck and Philippe C. Schmitter, 1–29. Beverly Hills, CA: Sage.

Strickland, Stephen. 1972. *Politics, Science and Dread Disease: A Short History of United States Medical Research Policy.* Cambridge, MA: Harvard University Press.

Suchman, Mark. 1995. "Localism and Globalism in Institutional Analysis: The Emergence of Contractual Norms in Venture Finance." In *The Institutional Construction of Organizations: International and Longitudinal Studies,* edited by W. Richard Scott and Søren Christensen, 39–63. Thousand Oaks, CA: Sage.

———. 1995b. "Managing Legitimacy: Strategic and Institutional Approaches." *Academy of Management Review* 20: 571–610.

———. 2000. "Constructed Ecologies: Reproduction and Structuration in Emerging Organizational Communities." In *Bending the Bars of the Iron Cage: Institutional Dynamics and Processes,* edited by Walter W. Powell and Daniel L. Jones. Chicago: University of Chicago Press.

Sutton, John. 1991. *Sunk Costs and Market Structure: Price Competition, Advertising, and the Evolution of Concentration.* Cambridge, MA: MIT Press.

Sylvester, David A. 1995. "Sequoia Hospital Seeking Partner." *San Francisco Chronicle,* October 12. p. A21.

Takagi, Junko. 1996. *Physicians in Transition: A Symbolic Framework Approach to Physician*

Autonomy and Satisfaction in Different Work Settings. Unpublished Ph.D. dissertation, Department of Sociology, Stanford University.

Thelen, Kathleen, and Sven Steinmo. 1992. "Historical Institutionalism in Comparative Politics." In *Structuring Politics: Historical Institutionalism in Comparative Analysis,* edited by Sven Steinmo, Kathleen Thelen, and Frank Longstregh, 1–32. Cambridge: Cambridge University Press.

Thomas, Lewis. 1977. "On the Science and Technology of Medicine." In *Doing Better and Feeling Worse: Health in the United States,* edited by John H. Knowles, 35–46. New York: W. W. Norton.

Thompson, Frank J. 1981. *Health Policy and the Bureaucracy.* Cambridge, MA: MIT Press.

Thompson, James D. 1967. *Organizations in Action.* New York: McGraw Hill.

Thornton, Patricia H. 1995. "Accounting for Acquisition Waves: Evidence from the U.S. College Publishing Industry." In *The Institutional Construction of Organizations,* edited by W. Richard Scott and Søren Christensen, 199–225. Thousand Oaks, CA: Sage.

Thornton, Patricia H., and Nancy Brandon Tuma. 1995. "The Problem of Boundaries in Contemporary Research on Organizations." Paper Presented at the Annual Meetings of the Academy of Management, Vancouver, Canada.

Thorpe, Kenneth E. 1997. "The Health System in Transition: Care, Cost, and Coverage." *Journal of Health Politics, Policy and Law* 22(2): 339–61.

Timmreck, Thomas, ed. 1982. *Dictionary of Health Services Management.* Owings Mills, MD: National Health Publishing.

Tom, Franklin. 1984. "Current Developments in Health Care Regulation under the Knox-Keene Act." *Whittier Law Review* 6: 625–31.

Topham, Edward. 1950. *St. Mary's Hospital and the Sisters of Mercy, 1903–1949.* San Francisco: Privately printed.

Topping, S., and S. Hernandez. 1991. "Health Care Strategy Research, 1985–1990: A Critical Review." *Medical Care Review* 48: 47–89.

Traugott, Elisabeth. 1996. "Medical Marriage: The Stanford/UCSF Merger Raises Questions about 'Academic Medicine.'" *Stanford Daily.* July 25.

Trauner, Joan B. 1983. *Preferred Provider Organizations: The California Experiment.* San Francisco: Institute for Health Policy Studies, University of California, San Francisco.

Tuma, Nancy B., and Michael T. Hannan. 1984. *Social Dynamics: Models and Methods.* New York: Academic Press.

Tushman, Michael L., and Elaine Romanelli. 1985. "Organizational Evolution: A Metamorphosis Model of Convergence and Reorientation." In *Research in Organizational Behavior,* edited by L. L. Cummings and Barry M. Staw, 7: 171–222. Greenwich, CT: JAI Press.

U.S. Bureau of Health Professions. 1990, 1995. *Area Resource File* [User Documentation and Computer Tapes]. Washington DC: Department of Health and Human Services.

U.S. Bureau of the Census. 1945a–96a. *Statistical Abstract of the United States.* Washington, DC: U.S. Department of Commerce, Economics, and Statistics Administration.

———. 1975b. *Historical Statistics of the United States, Colonial Times to 1970.* Washington, DC: U.S. Department of Commerce and Government Printing Office.

———. 1940c–1990c. *Census of the Population of the United States.* Washington, DC: Department of Commerce.

———. 1942d–1992d. *Census of Governments.* Volume 4: *Government Finances.* Washington, DC: Department of Commerce.

———. 1947e–1992e. *City and County Data Book*. Washington, DC: Department of Commerce.

———. 1995f. "Health Insurance Coverage Status by State—Number and Percent of Persons by Type of Coverage: 1987 to 1994." Report compiled from unpublished Current Population Survey data. Washington, DC: U.S. Department of Commerce, Income Statistics Branch/HHES Division.

U.S. Chamber of Commerce. 1984, 1985. *Directory of Business Coalitions for Health Action*. Washington, DC: Clearinghouse on Business Coalitions for Health Action.

U.S. Office of Management and Budget. 1997a. "Total Outlays for Grants to State and Local Governments by Function, Agency, and Program: 1940–2003." Table 12.3 from *The Budget For Fiscal Year 1999, Historical Tables*. [on-line report] Washington, DC: OMB.

———. 1997b. "Real Gross Domestic Product." Table 2A from *Summary National Income and Product Series, 1929–96*. [on-line report] Washington, DC: OMB.

U.S. Office of the Federal Register. 1950–95. *United States Government Manual*. Washington, DC: Government Printing Office.

U.S. Patent and Trademark Office. 1998a. *Cassis Patents BIB: Selected Bibliographic Information from U.S. Patents Issued 1969 to Present*. [CD-ROM data base] Washington, DC.

———. 1962–64. *Annual Report of the Commissioner of Patents*. Washington, DC: Department of Commerce.

———. 1977. *Technology Assessment & Forecast, Seventh Report, March 1977*. Washington, DC: Department of Commerce.

———. 1998b. *Cassis Patents CLASS: Current Classifications of U.S. Patents Issued 1790 to Present*. [CD-ROM data base] Washington, DC.

U.S. Senate Committee on Finance. 1974. *Background Materials Relating to Professional Standards Review Organizations (PSROs)*, May 8, 1974, Russell B. Long, Chairman. Washington, DC: Government Printing Office.

U.S. Superintendent of Documents. 1946–94. *United States Code, General Index*. Washington, DC: Government Printing Office.

UCSF (University of California, San Francisco). 1994. *Annual Report 1993–94*.

UCSF School of Medicine. 1940–94. *UCSF Medical School Courses of Instruction*. San Francisco: University of California.

USRDS (United States Renal Data System). 1996. *Annual Data Report: III. Treatment Modalities for ESRD Patients*. Bethesda, MD: NIH, National Institute of Diabetes and Digestive and Kidney Diseases.

Van de Ven, Andrew H., and David N. Grazman. 1994. "From Generation to Generation: A Genealogy of Twin Cities Health Care Organizations, 1853–1993." Paper Presented at the Annual Meetings of the Academy of Management, Dallas, Texas.

Van de Ven, Andrew H., and M. Scott Poole. 1995. "Explaining Development and Change in Organizations." *Academy of Management Review* 20: 510–40.

Via Christi Healthcare System. 1998. Internet site. URL: <www.viachristi.org>.

Visions and Progress: A Commemorative History of San Jose Hospital, 1923–1983. 1984. Unpublished booklet.

Walsh, John. 1970. "Medical Schools: Portents of National Health Insurance." *Science* 169: 267–68.

Wardwell, Walter I. 1992. *Chiropractic: History and Evolution of a New Profession.* St. Louis: Mosby-Year Book.

Wasserman, Elizabeth. 1996. "Kaiser Discussing Hospital Alliances." *San Jose Mercury News,* Saturday January 27, pp. 1B, 2B.

Waters, Yssabella. 1909. *Visiting Nurses in the United States.* New York: Charities Publications.

Weber, David J. 1994 "The Spanish-Mexican Rim." In *The Oxford History of the American West,* edited by Clyde A Milner II, Carol A. O'Connor and Martha A. Sandweiss, 45–77. New York: Oxford University Press.

Weeks, Lewis, and Howard Berman. 1985. *Shapers of American Health Care Policy: An Oral History.* Ann Arbor, MI: Health Administration Press.

Weick, Karl E. 1976. "Educational Organizations as Loosely Coupled Systems." *Administrative Science Quarterly* 21: 1–19.

Westphal, James, Ranjay Gulati, and Stephen M. Shortell. 1997. "Customization or Conformity: An Institutional and Network Perspective on the Content and Consequences of TQM Adoption." *Administrative Science Quarterly* 39: 367–90.

White, Charles H., and Cindy Arstein-Kerslake. 1983. "PPO Activity in California Hospitals." *CHA Insight* 7(May 26): 1–4.

White, William D. 1982. "The American Hospital Industry since 1900: A Short History." In *Advances in Health Economics and Health Services Research,* edited by Richard M. Scheffler, 3: 143–70. Greenwich, CT: JAI Press.

Whitley, Richard. 1992. "The Social Construction of Organizations and Markets: The Comparative Analysis of Business Recipes." In *Rethinking Organizations: New Directions in Organization Theory and Analysis,* edited by Michael Reed and Michael Hughes, 120–43. London: Sage.

Wholey, Douglas R., and Lawton R. Burns. 1993. "Organizational Transitions: Form Changes by Health Maintenance Organizations." In *Research in the Sociology of Organizations,* edited by Sam Bacharach, 11: 257–93. Greenwich, CT: JAI Press.

Wholey, Douglas R., and Susan M. Sanchez. 1991. "The Effects of Regulatory Tools on Organizational Populations." *Academy of Management Review* 16: 743–67.

Wilk, Chester A. 1996. *Medicine, Monopolies, and Malice: How the Medical Establishment Tried to Destroy Chiropractic in the U.S.* Garden City, NJ: Avery Publishing Group.

Williams, Greer. 1971. *Kaiser-Permanente Health Plan: Why it Works.* Oakland, CA: Henry J. Kaiser Foundation.

Williamson, Oliver E. 1975. *Markets and Hierarchies: Analysis and Antitrust Implications.* New York: Free Press.

———. 1981. "The Economics of Organization: The Transaction Cost Approach." *American Journal of Sociology* 87: 548–77.

———. 1985. *The Economic Institutions of Capitalism.* New York: Free Press.

Winslow, Ron. 1994. "Technology and Health: Kaiser Permanente will Allow Members to Get Care from Non-plan Physicians." *Wall Street Journal,* January 28, sec. B, p. 5.

Wolinsky, Frederic D., and William D. Marder. 1985. *The Organization of Medical Practice and Practice of Medicine.* Ann Arbor, Michigan: Health Administration Press.

Womack, James P., Daniel T. Jones, and Daniel Roos. 1990. *The Machine That Changed the World: The Story of Lean Production.* New York: Harper Perennial.

Yale Law Journal, eds. 1954. "The American Medical Association: Power, Purpose, and Politics in Organized Medicine." *Yale Law Journal* 63: 938–1022.

Yedidia, Avram. 1987. "History of the Kaiser Permanente Medical Care Program," an Oral History conducted in 1985 by Ora Huth, Regional Oral History Office, The Bancroft Library, University of California, Berkeley.

Zajac, Edward J., and Stephen M. Shortell. 1989. "Changing Generic Strategies: Likelihood, Direction and Performance Implications." *Strategic Management Journal* 10: 413–30.

Zipperer, Lorri A., ed. 1995. *The Health Care Almanac: A Resource Guide to the Medical Field.* Chicago: American Medical Association.

Zipperer, Lorri A., and Brian Pace, eds. 1993. *Healthcare: Resource and Reference Guide.* Chicago: American Medical Association, Division of Library and Information Management.

Zucker, Lynne G. 1989. "Combining Institutional Theory and Population Ecology: No Legitimacy, No History." *American Sociological Review* 54: 542–45.

Zuckerman, Howard S. 1979. "Multi-Institutional Systems: Their Promise and Performance." In *Multi-Institutional Hospital Systems,* edited by Lewis E. Weeks, 3–51. Chicago: Hospital Research and Educational Trust.

Zuckerman, Howard S., Arnold D. Kaluzny, and Thomas C. Ricketts III. 1995. "Strategic Alliances: A Worldwide Phenomenon Comes to Health Care." In *Partners for the Dance: Forming Strategic Alliances in Health Care,* edited by Arnold D. Kaluzny, Howard S. Zuckerman, and Thomas C. Ricketts III, 1–18. Ann Arbor, MI: Health Administration Press.

Zuckerman, Howard S., and Lewis E. Weeks, eds. 1979. *Multi-Institutional Hospital Systems.* Chicago: Hospital Research and Educational Trust.

Index